Proactive Support

Proactive Support of Labor

The Challenge of Normal Childbirth

Paul Reuwer
Hein Bruinse
Arie Franx

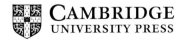

CAMBRIDGE UNIVERSITY PRESS
Cambridge, New York, Melbourne, Madrid, Cape Town, Singapore, São Paulo, Delhi

Cambridge University Press
The Edinburgh Building, Cambridge CB2 8RU, UK

Published in the United States of America by Cambridge University Press, New York

www.cambridge.org
Information on this title: www.cambridge.org/9780521735766

First published 2009

Printed in the United Kingdom at the University Press, Cambridge

A catalogue record for this publication is available from the British Library

Library of Congress Cataloguing in Publication data
Reuwer, Paul.
Proactive support of labor : the challenge of normal childbirth / Paul Reuwer, Hein Bruinse, Arie Franx.
p. ; cm.
Includes bibliographical references and index.
ISBN 978-0-521-73576-6 (pbk.)
1. Childbirth. 2. Obstetrics. I. Bruinse, Hein. II. Franx, Arie. III. Title.
[DNLM: 1. Maternal Health Services. 2. Delivery, Obstetric–methods. 3. Natural Childbirth.
4. Obstetric Labor Complications–prevention & control. 5. Pregnancy Outcome. WA 310.1 R448 2009]
RG524.R873 2009
618.2–dc22
2008049115

ISBN 978-0-521-73576-6 paperback

This book is dedicated to Kieran O'Driscoll, great obstetrician and distinguished teacher, forerunner in the development and evaluation of conceptual birth care. His fundamental insight and inspiring work provided the starting point of this treatise.

Contents

Foreword

Improvements in the care of the pregnant woman and fetal patient during the birthing process have been a success story for modern obstetrics. Less than a century ago maternal mortality during labor was commonplace in most developed countries, and fetal mortality and morbidity were even more common. The keystone of modern obstetrics was the introduction of hospital and safe cesarean deliveries in the early 20th century. However, too much of a good thing can sometimes lead to other problems.

In their book *Proactive Support of Labor*, Drs Reuwer, Bruinse and Franx make an important contribution to modern obstetrics by providing a critical counterbalance to technologic interference in labor and delivery. The authors introduce the concept of "Proactive Support of Labor" as an acceptable alternative to traditional labor and delivery management in order to shorten labor and ultimately ensure a safer delivery. They propose that results of improved labor and delivery management should be evaluated not only in physical terms (e.g., reduced morbidity and mortality) but also in terms of emotion and patient satisfaction. This concept is designed to not only improve the overall outcome but also patient satisfaction.

We agree that the perspective provided in this book should be carefully considered by all providers of healthcare to women in labor. The call for humanistic and evidence based obstetric care in labor and delivery by including the emotional needs of women in labor should be embraced throughout the world.

Amos Grunebaum
Director of Obstetrics, New York Weill Cornell
Medical College, New York Presbyterian Hospital

Frank A Chervenak
Chairman of Obstetrics and Gynecology,
New York Weill Cornell Medical College,
New York Presbyterian Hospital

Acknowledgments

Women's satisfaction with the childbirth experience, when caregivers have followed the strategy of
proactive support of labor, as well as the unremit-
ting enthusiasm of birth professionals who made
this approach their own, were the motivating
forces in writing this manual. The authors wish to
express their special gratitude and thanks to Vanessa
Stubbs, Simone Valk, Lo Pistorius, and Gerrit Jan
Noordergraaf for their help, advice, support, and
criticism.

Web-Forum

Readers are encouraged to share their opinions about *proactive support of labor* in the interactive web-forum: www.proactivesupportoflabor.com

General introduction

The natural process of birth increasingly involves medical intervention, but the benefits of this trend are questionable at best. The inexorable growth in operative delivery rates is not validated by tangible improvements in perinatal outcomes. Rather, maternal morbidity has risen significantly. Apart from its physical impact, giving birth is one of the most profound emotional experiences in a woman's life, but women's satisfaction with childbirth remains a cause for common concern. Despite all good intentions, modern maternity care is often perceived as professional but impersonal, and labor is not infrequently described as a traumatic or even "dehumanizing" experience.[1–3] This must be changed.

1.1 Purpose

The purpose of this manual is to present a cohesive, evidence-based plan for the care of the normal, healthy woman in labor, specifically designed to restore the balance between natural birth and medical intervention: *proactive support of labor*. The main target is to improve professional labor and delivery skills in order to promote spontaneous delivery and to enhance women's satisfaction with childbirth. *Proactive support of labor* is a carefully orchestrated and audited expert team approach involving the laboring woman, nurse, midwife, and obstetrician committed to a safe and normal delivery for both mother and baby. Emphasis is placed as much on the physical challenge as on the emotional impact of childbirth. The principles and proposed practices are universally applicable.

> *The objective is to enhance women's childbirth experience by improving professional labor and delivery skills and the overall quality of obstetrical care.*

1.2 Target readership

This manual is directed to:
- All professionals who are primarily responsible for the quality of childbirth: obstetricians, midwives, and labor room nurses. Obstetricians are in the prime position to improve all standards of care by creating the conditions for nurses and midwives to execute their labor support tasks properly.
- Medical students and student-midwives engaging in their first practical contacts with childbirth.
- All other health care providers involved in birth care such as family practitioners, childbirth educators, doulas, physiotherapists, sonographers, anesthesiologists, and home health nurses.
- Hospital administrators, health care policymakers, and health insurers, since high-quality care in labor requires a sound organization which should coincide with sound economics.
- Interested lay persons. No experience with childbirth is needed to understand the significance of *proactive support of labor*. Mothers-to-be have the most to gain from supportive care during

their labor and delivery effectively preventing everyday labor disorders. Although professional language is used, the text should be readily understandable to an educated lay-audience.

1.3 Presentation

This book is divided into three sections. The first section is a mirror for reflection, analyzing the mechanisms in everyday childbirth that explain excessive operative delivery rates and avoidable discontent of many women with their labor experience. The second section goes back to the basics and reviews the physiological prerequisites for a rewarding and safe birth that are all too often neglected in common childbirth practice. The third section proposes structural measures to solve most problems by introducing the principles and practice of *proactive support of labor*. Special attention should be paid to the subsection and paragraph headings as many address topics of critical importance that are seldom, if ever, discussed in standard textbooks.

Section 1: A wake-up call

To solve a problem, one must first admit that the problem exists and identify its causes. Inconsistencies in care, mismatches between women's expectations and practice, controversial midwifery and medical services, and unfounded concepts and dogmas on both sides of the aisle will all be identified and discussed in detail, as well as the self-sustaining mechanisms and stubborn nuisance values hampering structural improvements.

> *Many elements of care during pregnancy and childbirth can facilitate or jeopardize the successful accomplishment of this natural process.*

The numerous examples of preventable or overtly iatrogenic (provider-caused) birth disorders will be made undeniably apparent and will there-

fore confront childbirth professionals and even shock lay-readers. The defiant and provocative tone we adopt is by no means meant to question the integrity and devotion of obstetricians, midwives, and labor room nurses, or to belittle their efforts, but to promote debate. We wrote this section to serve as a mirror and an eye-opener, laying bare the fundamental problems plaguing modern childbirth practices all over the world.

Section 2: Back to basics

Many dogmas in mainstream childbirth practice have been relayed from teacher to student and from textbook to textbook without any serious attempt at verification until they have become the main impediments to improvements in everyday birth care. The critical reappraisals in this section will show that many conventional wisdoms about the physiology of labor are plain fallacies.

> *It is all too frequent in medicine to find ignorance about the most common events.*

The chapters in this section offer a fundamental reinterpretation of and ample material for deliberation on the biophysics dominating the natural process of birth. The basic biology is organized in a coherent manner, giving structure and direction to a scientifically based policy for the supervision of labor from its early start. We will challenge the classic understanding and teaching concerning the onset of labor and the course of normal cervical dilatation. We will clearly demonstrate that it is not the mechanics of delivery but primarily the dynamics of first-stage labor that provide the optimal chance for a successful birth. Furthermore, a basic knowledge of the biophysical changes in the uterus prior to birth is essential for an accurate understanding of the initiation of labor and for an understanding of the negative impact that induction of labor has on the birth process. Equally important is an accurate understanding of the physics of uterine contractions, dilatation, and expulsion. Crucial to the correct conduct and care of labor is recognition of the parasympathetic condition controlling birth and the negative impact that anxiety and stress have on the effectiveness of labor through adrenergic stimulation. These fundamental, universally valid aspects of labor and delivery are of such importance that each must be examined in considerable detail before genuine progress in labor supervision can be made.

Section 3: Proactive support of labor

The third section is the main emphasis of this book. It provides a step-by-step exposition of the policy framework for *proactive support of labor*. This method of supportive care is specifically designed to prevent everyday birth disorders and to detect and treat labor problems at an early stage, hence its name. This evidence-based concept of childbirth offers providers a foothold in negotiating the complexity of daily practice in the labor ward and guards them against clinical stalemates, inconsistent (non-) policies of care, and mismanagement of labor with self-created birth complications. If the strategy of *proactive support of labor* is followed, all elements of high-quality birth care will fall into place including fetal and maternal monitoring, pain relief measures, honoring women's needs and desires, and the prevention and timely correction of everyday labor complications.

> **Proactive support of labor**
>
> *A conceptual and evidence-based approach specifically designed to promote normal and rewarding labor and delivery. It is a cross-appeal to both obstetricians and midwives.*

The key points include a clear diagnosis of the onset of labor, early recognition and correction of dysfunctional labor, consistent conduct, personal attention and commitment, and continuous supportive care on a one-on-one basis extended to all women in labor. This method of care is founded on the pioneering work of Kieran O'Driscoll and Declan Meagher,[4] renowned leaders in the field of conceptual care during labor, but whose ideas have also been frequently misquoted, misunderstood, and abused. The present manual is an attempt to recreate interest in their original concept, now adding the clinical "evidence" from numerous studies all over the world.

Proactive support of labor encourages an active interest in the supervision of first-stage labor by all members of the delivery team and facilitates constant psychological support and good communication in labor. The central birth-plan promotes the development of team spirit between physicians, midwives, and nurses and dictates good labor ward organization which can improve labor care immensely. This well-defined policy at last makes possible a meaningful daily audit of all procedures in the supervision of childbirth, promoting and ensuring high-quality care. This approach effectively decreases operative delivery rates without any detrimental effects to the infants. Most importantly, this integrated, patient-centered care system invariably improves women's satisfaction with their childbirth experience.

1.4 Evidence grading

The grading of studies and the hierarchy of evidence used in this book are adapted from Eccles and Mason:[5]

Evidence Category	Source
Level I	Systematic review or meta-analysis of randomized controlled trials (Ia), or At least one randomized controlled trial (Ib).
Level II	At least one well-designed controlled study without randomization (IIa), or One other well-designed type of quasi-experimental study, such as a cohort study (IIb).

Evidence Category	Source
Level III	Well-designed non-experimental descriptive studies, such as comparative studies, correlation studies, case-control studies and case studies.
Level IV	Expert committee reports or opinions and/or clinical experience of respected authorities.

Hierarchy	Evidence
Level A	Directly based on category I evidence.
Level B	Directly based on category II evidence, and/or Extrapolation from category I evidence.
Level C	Directly based on category III evidence, and/or Extrapolation from category I or II evidence.
Level D	Directly based on category IV evidence, and/or Extrapolation from category I, II, or III evidence.

1.5 Advice for readers

Although childbirth is the same physiological process worldwide, childbirth services – even if confined to western countries – have proved to be strongly influenced by cultural differences and social pressures. For this reason, transcultural diversities in birth philosophies, childbirth practices, and care organizations should not be ignored and will be addressed throughout this book. Time and again, the principles and practice of *proactive support of labor* will be contrasted with ubiquitous but controversial approaches – ranging from midwifery-based care that eschews intervention to high-tech, fully medicalized childbirth – in order to illustrate the need for structural reforms in each type of care. Typical American or European issues should not distract from the universally valid observations, statements, and evidence-based policy proposals on the supervision of labor made here.

This book describes a cohesive and consistent concept of birth care universally applicable to all societal contexts. All aspects of normal and abnormal labor and delivery will be discussed, but emphasis is placed on redefining basic birth parameters, reinterpretation of physiological data, hard clinical evidence, consistent thought processes, and strict adherence to logic. For this reason we recommend reading the chapters of each section in the order in which they are presented.

1.6 Classification of birth professionals

Terminology with regard to childbirth professionals may be quite confusing as many physicians of unequal educational status are involved, ranging from junior residents to senior consultants. Likewise, the titles "nurse," "nurse-midwife," and "midwife" may cover dissimilar and often overlapping content, substance, and responsibilities. Sensitivity to status and emotion are involved here and a few terms as used in this book may therefore benefit from definition.

Obstetricians hold a specialist qualification in obstetrics and gynecology. They bear the ultimate responsibility for the medical well-being of their patients. They may also be called "consultants."

Residents are doctors in training to become a medical specialist. Senior residents are in their final years of training and largely function at a level equal to obstetricians after formal authorization.

Interns are undergraduate medical students performing their clinical rotations.

"Laborist" or "OB-hospitalist" is a new breed of caregiver still in its infancy but spreading fast.[6] The titles refer to medical officers who work exclusively in the hospital, keeping watch over women in labor and performing deliveries. The role should be compared with that of other and more familiar hospital-based doctors such as emergency room physicians. Confusingly, education and responsibilities vary widely, ranging from the level of junior residents to fully certified obstetricians. The titles are therefore avoided in this manual except in Chapter 26 on professional working relations and organization. It is for laborists/OB-hospitalists to decide how to recognize themselves in this book: either as residents or as fully qualified obstetricians.

Labor room nurses are general nurses with two years' additional training in maternity care. They support women in labor and assist midwives and doctors. Labor room nurses do not perform vaginal examinations or deliveries. Whenever the term "nurse" is used in this book, labor room nurses are meant unless indicated otherwise.

Midwives. The general term "midwife," as used in this manual, is a state-registered caregiver who has completed four years of vocational education at one of the official midwifery schools, including practice training programs in accredited hospitals and in home birth practices. They are regarded as specialists in the supervision of normal pregnancy and delivery. Midwives provide antenatal and postnatal care and supervise normal deliveries independently, mostly in the hospital and in some countries also in primary birth centers or still at the woman's home. They are trained in risk assessment and the detection of disease, at which point they will or should seek consultation and transfer the patient. A "clinical" or "senior midwife" is a postgraduate with two years' additional

education and medical training, often to the academic level of a masters degree in "advanced midwifery."

Family practitioners. Some primary care physicians (general practitioners) still attend births, mainly in the woman's home. Their childbirth services resemble those of community-based midwives. Although they are not specifically mentioned throughout this manual for reasons of readability, this group of primary care providers is not forgotten: whenever midwives are mentioned, readers may include family practitioners as well.

REFERENCES

1. Block J. *Pushed: The Painful Truth about Childbirth and Modern Maternity Care.* Cambridge, MA: Da Capo Press; 2007.
2. Wagner M. *Born in the USA: How a Broken Maternity System Must Be Fixed to Put Women and Children First.* Berkeley, CA: University of California Press; 2007.
3. Lake R, Epstein E. *The Business of Being Born.* A documentary film, 2007; www.thebusinessofbeingborn.com/about.htm.
4. O'Driscoll K, Meagher D, Robson M. *Active Management of Labour,* 4th edn. Mosby; 2003.
5. Eccles and Mason. How to Develop Cost-Conscious Guidelines. *Health Technology Assessment* 2001; 5: 16.
6. Weinstein L. The laborist: a new focus of practice for the obstetrician. *Am J Obstet Gynecol* 2003; 188(2): 310–12.

A wake-up call

"Not everything that is faced can be changed. But nothing can be changed until it is faced."

–James Arthur Baldwin

Medical excess in normal childbirth

The purpose of professional care during labor and delivery is to ensure that every child is born as healthy as possible while causing the least possible damage to the mother. For the most part this dual goal was realized during the twentieth century as demonstrated by the sharp decrease in maternal and perinatal mortality. In the past few decades, however, obstetrics has failed to maintain its objectives. The once-declining rate of maternal morbidity and mortality is now on the increase.[1] This untoward rise in maternal complications is due primarily to the ever-increasing cesarean birth rate without any benefits to overall neonatal outcome.[2,3] This is a trend that must be changed.

> *The rise in maternal morbidity and mortality rates, without any evidence of improvement in fetal outcomes, is indicative of the failure of modern childbirth practices.*

2.1 The cesarean pandemic

An ideal overall cesarean rate is not known, but on the basis of available databases little noticeable improvement in fetal outcome is observed once cesarean rates rise above 10–15%.[4,5] In the past decade, however, the cesarean birth rate in all western countries far exceeded these target figures.[6] By 1970, 5.5% of all babies in the USA were delivered through cesarean section. The rate doubled in five years and continued to increase until 1990 when it peaked at 22.7%. It remained stable and even declined slightly through the 1990s before picking up again in 1998. The temporary stabilization in the early 1990s can be explained by campaigns of national health officials and leading obstetricians who sounded the alarm and promoted a trial of vaginal birth after cesarean (VBAC) to avoid routine repeat procedures. However, liability concerns regarding uterine scar-related complications effectively sliced the American VBAC rate to 9.2% in 2004 and the old adage "once a cesarean, always a cesarean" again prevails. Today, one in three American babies is delivered by cesarean section. The rates of perinatal deaths and neonatal cerebral palsy, however, have remained steady over the past decades.[7,8] The "cesarean problem" that first seemed to be an American affliction is now international. The overall cesarean rates now range between 20% and 30% in most western countries and continue to climb.[9–11] In the private sector of India and Brazil even more shocking cesarean rates of between 50% and 80% have been reported.[12–14] Although relatively low in the Netherlands and Scandinavia, the overall cesarean rates in these countries also doubled in the past two decades and their cesarean rates in first pregnancies now exceed 20%.[15]

2.1.1 Operative solutions for failed labors

The cesarean pandemic is not the result of standard elective surgery for indications such as breech presentations, multiple pregnancies, or severely compromised pregnancies, since they represent only a small minority of all births. Neither do emergency interventions to rescue babies from neurological damage or death explain the rising cesarean excess.

The overall US cesarean rate for "fetal distress" has remained stable between 3.8% and 4.2% in the past decade.[16] The alarming observation is that the vast majority of cesarean deliveries today are performed as the easy-exit strategy for first-stage labor disorders in healthy women with a singleton term fetus in the cephalic presentation – the precise population presumed to be low risk. As could be expected, fetal outcome in this group has not improved at all during the past three decades of this trend.[1–8]

> *There is a growing tendency to resolve the problems of first-stage labor by surgical intervention.*

The American College of Obstetricians and Gynecologists (ACOG) clearly identified dystocia or failure to progress as the primary impetus for the dramatic expansion of cesarean deliveries, in particular in first labors. These failed labors and related repeat operations in next pregnancies account for two-thirds of all cesarean deliveries in the USA.[2] National statistics from all other countries with accurate obstetric records confirm similar trends worldwide. Faced with decreasing VBAC rates, a reduction in the primary cesarean section rate should have a significant effect on the need for subsequent surgical delivery and therefore a large impact on the overall cesarean delivery rate. Obviously, when trying to reduce undue cesarean rates one should focus on the supervision of low-risk first labors. That is precisely the emphasis of this manual (Sections 2 and 3).

> *Failure to progress accounts for the majority of cesarean deliveries in first labors and, by inference, for the largest proportion of elective repeat procedures.*

A detailed discussion regarding the recent trend of elective (planned) cesareans for no reason other than the patient's request falls outside the scope of this book, at least directly. Nonetheless, such requests must be considered in the overall context of current practice in which the appellant – upon denial of her request – still has a very high chance of a cesarean or an instrument-assisted vaginal delivery. In fact, most requests for elective cesarean relate to a previous traumatic labor experience or discouraging horror stories from others. Indeed, the overall cesarean rate is effectively determined – directly and indirectly – by the women-friendly conduct and care of first labors.

2.2 Instrumental delivery rates

With rising cesarean rates, fewer women reach the second stage of labor and the rates of instrumental vaginal deliveries should therefore decrease. However, this has not happened. In general, countries and hospitals with high cesarean rates also have high operative vaginal delivery rates.[17] The main indication is second-stage arrest. A forceps or vacuum delivery is not a trivial intervention either, as instrumental delivery is particularly damaging to a woman's pelvic floor[18–21] and potentially risky and certainly painful for her child. Instrumental delivery is strongly associated with serious perinatal birth injuries.[18–31]

First-time mothers-to-be (nulliparas) run the highest risks of operative delivery. Even when a nullipara manages to escape the major surgery of a cesarean, she still has a 25% chance of an instrument-assisted vaginal delivery – in most cases for failure to progress.[17,32] Of course, these are average figures as the rates vary greatly among hospitals and even among practitioners in the same institution. Overall, however, only half of all women in western countries deliver their first babies spontaneously by the normal route nowadays. There are only two possible explanations: either modern women are no longer capable of normal childbirth or modern childbirth services fail.

> *Currently, only about half of all first-time mothers in western countries give birth via the normal route without surgical or instrumental intervention.*

2.3 Conceptual flaws

High intervention rates in childbirth are often attributed to the supposedly changing needs of child-bearing women and their babies. Some authors suggest an association between increasing maternal age and weight and dysfunctional labor.[33–38] In reality, however, the predominant contributors to excessive operative delivery rates more likely relate directly to the caregivers and reflect birth philosophies, culture, organization, the extent to which doctors are paid on a "piecework" basis, their propensity for convenience and control, the extent to which malpractice litigation is feared, and so forth. It is impossible to express the relative impact of each of these factors in absolute numbers, but they all add up to current obstetric performance. The literature addressing these topics is extensive, but mostly vague, and it generally misses the point: the spiraling operative delivery rates actually reflect a progressive lack of normal labor and delivery skills of birth professionals.

> *At the core, high intervention rates originate in the lack of a consistent, scientifically based concept of childbirth and, consequently, absence of a structured labor management policy.*

2.3.1 Professional controversies

Professional birth care should be based on an astute comprehension of the fundamental processes of parturition such as the cervical and myometrial changes in late pregnancy, the onset of labor, the pattern of normal dilatation, and the length of normal labor. Although nature designed a biological blueprint for labor and delivery – fine-tuned over millions of years of evolution – appreciation of the basic biophysical processes controlling birth varies significantly among care providers. As a result, professional views range from understanding childbirth as a natural process, best supervised with the least possible interference, to the emphasis being placed on risks – leading to highly medicalized "management" of labor. This diversity in birth philosophies and practices echoes differences in opinion or lack of scientific knowledge, and the inexorable rise in failed labors seriously calls into question whether midwives and obstetricians still operate from valid concepts of childbirth, if from any.

> *Professional conduct and care of labor and delivery should be based on solid, scientific knowledge of the physiology of parturition.*

2.4 Counting the costs

The high failure rate of normal labor and delivery is more detrimental than meets the eye and includes severe psychological and physical harm to women, adverse maternal and neonatal outcomes, as well as serious economic and social damage.

2.4.1 Psychological harm

Ideally, women experience childbirth as an empowering and ultimately satisfying event in which the care providers are allowed to participate. Unfortunately, practice shows that this gratifying scenario is not achieved by many women, in particular not for their first labor. Apart from the physical burden of a stalled labor that ends in a forceps, vacuum, or cesarean delivery, the woman may sustain substantial emotional damage owing to a feeling of frustration and failure. An operative delivery denies her the unique experience of giving birth to her child by her own efforts as well as the sense of personal accomplishment from which she could gain further self-esteem and self-confidence. The harsh reality of daily practice is that current birth care turns many a birth into an ordeal. In the worst-case scenario the parturient ends up in a deplorable condition; after a whole day or more of exhausting labor she undergoes surgery or a difficult extraction. The psychological damage from such a mismanaged labor can be worse than the emotional impact of an emergency cesarean for acute fetal distress: a lasting aversion to all things related to birth maintained by recurring nightmares and complicated by feelings of inadequacy and (sub)conscious feelings of hostility toward her child.

> *The emotional impact of the labor experience remains a matter of common but underrated concern.*

The prevalence and severity of these life-lasting effects are generally underestimated as they mainly develop outside the field of vision of childbirth professionals. However, several prospective psychological studies indicate that a large group of women currently experience childbirth as a genuinely traumatic event. In a recent Dutch study among a low-risk midwifery population, only 16% of the mothers showed no symptoms of posttraumatic stress disorder (PTSD) at six weeks postpartum, whereas 42% reported symptoms on two clusters of PTSD, and 11% reported on all three clusters of PTSD.[39] In most international studies, 2–11% of new mothers suffer a full-blown PTSD as a consequence of childbirth.[40–43]

Instrumental deliveries strongly increase the risk of perinatal negative emotions, which in turn increase the risk of childbirth-related post-traumatic stress disorders.[44,45] Cesarean section is not a preventive intervention, as is shown by a structured meta-analysis;[46] mothers delivered by cesarean section express less immediate and long-term satisfaction with the birth process compared with mothers having a vaginal delivery, are less likely to breast-feed, experience a delay to first interaction with their infants, have less-positive reactions to them, and interact less with them at home (Evidence level B).

> *Childbirth-related depression and anxiety disorders are chronic conditions permeating throughout a woman's lifetime.*

2.4.2 Direct physical harm

Although a cesarean section is safer than ever before, it remains major abdominal surgery and the direct risks are far from negligible. The short-term complications, such as excessive blood loss, infectious morbidity, thromboembolic complications, longer recovery time, extended hospital stay, and chance of rehospitalization are all too well understood.[47–52] Moreover, the baseline maternal morbidity associated with cesarean delivery is severely increased in obese women, and obesity is another epidemic affliction of modern times.[53]

Generally less well-known is that the overall maternal mortality rate for cesarean section is more than four times greater than that for planned vaginal birth (relative risk [RR] = 4.9; 95% confidence interval [CI] = 3.0–8.0)[54] and the maternal death rate has been slowly but steadily increasing in western countries since the 1980s.[55,56]

The need for emergency hysterectomies has also increased: in about 1 per 200 cesarean deliveries as compared to 1 per 1000 vaginal deliveries.[57–59] More than 40% of postpartum emergency hysterectomies for massive hemorrhaging follow primary cesarean delivery.

> *Spiraling cesarean delivery rates dramatically increase rates of severe maternal morbidity.*

2.4.3 Medical harm to subsequent pregnancies

The negative implications for future childbirth are the most alarming although generally underrated. Firstly, the risk of unexplained stillbirth in women with a cesarean scar is doubled[60] and, secondly, up to 90% of American pregnant women with a previous cesarean undergo a repeat operation for fear of uterine rupture.[2] Many hospitals have actually banned VBACs. Inevitably, the more first cesarean deliveries performed today, the more repeat cesareans will be necessary tomorrow.

The most distressing, however, are the uterine scar-related complications as a result of placental implant in the uterine scar with placenta previa, accreta, or even percreta, leading to massive hemorrhaging. In effect, 2–3% of pregnant women with a cesarean scar – regardless of whether they are scheduled for elective cesarean or a vaginal birth – require massive blood transfusions, embolization therapy, or extensive surgery including emergency hysterectomies and post-treatment intensive care as a result of life-threatening uterine rupture or massive bleeding from the placental implantation site.[61–65] Too many women are severely harmed or even die because of these catastrophic complications in pregnancies that follow an unnecessary primary (first-time) cesarean delivery. These secondary calamities are, in fact, primarily iatrogenic in origin.

> *Since the 1980s, the maternal death rate has been on the increase in western countries, mainly owing to cesarean deliveries and the uterine scar-related complications in subsequent pregnancies.*

2.4.4 Increased neonatal mortality

In the past it was assumed that babies were delivered by cesarean because they were medically at risk, thereby explaining the higher infant and neonatal mortality rates typically associated with cesarean births. However, recent research of the US Centers for Disease Control and Prevention, analyzing over 5.7 million live births and nearly 12 000 infant deaths over a four-year period in the USA, suggested that the mechanism of cesarean birth itself induces an increased risk of neonatal mortality.[66] The study showed that for mothers at low risk, neonatal mortality rates are nearly three times higher among infants delivered by cesarean (1.77 per 1000 live births) than for those delivered vaginally (0.62 per 1000 live births). The increased risk for neonatal mortality related to cesarean delivery persisted even after adjustment for sociodemographic and medical risk factors.

The overall rate of babies delivered by cesarean among women with no formal indication (term births with no indicated medical risk factors or complications of labor and delivery) almost doubled in the USA between 1996 and 2004, and – although the neonatal mortality rate for this low-risk group remains low regardless of delivery method – the associated increase in the cesarean birth rate might inadvertently put a larger population of babies at risk for neonatal mortality.[66]

> *"Timely cesareans in response to medical conditions have proved to be life saving for countless babies. At present we are witnessing a different phenomenon: a nearly threefold increased risk for neonatal mortality in low-risk infants following cesarean birth with no formal medical indication."*[66]

2.4.5 Neonatal and long-term pediatric morbidity

No single scientific report indicates that newborns profit from cesarean delivery after an uneventful pregnancy. On the contrary, electively planned cesarean in uncomplicated pregnancies is associated with a threefold increase of short-term neonatal respiratory morbidity – necessitating admission to advanced care nurseries – compared with a trial of labor (RR 3.58, 95% CI 3.35–3.58).[67] Levine *et al.* also found a fivefold greater risk of persistent pulmonary hypertension for elective cesarean than for vaginal deliveries.[68] Older literature suggested that neonatal pulmonary hypertension, respiratory distress, and transient tachypnea in elective cesarean deliveries are the exclusive result of iatrogenic prematurity.[69] However, the latest evidence from well-dated pregnancies shows otherwise.[67] Apparently, labor itself benefits the newborn owing to less respiratory morbidity and mortality. Labor induces the release of fetal catecholamines and prostaglandins that promote lung surfactant secretion. In addition, epinephrine (adrenaline) release during labor and the physical compression of the infant help to remove fetal lung fluid and facilitate postnatal lung adaptation.[70] Moreover, babies born spontaneously are spared the potentially harmful effects of maternal anesthetic medication such as analgesics, antibiotics, and vasopressors.

A beneficial effect of vaginal birth might also hold true for other aspects of later health, as birth by cesarean is associated with a higher incidence of allergic diseases such as asthma and food intolerances[71] and even with an increased risk of psychosis in later life, possibly due to an altered perinatal adjustment of the dopamine metabolism.[72]

> There is no evidence whatsoever to indicate that elective cesarean after an uncomplicated pregnancy is of any benefit for the newborns. Rather, the reverse is true (Evidence level B–C).

2.4.6 Economic damage

Cesarean section has now achieved the dubious distinction of being the most frequently performed inpatient operation of any category. In the USA alone nearly 1.2 million cesareans are performed each year, relegating hysterectomy – perhaps not without a tinge of irony – into second place in the surgical league tables.[73,74] American hospitals charge on average about $14 200 for a cesarean section and $4500 for a non-complicated vaginal delivery (2004 prices) and these amounts do not include doctors' fees. A systematic review of health economic studies demonstrated that cesarean delivery costs a health service at least 3 to 5 times more than vaginal delivery.[75] This accounts for the direct expenses only, not those resulting from related repeat procedures and complications in subsequent pregnancies. Nearly a quarter of all US hospital stays are related to pregnancy and childbirth, but most people do not realize what a big chunk of hospital care that is: it involves approximately 4 million women and their babies each year in the USA alone. Cesarean deliveries cost more than $15 billion in the USA alone each year. Consumer watchdog group Public Citizen estimated that at least half of these are unnecessary and result in 25 000 extra infections and 1.1 million extra hospital days. Soon the costs of the cesarean pandemic will become unsustainable. Clearly, uncritical cesarean deliveries are a huge waste of resources, both financial and professional, and to the detriment of those who really need medical attention.

> The billions of dollars spent worldwide on inappropriate cesarean sections are an inexcusable assault on increasingly limited health care budgets.

2.4.7 Prejudice of future reproduction

Cesarean section decreases fertility.[76] A Scottish study followed over 25 000 women who had their first single child – multiple births were excluded – between 1980 and 1997 and found that women who had delivered their firstborn by cesarean were 9% less likely to conceive again compared with those who had a spontaneous natural delivery (66.9% versus 73.9%).[77] It was concluded either that women were avoiding second pregnancy because of the negative experience of cesarean delivery or that the surgery itself directly affected fertility. The latter explanation surely plays a role because women who have undergone cesarean section are more likely to suffer an ectopic pregnancy, with 9.5 occurring per 1000 pregnancies compared with women after spontaneous delivery, who suffer 5.7 per 1000 pregnancies.

2.4.8 Social damage

The social effects of obstetric excess are also disturbing. WHO consultant Marsden Wagner, an outspoken critic of medicalized childbirth, is intentionally provocative but essentially correct when he writes: "[A] woman giving birth is a human being, not a machine and just a container for making babies. Showing women – half of all people – that they are inferior and inadequate by taking away their power to give birth is a tragedy for all society." He concludes: "Respecting the woman as an important and valuable human being and making certain that the woman's experience while giving birth is fulfilling and empowering is not just a nice extra, it is absolutely essential as it makes the woman strong and therefore makes society strong."[78]

2.4.9 Dangerous export

Perhaps the most tragic result of the trend toward surgery-oriented obstetrics is its widespread export to developing countries from which so many graduates are trained in American and European institutes. In the third world a uterine scar is a far more dangerous condition than in the western world and extremely limited healthcare resources could be utilized far more wisely.

2.4.10 Declining overall quality of childbirth

Since most surgical interventions are performed to resolve problems of labor in low-risk pregnancies, spontaneous delivery rates are currently the most realistic objective measure of professional labor and delivery skills. By this criterion the overall standard of maternity care has declined markedly in recent times. Considering the impressive list of harms inflicted on mothers and the lack of evidence of any benefits for the newborns – rather the opposite is the case – the obstetrical establishment has some pertinent questions to answer about the explosive growth of operative deliveries in low-risk pregnancies.

> *Spontaneous delivery rates in low-risk pregnancies are the most realistic measure of the standard of care afforded to mothers.*

2.5 Summary

- The inexorably rising cesarean delivery rate without any evidence of improvement in maternal and fetal outcomes is indicative of the failure of modern obstetrics.

- Most operations are performed on healthy women – healthy, full-term women carrying their first child in cephalic presentation and single fetus, exactly those women presumed to be "low risk" – for the indication "dystocia" or "failure to progress."

- The effects are far more detrimental than is generally recognized and include not only severe physical and psychological harm to women but also increasing neonatal morbidity and mortality rates. In addition, there is a huge waste of resources, both financial and professional.

- The most worrying aspects of cesarean delivery are the serious uterine scar-related complications in subsequent pregnancy and childbirth.

- Inevitably, the more first neonates are delivered by cesarean today, the more repeat cesareans will be necessary tomorrow.

- Clearly, attempts to reduce inappropriate cesarean rates should focus on the supervision of first labors.

- Turning the tide requires a fundamental change in birth care: *proactive support of labor.*

REFERENCES

1. Centers for Disease Control and Prevention. www:cdc.gov/nchs/data/series/ (accessed October, 2007).

2. American College of Obstetricians and Gynecologists. *Task force on Cesarean Delivery Rates: Evaluation of Cesarean Delivery.* June, 2000.

3. Villar J, Valladares E, *et al.* Ceasarean delivery rates and pregnancy outcomes: the 2005 WHO global survey on maternal and perinatal health in Latin America. *Lancet* 2006; 367: 1819–29.

4. US Department of Health and Human Services. Public Health Service. *Healthy People 2000.* DHHS Publication No. 91–50213. Washington DC: US Government Printing Office; 1991: 378–79.

5. Enkin M, Keirse MJNC, Neilson J, *et al.* Cesarean section. In: *A Guide to Effective Care in Pregnancy and Childbirth*, 3rd edn. Oxford: Oxford University Press; 2000: 404–408.

6. Thomas J, Paranjothy S, RCOG Clinical Effectiveness Support Unit. *The National Sentinel Caesarean Section Audit Report.* London: RCOG Press; 2001.

7. Nelson KB. Can we prevent cerebral palsy? *N Engl J Med* 2003; 349: 1765–69.

8. Clark SL, Hankins GD. Temporal and demographic trends in cerebral palsy: fact and fiction. *Am J Obstet Gynecol* 2003; 188: 628–33.

9. National Collaborating Centre for Women's and Children's Health. *Caesarean section: Clinical Guideline*. RCOG Press, 2004.

10. Mammelle N, David S, Vendittelli F, *et al*. Perinatal health indicators in 2001 and its evolution since 1994. Results from the Audipog sentinel network. *Gynecol Obstet Fertil* 2002; 30: 6–39.

11. WHO website. www.who.int/whosis/database/ (accessed October, 2007).

12. Sreevidya S, Sathiyasekaran BW. High caesarean rates in Madras (India): a population-based cross sectional study. *Br J Obstet Gynaecol* 2003; 110: 106–11.

13. Belizan JM, Althabe F, Barros FC, Alexander S. Rates and implications of caesarean sections in Latin America: ecological study. *BMJ* 1999; 319: 1397–1400.

14. Rattner D. Sobre a hipotese de estabilizacio das taxas de cesareo do Estado de Sao Paolo. *Brasil Rev Saude Publica* 1996; 30(1): 19–33.

15. Odlind V, Haglund B, Pakkanen M, Otterblad Olausson P. Deliveries, mothers and newborn infants in Sweden 1973–2000. Trends in obstetrics as reported to the Swedish Medical Birth Register. *Acta Obstet Gynecol Scand* 2003; 82: 516–28.

16. Hendrix NW, Chaucan SP. Cesarean delivery for nonreassuring fetal heart rate tracing. *Obstet Gynecol N Am* 2005; 32: 273–86.

17. Stephenson PA, Bakoula C, Hemminki E, *et al*. Patterns of use of obstetrical interventions in 12 countries. *Paediatr Perinat Epidemiol* 1993; 7: 45–54.

18. Robinson JN, Norwitz ER, Cohen AP, McElrath TF, Lieberman ES. Episiotomy, operative vaginal delivery, and significant perineal trauma in nulliparous women. *Am J Obstet Gynecol* 1999; 181: 2105–10.

19. Christianson LM, Bovbjerg VE, McDavitt EC, Hullfish KL. Risk factors for perineal injury during delivery. *Am J Obstet Gynecol* 2003; 189: 255–60.

20. Johnson JH, Figueroa R, Garry D, *et al*. Immediate maternal and neonatal effects of forceps and vacuum-assisted deliveries. *Obstet Gynecol* 2004; 103: 513–18.

21. Casey BM, Schaffer JI, Bloom SL, *et al*. Obstetric antecedents for postpartum pelvic floor dysfunction. *Am J Obstet Gynecol* 2005; 192: 1655–62.

22. Williams MC, Knuppel RA, O'Brien WF, *et al*. Obstetric correlates of neonatal retinal hemorrhage. *Obstet Gynecol* 1993; 81: 688–94.

23. Uchil D, Arulkumaran S. Neonatal subgaleal hemorrhage and its relationship to delivery by vacuum extraction. *Obstet Gynecol Surv* 2003; 58: 687–93.

24. Johnson RB, Menon BK. Vacuum extraction versus forceps for assisted vaginal delivery. *Cochrane Database Syst Rev* 2000; (2): CD 00024.

25. Holroyde J, Woods JR Jr, Siddiqi TA, Scott M, Miodovnic M. Birth trauma: incidence and predisposing factors. *Obstet Gynecol* 1984; 63: 792–5.

26. Hughes CA, Harley EH, Milmoe G, Bala R, Martorella A. Birth trauma in the head and neck. *Arch Otolaryngol Head Neck Surg* 1999; 125: 193–9.

27. Gilbert WM, Nesbitt TS, Danielson B. Associated factors in 1611 cases of brachial plexus injury. *Obstet Gynecol* 1999; 93: 536–40.

28. Levine MG, Holroyde J, Woods JR Jr, *et al*. Birth trauma: incidence and predisposing factors. *Obstet Gynecol* 1984; 63: 792–5.

29. Gebremariam A. Subgaleal haemorrhage: risk factors and neurological and developmental outcome in survivors. *Ann Trop Paediatr* 1999; 19: 45–50.

30. Chadwick LM, Pemberton PJ, Kurinczuk JJ. Neonatal subgaleal hematoma: associated risk factors, complications and outcome. *J Paediatr Child Health* 1996; 32: 228–32.

31. O'Mahony F, Settatree R, Platt C, Johanson R. Review of singleton fetal and neonatal deaths associated with cranial trauma and cephalic delivery during a national intrapartum-related confidential enquiry. *Br J Obstet Gynaecol* 2005 May; 112(5): 619–26.

32. Royal College of Obstetricians and Gynaecologists. Clinical Green Top Guidelines. *Instrumental Vaginal Delivery: review*. October, 2000.

33. Main DM, Main EK, Moore DH 2nd. The relationship between maternal age and uterine dysfunction as a continuous effect throughout reproductive life. *Am J Obstet Gynecol* 2000; 182(6): 258–9.

34. Liu S, Rusen ID, Joseph KS, *et al*. Recent trends in caesarean delivery rates and indications for caesarean delivery in Canada. *J Obstet Gynaecol Can* 2004; 26: 735–42.

35. Ecker JL, Chen KT, Cohen AP, Riley LE, Lieberman ES. Increased risk of cesarean delivery with advancing age: indications and associated factors in nulliparous women. *Am J Obstet Gynecol* 2001; 185: 883–7.

36. Jensen H, Agger AO, Rasmussen KL. The influence of prepregnancy body mass index on labor complications. *Acta Obstet Gynecol Scand* 1999; 78(9): 799–802.

37. Usha Kiran TS, Hemmadi S, Bethel J, Evans J. Outcome of pregnancy in a woman with an increased body mass index. *Br J Obstet Gynaecol* 2005; 112: 768–72.

38. Cedergren MI. Maternal morbid obesity and the risk of adverse pregnancy outcome. *Obstet Gynecol* 2004; 103: 219–24.

39. Olde E, van der Hart O, Kleber RJ, *et al*. Peri-traumatic dissociation and emotions as predictor of PTSD symptoms following childbirth. *J Trauma Dissociation* 2005; 6: 125–42.

40. Ayers S, Pickering AD. Do women get posttraumatic stress disorder as a result of childbirth? A prospective study of incidence. *Birth* 2001; 28: 111–18.

41. Creedy DK, Shochet IM, Horsfall J. Childbirth and the development of acute trauma symptoms: incidence and contributing factors. *Birth* 2000; 27: 104–11.

42. Czarnocka J, Slade P. Prevalence and predictors of post-traumatic stress symptoms following childbirth. *Br J Clin Psychol* 2000; 39: 35–51.

43. Wijma K, Soderquist J, Wijma B. Posttraumatic stress disorder after childbirth: a cross-sectional study. *J Anxiety Disord* 1997; 11: 587–97.

44. Soet JE, Brack GA, DiIorio C. Prevalence and predictors of women's experience of psychological trauma during childbirth. *Birth* 2003; 30: 36–46.

45. Lyons S. A prospective study of post traumatic stress symptoms 1 month following childbirth in a group of 42 first-time mothers. *J Reprod Infant Psychol* 1998; 16: 91–105.

46. Dimatteo MR, Morton S, Lepper HS, *et al*. Cesarean childbirth and psychological outcomes: a meta-analysis. *Health Psychol* 1996; 15: 348–53.

47. Jackson N, Paterson-Brown S. Physical sequelae of cesarean section. *Best Pract Res Clin Obstet Gynaecol* 2001; 15: 883–92.

48. Ham van MA, Dongen van PW, Mulder J. Maternal consequences of cesarean section. A retrospective study of intraoperative and postoperative maternal complications of cesarean section during a ten year period. *Eur J Obstet Gynecol Reprod Biol* 1997; 74: 1–6.

49. Goepfert A for the NICHD Maternal-Fetal Medicine Units Network: The MFMU cesarean registry. Infectious morbidity following primary cesarean section. *Am J Obstet Gynecol* 2001; 185: S192.

50. Burrows LJ, Meyn LA, Weber AM. Maternal morbidity associated with vaginal versus cesarean delivery. *Obstet Gynecol* 2004; 103: 907–12.

51. Rajasekar D, Hall M. Urinary tract injuries during obstetric intervention. *Br J Obstet Gynaecol* 1997; 104: 731–4.

52. Lydon-Rochelle M, Holt VL, Martin DP, Easterling DP. Association between mode of delivery and maternal rehospitalization. *JAMA* 2000; 283: 2411–16.

53. Myles TD, Gooch J, Santolaya J. Obesity as an independent risk factor for infectious morbidity in patients who undergo cesarean delivery. *Obstet Gynecol* 2002; 100: 959.

54. National Collaborating Centre for Women's and Children's Health. *Caesarean Section. Clinical Guideline*. RCOG Press, 2004.

55. Hall MH, Bewley S. Maternal mortality and mode of delivery. *Lancet* 1999; 354: 776.

56. Harper MA, Byington RP, Espeland MA, *et al*. Pregnancy-related death and health care services. *Obstet Gynecol* 2003; 102: 273.

57. Shellhaas for the NICHD MFMU Network: The MFMU cesarean registry: Cesarean hysterectomy – its indications, morbidities, and mortality. *Am J Obstet Gynecol* 2001; 185: S123.

58. Kastner ES, Figueroa R, Garry D, *et al*. Emergency peripartum hysterectomy: experience at a community teaching hospital. *Obstet Gynecol* 2002; 99: 971.

59. Knight M, Kurinczuk JJ, Spark P, Brocklehurst P; United Kingdom Obstetric Surveillance System Steering Committee. Cesarean delivery and peripartum hysterectomy. *Obstet Gynecol* 2008; 111(1): 97–105.

60. Smith GC, Pell JP, Dobbie R. Caesarean section and risk of unexplained stillbirth in subsequent pregnancy. *Lancet* 2003; 362: 1779–84.

61. Green R, Gardeil F, Turner MJ. Long-term effects of cesarean sections. *Am J Obstet Gynecol* 1996; 176: 254–5.

62. Kwee A, Bots ML, Visser GH, Bruinse HW. Obstetric management and outcome of pregnancy in women with a history of caesarean section in The Netherlands. *Eur J Obstet Gynecol Reprod Biol* 2007; 132(2): 171–6.

63. Kwee A, Bots ML, Visser GH, Bruinse HW. Uterine rupture and its complications in the Netherlands: a prospective study. *Eur J Obstet Gynecol Reprod Biol* 2006; 128(1–2): 257–61.

64. Kwee A, Bots ML, Visser GH, Bruinse HW. Emergency peripartum hysterectomy. A prospective study in the Netherlands. *Eur J Obstet Gynecol Reprod Biol* 2006; 124: 187–92.

65. Guise JM, McDonagh MS, Osterwell P, *et al.* Systematic review of the incidence and consequences of uterine rupture in women with a previous cesarean section. *BMJ* 2004; 329: 1–7.

66. MacDorman MF, Declercq E, Menacker F, Malloy MH. Infant and neonatal mortality for primary cesarean and vaginal births to women with "no indicated risk," United States, 1998–2001 birth cohorts. *Birth* 2006; 3: 175–82.

67. Fogelson NS, Menard MK, Hulsey T, Ebeling M. Neonatal impact of elective repeat cesarean delivery at term: A comment on patient choice cesarean delivery. *Am J Obstet Gynecol* 2005; 192: 1433–6.

68. Levine EM, Ghai V, Barton JJ, Strom CM. Mode of delivery and risk of respiratory diseases in newborns. *Obstet Gynecol* 2001; 97: 439–42.

69. Bowers SK. Prevention of iatrogenic respiratory distress syndrome: elective repeat section and spontaneous delivery. *Am J Obstet Gynecol* 1982; 143: 186–9.

70. Doherty EG, Eichenwald EC. Cesarean delivery: emphasis on the neonate. *Clin Obstet Gynecol* 2004; 47: 332–41.

71. Laubereau B, Filipiak-Pittroff B, von Berg A, *et al.* Caesarean section and gastrointestinal symptoms, atopic dermatitis, and sensitisation during the first year of life. *Arch Dis Child* 2004; 89(11): 993–7.

72. Seeman P, Weinshenker D, Quirion R, *et al.* Dopamine supersensitivity correlates with D2High states, implying many paths to psychosis. *Proc Natl Acad Sci USA* 2005; 102(9): 3513–18.

73. Agency for Healthcare Research and Quality's Healthcare Cost and Utilization Project. *Nationwide Inpatient Sample 2003.* www.hcup.ahrq.gov/.

74. Ventura SJ, Martin JA, Curtin SC, Mathews TJ, Park MM. Births: Final data for 1998. *Natl Vital Stat Rep* 2000; 48(3): 1–10.

75. Henderson J, McCandlish R, Kumiega L, Petrou S. Systematic review of economic aspects of alternative modes of delivery. *Br J Obstet Gynaecol* 2001; 108: 149–57.

76. Murphy DJ, Stirrat GM, Heron J; ALSPAC Study Team. The relationship between Cesarean section and subfertility in a population-based sample of 14 541 pregnancies. *Hum Reprod* 2002; 17: 1914–17.

77. Mollison J, Porter M, Campbell D, Bhattacharya S. Primary mode of delivery and subsequent pregnancy. *Br J Obstet Gynaecol* 2005; 112: 1061.

78. Wagner M. Fish can't see water: the need to humanize birth. *Int J Gynaecol Obstet* 2001; 75: S25–S37.

3

Iatrogenic causes of failed labors

Dysfunctional labor is the primary indication for cesarean delivery in first pregnancies and therefore the indirect cause of most repeat operations.[1] The terminology generally favored to describe the problem is "failure to progress," or "dystocia," from the Greek meaning abnormal labor as opposed to "eutocia" meaning normal labor. These medical terms, however, serve as a cloak to obscure lack of true meaning because they relay little if any information about the underlying problems. Similarly, we can describe patients with thyroid disease as euthyroid or dysthyroid, but it gives no information whatsoever for institution of treatment. Obviously, we cannot hope to tackle the problem of failed labors without resorting to cesarean delivery, unless we explore the pathophysiological heterogeneity of the condition and attempt to define causal diagnoses.

> *Dystocia or failure to progress is not a diagnosis but an observation.*

3.1 Dynamic labor disorders

Basically, the ability of the fetus to negotiate the birth canal depends on *the powers, the passage*, and *the passenger*. This leaves, in essence, only two main explanations when labor stalls:

1. Mechanical obstruction, resulting from fetopelvic disproportion or fetal malposition.
2. Dynamic labor disorders in which the uterine force or the remaining strength of the birthing

woman is insufficient: δυναμις (dynamis) is the Greek word for "force."

Faced with the virtual disappearance of pelvic anatomical deformities since the elimination of rickets ("*the passage*") and with a stable mean birthweight ("*the passenger*"), the only possible explanation for the rise in operative deliveries for "dystocia" must be an increase in the incidence of dynamic labor disorders ("*the powers*") that arise in initially normal cases. If scrutinized, dynamic dystocia in turn consists of a large group of specific and identifiably distinct labor disorders (Sections 2 and 3), which too frequently pass unnoticed and are therefore treated after the fact with surgery. In many cases dynamic labor disorders are even plainly iatrogenic (physician-caused) from the outset, in particular when labor is induced.[2–13] These are harsh but at the same time hopeful conclusions, because they implicitly carry the real possibility of decreasing operative delivery rates and enhancing women's labor experience by improving the professional conduct and care of normal labor.

> Fundamental problem 1
>
> *High operative delivery rates are provoked by high rates of (iatrogenic) dynamic labor disorders.*

3.1.1 Symptom-based interventions

Even dynamic dystocia is not a diagnosis but a syndrome of a variety of labor problems. A true and specific diagnosis allows for other measures rather than the easiest way out using surgery or traction. Clearly, as long as the pathophysiology of the daily problems in the delivery room is not recognized and the various dynamic labor disorders are not properly defined and diagnosed, one cannot begin to formulate an effective policy to reduce undue operative delivery rates. Such detailed analyses will be provided in Sections 2 and 3 of this manual. In effect, accurate diagnosis is the most important single factor in responsible care of labor.

Fundamental problem 2

Failure to submit "dystocia" to detailed analysis and diagnosis renders a structured policy for the reduction of operative delivery rates virtually impossible.

3.1.2 Lack of definitions

The widely differing criteria for dystocia manifest the lack of a scientific foundation for current childbirth. Scientific disciplines are based on universally valid definitions, but within obstetrics and midwifery one will search in vain for a common set of definitions, even for the most elementary parameters of birth. The onset of labor, the normal progression and duration of labor, and objective criteria distinguishing between a normal and an abnormal course of labor are actually poorly defined. The development and evaluation of a system of high-quality care is hampered by a pseudo-exact understanding of basic concepts such as the latent phase of labor compared with false labor, efficient compared with inefficient contractions, normal progression compared with prolonged labor, pelvic adequacy compared with fetopelvic disproportion, and fetal reserves compared with fetal distress. This imprecision results in subjective and thus arbitrary care, based on beliefs and doctrines rather than evidence-based norms. Consequently, both

the chance of intervention and the form it takes are determined more by the personal perspective of the caregiver than by the specific obstetric situation.

Fundamental problem 3

The main obstacle for quality birth care is a lack of strict definitions and, consequently, absence of objective and prospective criteria for the distinction between "normal" and "abnormal" labor.

3.2 Lack of an overall plan

The lack of commonly held definitions leads to a lack of consistent standards for the conduct and care of normal childbirth. Rates of induction, labor augmentation, and operative delivery vary by more than a factor of 4 between hospitals within the same region, even after correcting for differences between populations.[14] The consequences of such arbitrariness are enormous for the pregnant woman: she does not know that she is 4 times more likely to have a cesarean or instrumental delivery in one hospital than in another, without a shred of evidence of any benefit to herself or her child.

3.2.1 Non-management of first-stage labor

The most influential textbook *Williams Obstetrics* (2005) argues: "It is generally agreed that dystocia leading to cesarean delivery is overdiagnosed in the USA and elsewhere. Factors leading to increased use of cesarean delivery for dystocia, however, are controversial. Those implicated have included incorrect diagnosis of dystocia, fear of litigation and even clinician convenience."[15] But it could be stated with even stronger arguments that dystocia is generally underdiagnosed, that is to say, not timely recognized, not causally specified, and not corrected in a due manner, which leaves surgery as the only solution after the fact. In other words:

> *The current high rates of operative deliveries in low-risk pregnancies are the result of the widespread disregard for a systematic childbirth policy aimed at short labor and a spontaneous, safe delivery.*

3.2.2 Lack of professional interest

Unfortunately, many obstetricians show little interest in the prevention of labor disorders, which is surprising as labor is the final common pathway for all pregnancies entrusted to their care. In private care the doctor is often not in the hospital and must be called in by the nurse when trouble develops. Or private doctors typically come in only when the head is about to be born in order to witness birth and to congratulate their patient (and write the bill). Women in public hospitals often do not see the obstetrician at all or not until the birth is definitely deemed not to be progressing. The busy obstetrician has other things to do. Thus, nurses, midwives, and the least experienced interns and residents are the main attendants of the tedious hours of first-stage labor. If the labor becomes increasingly difficult, it is these attendants – not the physician-specialist who is ultimately responsible and accountable – who must sell the decision of waiting to the helpless patient and her desperate partner. Obstetricians confidently approve epidural analgesia or large amounts of opioid drugs, far out of harm's way from behind a desk or from their beds over the telephone. Since a call schedule of two nights a week is the rule rather than the exception, many obstetricians try to lessen this nightly inconvenience by coming to the labor room only when strictly necessary. Their attitude to labor might very well be the reverse in the daytime, especially in busy maternity units where there is constant pressure to keep patients moving through. In the late afternoon obstetricians (on duty that night) may advise speeding up labor or considering

a cesarean, often without having seen the patient at all.

> *In many childbirth settings the care provided during labor depends strongly on the time of day labor happens to begin.*

In many hospitals the responsibility for the management of labor is generally passed on to nurse-midwives and residents, who are often allowed to act unsupervised after only a few weeks on the labor and delivery ward. Close supervision by an obstetrician is indeed available for acute problems or the actual (assisted) birth, but proactive supervision during the first stage of labor is usually nonexistent. The lack of consistent guidelines on how to proceed when a labor gets tough exposes the resident or midwife to the possibility of unfair criticism from both the patient and the distant supervisor. Such grievances contribute to the low morale and lack of team spirit that is characteristic of all too many delivery wards all over the world. "And whenever there is a lack of trust, decisions are avoided, care is not pursued effectively, and cesarean deliveries are performed unnecessarily because surgery provides a soft option for those anxious to avoid blame."[16]

> *Lack of team spirit in the labor and delivery ward is detrimental to the quality of birth care.*

Many consultant gynecologists enter the delivery room only when they are needed to solve problems, honing their skills in the "tricks of the trade": vacuum, forceps, and cesarean. They are often involved in other subspecialties and regard obstetrics as a simple but burdensome part of a much broader profession. It is for this reason that most gynecologists typically seek intellectual fulfillment outside the labor room. As a result, birth attendance and care are left in the hands of lower-qualified personnel and when there is a problem the specialist quickly performs an instrumental or cesarean delivery in the midst of all his or her other work obligations. These common practices emphasize the need for a new, inspiring childbirth system that encourages an active interest in first-stage labor by all professional staff, including the obstetricians who must actually take the initiative (Section 3).

Fundamental problem 4

Lack of direct involvement at consultant level in the supervision of first-stage labor is indicative of the state of apathy within the obstetric establishment regarding the supervision of first-stage labor.

3.2.3 Discontinuous care

Women have several caregivers over the length of their labor because of the 8-hour work shifts. This turnover in personnel during one birth makes it difficult to maintain consistent and high-standard birth care as long as a central policy of care is not formulated and implemented. What one attendant regards as normal another finds abnormal and vice versa. This inevitably results in inconsistencies in care and a lack of clarity at the bedside. Furthermore, the lack of agreement regarding criteria for normal progress of labor results in heated, endless discussions between nurse-midwives and obstetricians and, most importantly, it stands in the way of effective cooperation.

Fundamental problem 5

Impersonal and discontinuous labor care can be attributed to the general lack of a central birth-plan.

In some western countries autonomous, community-based midwives still attend births at the woman's home or in alternative, primary birth centers, claiming to provide more personal care. But practice shows that it is typical for these midwives to remain with a parturient only when approaching full dilatation. In the long first stage of labor it is presumed that intermittent care with periodic visits at three-hourly intervals will suffice (Chapter 5). As a result, many women giving birth at home go through the greatest part of their dilatation stage unattended and unsupported by professional help.

3.2.4 The expectant approach

The midwifery approach to labor is to wait for the natural process to unfold. This method originates in the fundamental philosophy that the natural process of birth neither can be improved nor needs improvement. As a result, conservative caregivers see no alternative to waiting, even when labor takes a very long time. In this tradition of care, which is passed on from generation to generation without question, the main task of the midwife is to ensure that no direct problem arises to make intervention necessary. If Mother Nature fails, there is always the obstetrician as back-up, solving the problem after the fact. It should be noted, however, that midwives are not alone in defending this passive wait-and-see attitude; it is one that is conveniently shared by many obstetricians.

In effect, there is too little attention given to the relationship between the length of labor and the woman's exhaustion. When the patience of birth attendants exceeds the stamina of a laboring woman, a cascade of unmanageable complications is the result. After an unnecessarily long first stage, most women can no longer push, no longer want to push, or may not reach the point of pushing. Thus, the decision to intervene is belatedly motivated by compassion. This passive approach toward first-stage labor, together with women's increasing unwillingness to tolerate protracted pain and stress, and the public's general trust in the presumed safety of surgery are accountable for the greater proportion of the increase in cesarean births. These operations are in fact emergency solutions that could have been prevented by much earlier and far less invasive measures.

> *After an unnecessarily long first stage of labor, women can no longer push, no longer want to push, or may not reach the point of pushing.*

3.2.5 The interventional approach

The patience of many providers during labor contrasts sharply with practitioners' impatience during late pregnancy. About 20–40% of all women in western countries give birth after having their labor induced.[17–19] Labor may be induced because of a supposed medical indication or because of opportunistic reasons on the part of the obstetrician – those who deliver during the day are not, after all, delivering at night – or at the request of the pregnant woman herself. An induced uterus is not yet ready for labor and so must be coerced into contractions. It is for this reason that a woman's labor, if induced, is often less effective than if one had waited for spontaneous onset to occur. Induction increases the chance of a long labor due to inefficient and thus ineffective contractions and seriously increases the risk of cesarean delivery because of non-progressing dilatation. Induction also increases the likelihood of a forceps or vacuum delivery owing to the woman's exhaustion and heightens the risk of fetal distress as a result of overstimulation (Chapters 8 and 22). Other prevalent but unnecessary procedures that lead to dysfunctional labor will be highlighted in Chapter 4.

> **Fundamental problem 6**
>
> *Induction is one of the leading causes of iatrogenic labor disorders.*

3.2.6 The paradox

In the final analysis, avoidable cesarean section and other operative deliveries are the result of two common policies that are strangely practiced side by side: the interventional approach with the use of inductions and other interventions leading to long labor and all of its associated complications, and the passive approach in spontaneous labor in which a protracted first stage is not recognized in a timely manner so that it is only possible to attend to the problems after the fact. The fundamental explanation of this paradox is the still widely prevailing mechanistic view of birth in which second-stage mechanics rather than first-stage labor dynamics is the main focus of professional attention.

> *There is a direct relationship between the length of labor and surgical interventions.*[20,21]

3.3 Mechanics-oriented view of childbirth

To reiterate, the mechanism of labor is basically simple and classically dependent on the interaction of three factors:

- *The passenger*, meaning the dimensions and the position and attitude of the fetus's head
- *The passage*, meaning the shape and size of the woman's pelvis
- *The powers*, meaning the efficacy of uterine contractions

The first two factors represent the mechanical condition and the third variable represents the dynamic prerequisite for a successful birth. By and large, the mechanical factors are widely overrated, while the true dominance of the dynamic factor is generally unrecognized or underestimated. Undue preoccupation with the mechanics of birth dates from historical times when nothing could be done to improve uterine performance, whereas pelvic deformations and fetal malformations were a frequent cause of birth obstruction. Although these conditions now belong to ancient history, the general view of birth is still mechanistic, viz. focused on the mechanics of parturition.

Fundamental problem 7

Obstetrics and midwifery still focus more on the mechanics of second-stage labor rather than on the dynamics of first-stage labor.

Traditionally, obstetrics has been strongly oriented toward the mechanics of birth and manual skill. The word "obstetrics" comes from the Latin verb *obstāre*, to stand in front of. This is an etymological explanation for the language of obstetrics, in which the doctor or midwife "delivers" the baby or "does" the delivery instead of the mother herself. The word midwife literally means "the woman standing by women." If labor is slow and increasingly difficult, the orthodox midwife, however, then typically feels there is nothing she can do beyond tender loving care to resolve an admittedly unpleasant situation without the introduction of presumed extraneous hazards to mother or child. From her mechanistic point of view, the midwife is patiently waiting for . . . full dilatation.

In hospitals, long and difficult labor is regarded as a burden but one that is acceptable and can be relieved by an epidural – if such a service is available 24/7 – or by large amounts of opioid drugs. Augmentation of labor is generally not considered before 3 cm dilatation is reached ("active labor established") or, even worse, until a woman shows the first signs of exhaustion. What is more, in many hospitals augmentation of labor often is an option during business hours only. For the woman whose cervix dilates unsatisfactorily late at night, sedation is typically the course of action and in the morning the restless and distressing night is followed by the "total package" of an epidural, electronic fetal monitoring, an intrauterine pressure catheter, and an oxytocin drip. At this point, meconium is present in the amniotic fluid and the uterus is already beyond stimulation. Morale crumbled hours before and the now emotionally drained patient shuts herself off from her attendants, in whom she has progressively lost all trust. All the same, orthodox care providers eagerly await

and expect the achievement of the ultimate goal: . . . full dilatation.

Fundamental problem 8

The dilatation stage of labor comprises more than 90% of the total time of a birth, but it is insufficiently recognized that the majority of birth disorders arise or are created during exactly this first stage.

3.3.1 The mechanistic paradox

As soon as the cervix no longer presents an obstacle, the attitude of orthodox birth attendants undergoes a change as sudden as it is radical; there is a strict time limit on pushing and nearly every invasive intervention seems permissible to force a vaginal birth. Conventional care providers do not seem to realize that if a baby can safely be pulled through the birth canal by forceps or vacuum extractor then delivery should, in principle, be possible by the expulsive force of the woman herself – provided she has enough strength remaining.

The sudden transition from an extremely expectant approach during the first stage to an equally aggressive approach in the second stage epitomizes the widely prevalent mechanistic view of birth.

Obstetricians spend a great deal of their training in learning manual and operative skills to solve an arrested birth, while little or no attention is given to the possibility of preventing the situation. In many textbooks there is still more attention paid to abnormal fetal presentations and deviant pelvic structures than to the dynamics of normal birth, the physics of effective uterine contractions, and the proactive, early correction of slow labor.

Characteristic of the passive attitude toward the first stage of labor – known in French as *la période du désespoir* or the period of despair and hopelessness – is the manner in which patience has been elevated to the level of a professional ethic in midwifery and conventional obstetrics alike. Orthodox publications discuss the idea of "masterly expectancy" and claim that "patience is not a weakness but a controlled force" and that "the clock is the midwife's enemy." Each of these expressions highlights the focus on "the main event," the expulsion of the fetus, while the importance of a smooth first stage of labor is neglected. This oversight is the core of a multitude of problems that will be addressed in detail in the next chapters. In reality, physical and emotional exhaustion are the most frequent and most underrated complications of birth nowadays and attention to the prevention of long labor is far more worthwhile than the attention which is usually devoted to its operative resolution.

> *Physical and emotional exhaustion is the most frequent and most underrated complication of first labors. Women declare their intolerance of long labors by increasingly requesting cesarean delivery.*

3.4 Summary

- Most operative deliveries are performed for the indication "dystocia," which actually represents a poorly defined container term for a multitude of distinct birth disorders for which there are often much less intrusive solutions.
- Obviously, tackling the problem of failed labors requires precise definition of the underlying pathophysiology and attempts to make a specific, causal diagnosis.
- The marked variations that exist between the types of care women receive depend more on which maternity unit they go to, which professionals they consult, and what time labor happens to begin than on their individual needs or preferences.
- This diversity in care echoes disagreement in appreciation of first-stage labor physiology.

- Inconsistent management of labor originates in a lack of universal definitions for elementary birth parameters. This shortcoming blocks the determination of objective criteria for normal versus abnormal labor.
- The chance of a traumatic birth experience and operative delivery correlates strongly with the length of labor. Physical and emotional exhaustion is the most frequent and most underrated complication of birth. Women have declared their intolerance of long labors by increasingly requesting intrapartum cesarean section.
- Widespread tolerance of long labor originates in the traditional mechanistic view of childbirth which focuses on the expulsion stage, whereas first-stage labor disorders are either created or go undetected for too long.
- Undue preoccupation with the mechanics of birth has prevented progress in rational labor management for a very long time. In reality, it is labor dynamics rather than mechanics that determines the chance of a successful and safe vaginal delivery.
- The majority of problems surrounding childbirth can be attributed to the widespread lack of a consistent and cohesive policy framework for the conduct and care of normal labor.
- As effective uterine contractions are the key to normal labor and delivery, the central problem of dystocia can be solved by much simpler methods than resorting to cesarean delivery.
- Turning the tide of ever-increasing operative delivery rates requires a fundamental change in the conduct and care of normal labor: *proactive support of labor* (Section 3).

REFERENCES

1. American College of Obstetricians and Gynecologists. Task force on Cesarean Delivery Rates: Evaluation of Cesarean Delivery. June 2000.
2. Heffner LJ, Elkin E, Fretts RC. Impact of labor induction, gestational age and maternal age on cesarean delivery rates. *Obstet Gynecol* 2003; 102: 287–93.

3. Seyb ST, Berka RJ, Socol ML, Doodley SL. Risk of cesarean delivery with elective induction of labor at term in nulliparous women. *Obstet Gynecol* 1999; 94: 600–7.

4. Macer JA, Macer CL, Chan LS. Elective induction versus spontaneous labor: a retrospective study of complications and outcome. *Am J Obstet Gynecol* 1992; 166: 1690–6.

5. Cammu H, Marten G, Ruyssinck G, Amy JJ. Outcome after elective induction in nulliparous women: a matched cohort study. *Am J Obstet Gynecol* 2002; 186: 240–4.

6. Luthy DA, Malmgren JA, Zingheim RW. Increased Cesarean section rates associated with elective induction in nulliparous women; the physician effect. *Am J Obstet Gynecol* 2004; 191: 1511–15.

7. Dublin S, Lydon-Rochelle M, Kaplan RC, Watts DH, Critchlow CW. Maternal and fetal outcomes after induction without an identified indication. *Am J Obstet Gynecol* 2000; 18: 986–94.

8. Van Gemund N, Hardeman A, Scherjon SA, Kanhai HH. Intervention rates after elective induction of labor compared to labor with a spontaneous onset: a matched cohort study. *Gynecol Obstet Invest* 2003; 56(3): 133–8.

9. Maslow AS, Sweeny AL. Elective induction of labor as a risk factor for cesarean delivery among low-risk women at term. *Obstet Gynecol* 2000; 95: 917–22.

10. Smith KM, Hoffman MK, Sciscione A. Elective induction of labor in nulliparous women increases the risk of cesarean section. *Obstet Gynecol* 2003; 101: S45.

11. Kauffman K, Bailit J, Grobman W. Elective induction: an analysis of economic and health consequences. *Am J Obstet Gynecol* 2001; 185: S209.

12. Vahratian A, Zhang J, Troendle JF, *et al.* Labor progression and risk of cesarean delivery in electively induced nulliparas. *Obstet Gynecol* 2005; 105: 698–704.

13. Hamar B, Mann S, Greenberg P, *et al.* Low-risk inductions of labor and cesarean delivery for nulliparous and parous women at term. *Am J Obstet Gynecol* 2001; 185: S215.

14. Main EK. Reducing Cesarean birth rates with data-driven quality improvement activities. *Pediatrics* 1999; 103: 374–83.

15. Cunningham FG, Leveno KJ, Bloom SL. Section IV. Labor and Delivery. In: *Williams Obstetrics*, 22nd edn. New York: McGraw-Hill; 2005: 496.

16. O'Driscoll K, Meagher D, Robson M. *Active Management of Labour*, 4th edn. Mosby; 2003.

17. O'Connell MP, Lindow SW. Trends in obstetric care in the United Kingdom. *J Obstet Gynaecol* 2000; 20: 592–3.

18. Goffinet F, Dreyfus M, Carbonne B, Magnin G, Cabrol D. Survey of the practice of cervical ripening and labor induction in France. *J Gynecol Obstet Biol Reprod* 2003; 32(7): 638–46 (article in French).

19. Humbert R, Clerson P, Philippe HJ, Breart G, Cabrol D. National survey on the use of induced labor by obstetricians. *J Gynecol Obstet Biol Reprod* 1999; 28(4): 319–29 (article in French).

20. Cardozo LD, Gibb DM, Studd JW, Vasant RV, Cooper DJ. Predictive value of cervimetric labour patterns in primigravids. *Br J Obstet Gynaecol* 1982; 89: 33–8.

21. Chelmow D, Kilpatrick SJ, Laros RK Jr. Maternal and neonatal outcomes after prolonged latent phase. *Obstet Gynecol* 1993; 81(4): 486–91.

4

Harmful birth care practices

There is an undeniable trend worldwide toward the acceptance and even the pursuit of medicalized childbirth. Giving birth is increasingly perceived as a risky experience for which only the medical practitioner seems to have the proper answers. Technological advances and possibilities are highlighted in the media and appear unlimited. Supply generates demand and the client demands as much security as possible. To this end, patients and many care providers have the false assumption that the utmost in diagnostic and medical precautions guarantees the best chance of health. The extent to which the reverse is true is largely underestimated. Along with the benefits resulting from the proper use of technology for women with real pregnancy and birth complications (the minority of pregnant women) have come the unnecessary medicalization and the high price of iatrogenic complications in healthy pregnancies (the majority of pregnant women). Undue medicalization of birth causes anxiety and stress, thereby directly and indirectly creating problems in the dynamics of labor and delivery (Chapter 7). In this way, doctors create and maintain their own patient population.

The Medical Paradox

For women with a complicated pregnancy (the minority) there is no better place to give birth than a hospital. For healthy women with a normal pregnancy (the majority) hospitals can be very dangerous.

4.1 Idle faith in technology

Obstetricians often claim that the use of high-tech maternity care equates with real progress, but the scientific evidence indicates otherwise. Over the past 30 years no significant improvement has been demonstrated in highly industrialized countries in the incidence of low-birth-weight babies or cerebral palsy.[1] The slight reduction in the perinatal mortality rate in these countries during the past three decades is attributable not to obstetrical improvements or to any decrease in fetal mortality but to a slight decrease in neonatal mortality associated with neonatal intensive care. Indeed, all attempts to associate lower perinatal mortality rates with the higher obstetrical intervention rates in developed nations have failed.[2] Notzon comments in a US National Center for Health Statistics study that "the comparisons of perinatal mortality ratios with cesarean and with operative vaginal rates find no consistent correlations across countries."[3] A review of the scientific literature on this issue by Lomas and Enkin for the Oxford National Perinatal Epidemiology Unit states: "A number of studies have failed to detect any relation between crude perinatal mortality rates and the level of operative deliveries."[4] The US Centers for Disease Control and Prevention actually demonstrated a threefold risk of neonatal death for infants born by cesarean section to low-risk mothers and an alarming rise in US maternal mortality rates.[5,6] These findings suggest that we have now passed the point at which the benefits of development and technology outweigh the negative effects.

High-tech childbirth is thought to be real progress, but the scientific evidence indicates otherwise.

4.1.1 The cesarean boomerang

In the past, cesarean section was used exclusively in perilous situations to save mother or infant from injury or death. Today, as indications broaden and rates continue to go up, lives are saved in a smaller and smaller proportion of all cesarean deliveries. But the risks of this major surgical procedure do not decrease with increasing rates and consequently a rate has been reached at which cesarean section inevitably inflicts more harm on babies and mothers than it prevents. The remedy has become its own disease.

Uncritical use of cesarean delivery eventually kills more women and babies than it saves.

4.1.2 Technical excess and harmful rituals

So far, mainstream obstetrics has not been able to exploit the advantages of medicalized pregnancy while avoiding the disadvantages such as the drift to medical excess. Technological advance has led to the almost automatic use of new, primarily diagnostic techniques without any concomitant therapeutic options. Aside from misinterpretation, prenatal diagnosis, routine ultrasound, and routine electronic fetal monitoring have also led to new questions and problems that may become unmanageable for patients and providers. The latter must translate their findings into practice and dubious information often creates more insecurity than confidence in both mothers and caregivers. This leads to the unnecessary medicalization of essentially healthy women.

Routine rituals in the labor ward such as repeatedly taking blood pressure and temperature, restricting fluids and food, prohibiting a woman from wearing her own nightgown, restricting movement, routine insertion of fetal scalp electrodes and intrauterine lines, use of enemas, shaving the perineum, requiring personnel to wear scrubs, cap, and masks, and so forth, greatly increase the stressfulness of labor. Many birth disorders are indirectly caused by these routines with no recognition of the negative effects of this clinical excess on the dynamics of the parasympathetic birth process. Stress inhibits labor (Chapter 7). Moreover, systematic reviews incontestably demonstrate that all the routines listed above lack any clinical benefit and should therefore be abandoned.[7]

Even simple procedures during prenatal care as seemingly innocent as a routine vaginal examination in late pregnancy to determine whether the cervix is "ready for labor" or "stripping" the membranes (digital separation of the fetal membranes from the lower uterine segment), cause more problems than one realizes. False labor, from the anticipation created when a vaginal examination reveals "cervical ripeness" or from sweeping the membranes, is rarely recognized as iatrogenic (Chapter 23).

4.2 Negative psychology

Generally, the detrimental influence of negative psychology on the course and outcome of labor is greatly underestimated. Providing the patient with explanations and guidance is a must, but the manner in which they are presented is everything. Well-meaning information regarding possible risk factors, when presented without professional tact, casts a shadow of doubt on a woman's trust in a good outcome. When a woman becomes alarmed, her anxiety progressively undermines the motivation and self-confidence that are vitally important for creating the best environment for a safe and spontaneous birth (Chapter 7).

The "Black Cloud" Phenomenon

Negative psychological influences undermine the self-confidence and mental conditions necessary to create the best possible chance of an uncomplicated birth.

4.2.1 Discouraging stories

As it is now, negative psychological stimuli are freely spread through the woman's everyday surroundings. One out of two of her friends is likely to be an expert-by-experience in an operative delivery and is only too happy to share: "A whole day of suffering, and still a cesarean." What about sensational tabloid headlines such as "Actress's Baby Dead," or the pseudo-informative division of serious media, "The Truth about Uterine Rupture," or the flatly distasteful reality-TV show "A Birth Story," which spends two minutes on the dilatation stage and three-quarters of an hour on misrepresentative and demeaning shrieks and growls in the second stage?

4.2.2 The culture of fear

Beyond this, it is really the care providers themselves who generate the darkest clouds. Routine ultrasound often leads to dubious interpretations of supposedly "abnormal" findings. This has been described by a leading expert in sonography as "the best way to terrify pregnant women."[8] Unnecessary uncertainty is aroused when the estimated fetal weight (generally inaccurate) is printed on the sonography report that the parents take home – a prediction taken as an indication of likely birth outcome. A large baby diagnosed and a worried look on the doctor's face during the pelvic examination are not motivating. The "trial of labor" is likely to fail, not because of fetopelvic disproportion but because of ineffective uterine action triggered by anxiety and the induction procedure.

> *Unfavorable predictions often are self-fulfilling prophecies.*

Similarly, it does not build a woman's confidence when her providers schedule preparations for induction of labor when pregnancy is only one week overdue "because your baby is at risk." Other findings such as a small belly, low-lying placenta, low amniotic fluid level, and so forth often lead to intensive observation by medical staff and readying

of cross-matched blood and an IV line during labor as well as food restriction, "just in case." None of these actions have proven therapeutic benefits.[7] Instead, when performed thoughtlessly or with negative body language these precautionary actions generate undue stress and anxiety, which is the best way to provoke undesirable interventions and outcomes.

Likewise, well-meaning warnings in the woman's chart, such as "BEWARE" or "low-threshold for C section," are not conducive to the creation of a positive attitude among the on-duty staff who must convey to the woman in labor that she is perfectly capable of a spontaneous delivery. It is much easier to confirm the prediction of a problematic birth that it is to prevent it. Women in labor do not benefit from the insecurities created by the overt anticipation of problems that have yet to occur. A risk factor is still not an illness – a distinction that is not immediately clear to most patients and some care providers.

> *The darkest clouds are produced by the care-givers themselves.*

There is considerable evidence of the harmful effects of iatrogenic anxiety in clinical practice worldwide. For example, an American trial showed that false positive prediction by ultrasound of fetal macrosomia provoked a 50% increase in cesarean delivery of same-weight babies.[9] A Canadian trial revealed that labeling a woman as gestational diabetic conferred a doubled cesarean delivery rate, regardless of the fetal or maternal condition and with no relationship to birth weight.[10] In a German study, the label "growth retardation" biased interpretation of and action taken for fetal monitoring and led to twice as many cesarean sections as occurred in undetected cases of growth restriction.[11] A twin study from Iceland and Scotland revealed no difference in outcome of "naturally conceived" twins as compared to twins after "assisted conception," except that the cesarean rate was twice as high in the assisted-conception group.[12] In a Swedish study, older nulliparas had dramatically increased odds of cesarean delivery regardless of maternal or fetal condition.[13] A Canadian study of the definition and management of dystocia found that among the strongest determinants of a decision for cesarean delivery were acquisition of a dystocia perception and label in the mind of the physician, although a significant proportion of such decisions were made during the "latent phase" of labor.[14]

4.2.3 Professional daunting

Downright discouragement of vaginal birth may be part of prelabor counseling to protect the hospital against liability suits. A woman has to sign a document of consent after being informed that she is likely to have an episiotomy, that she might severely tear her vulva and pelvic floor, that she might bleed profusely, that she might need an emergency surgical delivery, and that she might lose her baby. Little wonder some people feel hospitals try to bully them into cesarean delivery.

4.3 Clinical ambiance

For many women pregnancy is the most amazing and wonderful time of their lives and its conclusion by giving birth should be an intimate experience leading to an ultimate sense of accomplishment and satisfaction. The great majority of women in labor, however, are not properly educated (Chapter 19) and thus not properly prepared for this job; they are just told by staff to "get on with it." In many hospitals, routine procedures more often give rise to ambiguity and the feeling that one is neither being heard nor taken seriously. Added to this, the clinical outfit and attitude of providers and the "functional" and sterile furnishing of many delivery rooms may often act as potent tocolytic methods. Stress inhibits labor (Chapter 7). The result is iatrogenic dysfunctional labor.

4.3.1 Women's sense of isolation

The more efficiently the hospital seems to be organized, the more rapidly women feel reduced to a number. From time to time a nurse looks in, but most of the time women lie alone enduring the first stage of labor. Many caregivers do not realize how lonely women in labor may feel, especially in a busy labor unit, and how frightful loneliness can be. The women's partners, if in attendance, feel equally helpless. The sense of isolation and the reality of being left alone, even momentarily, are often compounded by the appearance and disappearance of a rapidly changing cast of students, midwives, interns, residents, and occasionally consultants. Several survey studies report that a low-risk mother having her first child is attended by from 5 to 15 unfamiliar people (dubbed by one author as "masked intruders") but is still left alone most of the time.[7]

Medical equipment is used simply because it is present or for reasons of efficiency only. Personal attention and supportive care are replaced by watching the fetal monitor screen in the coffee room. This method of care requires fewer personnel. This is convenient from a budget perspective but disastrous to the provision of real care. It seems that the main "advantage" of the introduction of routine electronic fetal monitoring has been that women in labor can be left unattended by nursing care.

> "It is not too fanciful to compare the state of laboring women nowadays with that of the absolutely terrified pregnant monkeys so often cited in relation to psychological stress, failed deliveries, and fetal distress."[15]

4.3.2 Frustratingly casual attitudes

In orthodox medical circles, recognition has come slowly that women may experience medicalized childbirth as genuinely traumatic. Failure to pay nearly enough attention to this important issue has been attributed to the fact that until recently obstetricians were mostly men, although the current, rapid feminization of the obstetric profession has not, as it seems, resulted in more woman-friendly provisions, attitudes, and approaches. Rarely is human consciousness more susceptible to impressions than during labor, and the all-too-common casual approach by professionals – both male and female – burdens women with frustrated feelings of dismissal.[16,17] Things as seemingly trivial as leaving the woman lying naked after an examination, thoughtless remarks, conversations about other patients in her presence, blood-stained clothing, unconsidered answers, inconsistent explanations by ever-changing staff, delays in giving her test results, concealing one's actual intentions, leaving her alone for long periods of time, not keeping appointments – to the woman, all these seem like personal insults. For obvious reasons she interprets this behavior as indifference on the part of precisely the people in whom she has put her trust during the most vulnerable hours of her life.

In reality, however, indifference is not the problem. The majority of birth care providers are devoted to the patients in their care. Many seemingly thoughtless actions are rather the result of the lack of a central plan of childbirth and unnecessarily long labors. For example, many conservatively supervised first births take far longer than the length of one work shift. This means that it is increasingly rare for women to have continuous and personal attention from one and the same care provider throughout their labor. What is more, an unclear perspective on how to proceed when slow labor becomes increasingly difficult has a demoralizing effect not only on the patient and her partner but also on the nursing staff. As a result, labor room staff consciously or unconsciously avoid the birthing room and frequent the coffee room.

> *Deficient nursing care is the inevitable result of unnecessarily long labors.*

4.3.3 Divided attention

A labor room nurse must equally divide her attention among more patients while frequently attending to responsibilities that have nothing to do with birth but by which nearly every labor ward is plagued, such as (semi)emergency consultations, small tasks, antenatal non-stress tests, external cephalic versions of breech, etc. And many a labor and delivery ward is abused as a gynecological first-aid facility. The personal attention the midwife or labor room nurse can provide to women in labor is further hampered by modern hospital rules regarding "quality assessments," which essentially require the keeping of extensive records of mostly irrelevant data at the expense of basic care. Defensive medicine dictates silly administration: "If you don't document it, preferably in triplicate, it wasn't done." In addition, understaffing in the interest of efficiency has taken over hospital policies. It is in this way that the backlash of budget cuts (so-called "managed care") and supposed but irrelevant "quality demands" are felt most profoundly in labor rooms. Managers and policymakers seldom realize that indispensable personal attention throughout labor requires sufficient personnel at the bedside whose focus should be on direct supportive care for each woman in labor.

> Fundamental problem 9
>
> *Personal and continuous one-on-one support extended to all women in labor is critical to providing quality care, but it is a requirement that hardly any hospital meets.*

4.4 Care of fetus versus care of mother

Obstetrics has evolved from maternity care toward perinatology and prevention of perinatal morbidity and mortality is at present its dominant benchmark. However, this also poses a significant risk to women. In the words of Kieran O'Driscoll: "Somehow the idea has gained ground that a conflict of interest exists between mother and child during labor and that mothers can be subjected to almost any form of indignity or discomfort provided it is well intentioned and undertaken on behalf of her baby."[18] Additional concerns about liability, whether real or remote, play an increasingly greater role in the defensive interpretation of indications used to justify aggressive interventions. As the saying goes: "When in doubt, get it out." Numerous inductions of labor or cesarean deliveries are performed on the basis of "fetal compromise," with the nature and validity of that generalization undefined. The majority of the supposedly compromised fetuses most likely are not, but are "rescued from normalcy" by induction of labor and/or operative delivery for enhanced provider and patient anxiety (Chapter 24).[19]

4.4.1 Fetal trauma

Augmentation of slowly progressing labor is often postponed because of a supposed negative effect on fetal oxygen supply, as though the interests of mother and child were opposed. This widespread misconception leads to therapeutic paralysis. On the one hand caregivers are hesitant to accelerate slow labor, especially in the so-called "latent phase" of labor, but on the other long labor does not benefit the fetus either. On the contrary, exhaustion after too long a labor is strongly associated with instrumental vaginal delivery and these interventions are the predominant cause of severe fetal injuries such as fetal skin lacerations, bone fractures, bleeding, paralyses, and lethal rupture of tentorium cerebelli. Strangely, a paradoxical discrepancy continues to exist between the fear of fetal hypoxia and the failure to anticipate mechanical birth injuries. These obstetrical traumas are rarely seen in children delivered spontaneously but are nearly always the result of forced instrumental delivery.[20–26]

The trauma paradox

The aggressive precautions taken to prevent fetal hypoxic damage are in sharp contrast to the

---

failure to foresee the fetal birth traumas caused by instrumental traction with vacuum extractor or forceps.

4.4.2 Parallel interests

In essence, fetal trauma can be discussed under the same heading as severe birth injuries to the mother such as cervical laceration, vault rupture, and fourth-degree lacerations that need extensive surgical repair as well as damage to the pudendal nerve, the levator ani muscle, the fascial pelvic organ supports, and the anal sphincter, which may result in life-long dyspareunia and urinary or fecal incontinence. These injuries occur in second-stage labor and the circumstances that give rise to severe maternal trauma are essentially the same as those which give rise to severe fetal trauma – i.e., forced traction.[27–36] In reality, the interests of mother and child are parallel in that both profit from a strategy of care that is specifically focused on preventing an overly long labor that ends in a forced instrumental delivery: *proactive support of labor* (Section 3).

Proactive support of labor serves the best interests of both mothers and their babies.

4.5 Summary

- Many elements of care during pregnancy and childbirth can foster or jeopardize the successful conclusion of this natural process.
- Overmedicalization of childbirth has numerous adverse effects on women's labor experiences and the objective outcomes of labor and delivery.
- Technical excess, clinical routines, discontinuous care, and negative psychology create physical and emotional stress leading to numerous negative domino effects that are hardly ever recognized for what they are: iatrogenic birth disorders.

- Structural improvements require a new approach and an overall plan for normal childbirth: *proactive support of labor.*

REFERENCES

1. National Center for Health Statistics. http//www.cdc.gov/nchs/.
2. Matthews TG, Crowley P, Chong A, *et al.* Rising caesarean section rates: A cause for concern. *Br J Obstet Gynaecol* 2003; 110: 346–9.
3. Notzon FC. International differences in the use of obstetric interventions. *JAMA* 1990; 263(24): 3286–91.
4. Lomas J, Enkin M. Variations in operative delivery rates. In Chalmers I, Enkin M, Keirse MJ, eds. *Effective Care in Pregnancy and Childbirth*. Oxford: Oxford University Press; 1998.
5. MacDorman MF, Declercq E, Menacker F, Malloy MH. Infant and neonatal mortality for primary cesarean and vaginal births to women with "no indicated risk," United States 1998–2001 birth cohorts. *Birth* 2006; 3: 175–82.
6. Centers for Disease Control and Prevention. http//www:cdc.gov/nchs/data/series/ (accessed October, 2007).
7. Enkin M, Keirse MJNC, Neilson J, *et al.* Hospital practices. In: *A Guide to Effective Care in Pregnancy and Childbirth*, 3rd edn. Oxford: Oxford University Press; 2000.
8. Filly RA. Obstetrical ultrasonography: the best way to terrify a pregnant woman. *J Ultrasound Med* 2000; 19: 1–5.
9. Levine AB, Lockwood CJ, Brown B, Lapinski R, Berkowitz RL. Sonographic diagnosis of the large for gestational age fetus at term: does it make a difference? *Obstet Gynecol* 1992; 79: 55–8.
10. Naylor CD, Sermer M, Chen E, Sykora K. Cesarean delivery in relation to birth weight and gestational glucose tolerance: pathophysiology or practice style? *JAMA* 1996; 275: 1199–2000.
11. Jahn A, Razum O, Berle P. Routine screening for intrauterine growth retardation in Germany: low sensitivity and questionable benefit for diagnosed cases. *Acta Obstet Gynecol Scand* 1998; 77: 643–8.
12. Agustsson T, Geirsson RT, Mires G. Obstetric outcome of natural and assisted conception twin pregnancies is similar. *Acta Obstet Gynecol Scand* 1997; 76: 45–9.
13. Cnattingius R, Cnattingius S, Notzon FC. Obstacles to reducing cesarean rates in a low-cesarean setting: the effect of maternal age, height and weight. *Obstet Gynecol* 1998; 92: 501–6.
14. Stewart PJ, Duhlberg C, Arnett AC, Elmslie T, Hall PF. Diagnosis of dystocia and management with cesarean section among primiparous women in Ottowa Carleton. *CMAJ* 1990; 142: 459–63.
15. Enkin M, Keirse MJNC, Neilson J, *et al. A Guide to Effective Care in Pregnancy and Childbirth*, 3rd edn. Oxford: Oxford University Press; 2000.
16. Simkin P. Just another day in a woman's life? Women's long-term perceptions of their first birth experience. Part I. *Birth* 1991; 18: 203–10.
17. Simkin P. Just another day in a woman's life? Women's long-term perceptions of their first birth experience Part II. *Birth* 1991; 19: 64–81.
18. O'Driscoll K, Meagher D, Robson M. *Active Management of Labour*, 4th edn. Mosby; 2003.
19. Menticoglou SM, Hall PF. Routine induction of labour at 41 weeks gestation: nonsensus consensus. *Br J Obstet Gynaecol* 2002; 109: 485–91.
20. Holroyde J, Woods JR jr, Siddiqi TA, Scott M, Miodovnic M. Birth trauma: incidence and predisposing factors. *Obstet Gynecol* 1984; 63: 792–5.
21. Menticoglou SM, Manning F, Harman C, *et al.* Perinatal outcomes in relation to second-stage duration. *Am J Obstet Gynecol* 1995; 173: 906–12.
22. Menticoglou SM, Perlman M, Manning FA. High cervical spinal cord injury in neonates delivered with forceps: Report of 15 cases. *Obstet Gynecol* 1995; 86: 589–94.
23. Williams MC, Knuppel RA, O'Brien WF, *et al.* Obstetric correlates of neonatal retinal hemorrhage. *Obstet Gynecol* 1993; 81: 688–94.
24. Johnson JH, Figueroa R, Garry D, *et al.* Immediate maternal and neonatal effects of forceps and vacuum-assisted deliveries. *Obstet Gynecol* 2004; 103: 513–18.
25. Uchil D, Arulkumaran S. Neonatal subgaleal hemorrhage and its relationship to delivery by vacuum extraction. *Obstet Gynecol Surv* 2003; 58: 687–93.
26. Johnson RB, Menon BK. Vacuum extraction versus forceps for assisted vaginal delivery. *Cochrane Database Syst Rev* 2000; (2): CD 00024.
27. Casey BM, Schaffer JI, Bloom SL, *et al.* Obstetric antecedents for postpartum pelvic floor dysfunction. *Am J Obstet Gynecol* 2005; 192(5): 1655–62.
28. Dietz HP, Wilson PD. Childbirth and pelvic floor trauma. *Best Pract Res Clin Obstet Gynaecol* 2005; 19 (6): 913–24.

29. Rortveit G, Kjersti Daltveit A, Hannestad YS, Hunskaar S. Urinary incontinence after vaginal delivery or cesarean section. *N Engl J Med* 2003; 348: 900–7.

30. Lal M. Prevention of urinary and anal incontinence: role of elective cesarean delivery. *Curr Opin Obstet Gynecol* 2003; 15(5): 439–48.

31. Bahl R, Strachan B, Murphy DJ. Pelvic floor morbidity at 3 years after instrumental delivery and cesarean delivery in the second stage of labor and the impact of a subsequent delivery. *Am J Obstet Gynecol* 2005; 192 (3): 789–94.

32. Wang A, Guess M, Connell K, *et al.* Fecal incontinence: a review of prevalence and obstetric risk factors. *Int Urogynecol J Pelvic Floor Dysfunct* 2006; 17 (3): 253–60.

33. Kearney R, Miller JM, Ashton-Miller JA, DeLancey JO. Obstetric factors associated with levator ani muscle injury after vaginal birth. *Obstet Gynecol* 2006; 107(1): 144–9.

34. Andrews V, Sultan AH, Thakar R, Jones PW. Risk factors for obstetric anal sphincter injury: a prospective study. *Birth* 2006; 33(2): 117–22.

35. Buhling KJ, Schmidt S, Robinson JN, *et al.* Rate of dyspareunia after delivery in primiparae according to mode of delivery. *Eur J Obstet Gynecol Reprod Biol* 2006; 124(1): 42–6.

36. Hicks TL, Goodall SF, Quattrone EM, Lydon-Rochelle MT. Postpartum sexual functioning and mode of delivery: summary of the evidence. *J Midwifery Women's Health* 2004; 49: 430–36.

5

Destructive territorial disputes

Women's critique of the excessive medicalization and related "dehumanization" of childbirth has led to calls for the return of independent midwifery care and even home births.[1–3] The question is whether this post-modern trend will provide proper solutions. Answers can be found by examining western childbirth systems that formally include autonomous midwifery care. In this context some fundamental differences between midwifery care and the medical approach must be illuminated. Strong prejudices and emotions are involved here and disputes are often characterized more by heat than by light: the debate is usually about choice of caregiver and place of birth, rather than about labor.

5.1 Controversial birth philosophies

Unlike obstetricians and hospital managers, who generally see childbirth as a standard medical problem subject to the modern paradigm of "managed care," midwives typically approach labor and delivery as a natural process and a highly individual experience, sometimes even compounded with a spiritual, nigh-mystical atmosphere. An exemplary quote: "[labor,] . . . it is predictable that it will occur, but unpredictable and idiosyncratic in its actual occurrence. Despite attempts to package labor into discrete phases and stages, it is better understood as a whole, with an ebb and flow and rhythms of its own. It is intensely physical and emotional, consuming all of one's attention and energy; yet life-giving and empowering in that intensity. How then is it possible to 'manage' labor?"[4]

5.1.1 Adverse working relations

The typical role of the midwife is to provide strong supportive care in labor and to preserve a woman's place in the group categorized as "normal" for as long as possible without intervention. In contrast, obstetricians focus on risks and pathological conditions, want to be in control, and put trust in technology. The differing starting points that typically characterize the two professions have often made for tense and even hostile working relations. Obstetricians accuse midwives of backwardness, blocking progress, and trusting recklessly in biology. One obstetrician best summarizes the general sentiment of many: "Nature is a lousy obstetrician." On the other hand, midwives reproach obstetricians for providing interventional, impersonal, and technocratic birth care, for having a lack of faith in nature, for disempowering women, and for overriding biology. In such adversarial circumstances it is the patients who draw the shortest straws. In reality, women's preferences and needs contain many elements of both midwifery and medical styles of care and all laboring women should benefit from what are, in fact, the complementary skills of both professional groups. Clearly, both obstetricians and midwives – and above all laboring women – have much to gain from a childbirth system that combines the best of midwifery and medicine: *proactive support of labor* (Section 3)

> *Women's preferences and needs contain many elements of both midwifery and medical styles of care.*

5.2 Cross-cultural differences

Reforming childbirth services is not an easy task. No single component of health care is influenced more by culture, tradition, social pressures, politics, and litigation issues than pregnancy care. Consequently, there are three established forms of maternity services in the western world: the fully medicalized, doctor-centered childbirth system typically found, for example, in the USA, France, and Spain; the midwife-centered system almost exclusively found in New Zealand, the Scandinavian countries, and the Netherlands; and a mixture of both systems, found, for example, in the UK, Canada, Australia, Germany, and Japan. Clearly, the defined role of midwives varies significantly throughout the western world. As a result, the disputes between midwives and obstetricians are at different levels in different countries. We will briefly discuss the extremes of the spectrum at the risk of caricaturing.

> *For a detached woman having her first baby, it can be difficult to believe how culturally shaped the childbirth service can be.*

5.2.1 Disputes in medicalized countries

Strikingly, the term "midwife" is not mentioned once in the 1441 pages of the authoritative US textbook *Williams Obstetrics* (2005). Home births are actively discouraged and 99% of all US births take place in hospitals. Independent, community-based midwives have been marginalized or even pushed into illegality, situations that in turn attract women who are fed up with the medicalized system. Birth in

the USA is the responsibility of doctors. Auxiliary personnel are called "labor and delivery nurse" or "nurse-midwife." American midwives practice under the strict authority of the obstetricians, but for the convenience of the doctor are given a high degree of responsibility. "Nurse-midwives" assess the patient and then contact the obstetrician, who is mostly not in the hospital, seeing patients in his office. The midwife, of course, knows the proclivity of each individual doctor and so how she presents her findings is influenced by this knowledge. Despite the claim that they are "a team" they all know that the obstetrician is the boss. An insider explained it thus: "It is like a marriage where the husband and wife are a 'partnership' but the husband is ultimately in charge. The wife resorts to all kinds of trickery and manipulation to get the husband to do what she wants. That is what the relationship is like in the USA between nurse-midwives and obstetricians." Midwives have to fight for every inch of bringing midwifery care back to American childbirth. In practice, many resort, as it seems, to everyday acts of resistance to put off unnecessary interventions by practitioners. Clearly, there is an urgent need to redefine the professional relationships between US obstetricians and midwives (Chapter 26).

5.2.2 Disputes in midwife-centered systems

An example at the other end of the spectrum is the Dutch childbirth system. Midwifery has a long history as an established and independent profession in the Netherlands. Midwife-led home birth is still valued as part of a cultural heritage, not only by the midwives but also by a considerable percentage of Dutch women. The midwives stake their claim to an autonomous existence in isolation from the medical department on the premise that pregnancy and birth are natural processes, not illnesses. Thus, in those midwives' eyes, the pregnant woman is not a patient but a client. Since midwives attend only "normal labor" and are not allowed to intervene, the bounds of "normal" are then widely overstretched. In this way the strict separation between midwifery and medical obstetrics creates illogical barriers against the small and timely corrections of slow labor that could forestall far more intrusive interventions at a later stage. Typically, a woman is transferred to the hospital only if she and the midwife no longer see the possibility of a natural end to labor. In this way, Dutch obstetricians function as a safety-net and obviously address problems only after the fact. Too many out-of-control labors – often dubbed "a total loss" or "a train wreck" – are offered. What essentially was a dynamic problem is then solved mechanically: by an operative delivery.

> *Autonomous midwifery creates a barrier to minor and timely corrections of slow labor that can prevent the need for far more invasive interventions at a later stage.*

Unlike the situation in the USA – where midwives have not reached the point of practicing independent midwifery and quality of childbirth might surely benefit from a reappraisal of some aspects of midwifery care – the debate in the Netherlands is at a different level. Dutch obstetricians feel the need to have more input in the decision making about when a parturient has crossed the line from normal to abnormal labor. Clearly, in both doctor- and midwifery-centered systems much better co-operation is needed.

5.3 Myths and facts of autonomous midwifery

While most readers will be familiar with medicalized childbirth systems and recognize the urgent need for reforms, most are unaware of the ins and outs of a formal midwifery-centered system. Since the childbirth system in the Netherlands is often extolled as a "midwives' Mecca" that deserves to be copied elsewhere, the facts and myths of

its childbirth system need to be put into proper perspective.

5.3.1 Autonomous gate-keepers

The Dutch system seems to embody what many midwives worldwide are struggling for and that is acknowledgment of the appropriateness and self-proclaimed superiority of midwifery care for normal pregnancy and birth. In the Netherlands primary (midwifery) care has a gate-keeper role: healthy women expecting a normal birth are directed into primary care, whereas women facing some kind of risk are referred to secondary (medical) care.[5] A formal list of indications defines the conditions that require a referral from primary to secondary care.[6] Primary (midwifery) care is practiced independently in a primary birth center or at the birthing woman's home.

Only a minority of Dutch midwives work in hospitals as "clinical midwives" and report to an obstetrician as is typical in most countries. The majority of Dutch midwives still work independently in that they are self-employed, work outside of the hospital, carry independent insurance, and are paid directly through their clients' insurance. Although all Dutch midwives are well trained and legally certified, their training in the supervision of labor is in the traditional philosophy of expectancy. As a matter of principle, labor and delivery are approached conservatively. The Dutch government assures the midwives' job security. Under health insurance law, healthy pregnant women are reimbursed only if they see a midwife for their care. In other words, midwifery is the system for normal childbirth in the Netherlands.[7] Dutch obstetricians supposedly are not involved in the care of normal pregnancy and childbirth, unless the midwife requests their help. That is the story, now the facts.

> *There are many misguided ideas about the benefits of autonomous midwifery.*

5.3.2 Transfer rates

Serious doubts must be raised about the efficacy and safety of the gate-keeper role of primary care, in particular with regard to first pregnancies. In reality, the primacy of Dutch midwifery does not prevent the medicalization of birth: 77% of all primigravidas eventually end up in the secondary care division;[8] 18% begin their antenatal care with an obstetrician because of a preexisting condition or risk factor; 40% are referred during pregnancy; and of the remaining 42% who start labor at home, nearly 50% are transferred to the hospital where an obstetrician (or rather the youngest resident) takes over their care. The main indications for intrapartum referral include failure to progress in the first stage (but often quite late), meconium, abnormal fetal heart beat counts, second-stage arrest, and afterbirth disorders. These transfer rates seriously question the cost-to-benefit ratio of primary birth care by autonomous midwives for first-time mothers. What is more, women who are transferred to the hospital during labor report significantly less satisfaction with childbirth than those who planned a hospital birth in advance.[9]

5.3.3 Discontinuous and unsafe care

Unlike the midwives of earlier times – who worked around the clock and stayed with their parturient clients from beginning to end – contemporary midwives have their own family life, often disallowing continuous labor attendance with their clients. As a result, periodic visits at intervals of three hours or more during the first stage of labor are now standard practice in Dutch home midwifery. Labor support and care – and thus responsibility for maternal and fetal well-being – are left to the woman's partner, a relative, or a friend. Clearly, this situation is far from ideal and, in fact, is irresponsible. The perinatal mortality rate for term babies in Holland, albeit low, now exceeds that of most other European countries[10] and this reflects, at least in part, its midwifery-centered childbirth

system. Fifty percent of all term stillbirths in Holland occur under "low-risk," autonomous midwifery care.[11] Added to that, 50% of all term babies admitted to Dutch neonatal intensive care units – in most cases for meconium aspiration, post-asphyxia syndrome, or neonatal sepsis – are born to women whose "low-risk labor" at home or in alternative birth centers was – initially or until the end – attended by independent midwives.[11] Evidently, when professional labor attendance is intermittent, many a serious perinatal complication in so-called "low-risk pregnancies" cannot be predicted and are not assessed in time for safe and timely transferral to the hospital.

> *Advocates of home births should be cautioned not to replace obstetric excess by non-attendance and undertreatment.*

However, those who advocate the spread of the midwife-centered system to other countries never mention these key figures. The self-proclaimed superiority of Dutch midwifery care resembles the story of the emperor's new clothes. A 50% emergency transfer rate during childbirth – not infrequently compounded with a nerve-racking ambulance drive – whereby the care is definitively taken over by strangers no longer supports the proposition that a trial of first-time childbirth at home is a positive life event, an empowering experience, enhancing women's self-esteem and self-confidence. It also does not support the assumption that midwifery care during a first childbirth at home is personal, superior, and safe. The unique Dutch system is actually on the verge of a breakdown unless the working relationships between midwives and obstetricians change drastically (Chapter 26).

> *Autonomous midwifery does not prevent the medicalization of birth, whereas safety issues are insufficiently appreciated.*

An autonomous midwifery service for normal pregnancy and childbirth is often claimed to have psychological advantages, but the Dutch reality developed into the opposite in recent decades: 77% of all primigravidas eventually end up in the secondary care division and are implicitly told they have to deliver in the hospital because their pregnancy or labor is now "at risk" or "abnormal." The mismatch between prior expectations and actual place of birth surely contributes to women's dissatisfaction.[9]

5.4 Universality of childbirth

Although normal childbirth is the same physiological process worldwide, there are important cross-cultural differences in childbirth systems. Territorial disputes – prevalent all over the western world, albeit on different levels – are destructive of the quality of birth care and block improvements. The universality of childbirth and solid science should eliminate territorial struggles and refocus attention on the real issue: the interests of pregnant women whose needs and preferences include many elements of both midwifery and medical styles of care. Both the exclusively medical, typically interventional approach and the orthodox midwifery approach unsupported by congenial medical back-up lack a scientific basis. Many conclusions from clinical studies in high-risk pregnancies have been inappropriately extrapolated to low-risk care, mostly resulting in medicalization of normal childbirth without improving outcomes. Fully medicalized obstetrics easily results in *mismanagement* of labor with spiraling cesarean rates. On the other hand, independent midwifery care that eschews intervention may easily result in *non-management* of labor with equally unintended effects. Clearly, drastic reforms at both ends of the spectrum are needed. Cultural prejudices and entrenched positions must be overcome. The interests of birthing women are universally the same. Maternity care anywhere should be woman-centered instead of provider-centered in its approach (Chapter 26).

> *Both the interventional medical care and the non-interventional midwifery care must be seen as two opposite but equally uninformed and unscientific approaches. A compromise is urgently needed.*

5.4.1 In search of the evidence

Debates are being dominated by emotions clouding facts. Until now most midwives have not been educated in the creation and critical review of scientific studies, resulting in a paucity of scientific work originating at the level of primary care. This has hindered the achievement of scientifically founded professional midwifery standards. In fact, evidence-based guidelines on labor supervision of initially low-risk pregnancies are non-existent. Dutch midwives' claims of providing superior care in normal childbirth are not supported by higher spontaneous delivery rates and/or better fetal outcomes of women who begin their first labor under their care. Quality assessments reliably exploring women's satisfaction with midwife-led childbirth are not available either. One must conclude that home delivery is advocated by reactionary midwives and home-birth activists on the basis of biased sentiments rather than solid arguments. There are no valid reasons to support initiatives for introduction of the Dutch system in other western countries. The Dutch system is a vestige rather than a vanguard. That is not to say that the fully medicalized systems of other western countries perform any better.

> Fundamental problem 10
>
> *Unfortunately, debate is usually about choice of caregiver and place of birth, rather than about labor.*

The advantage of a reappraisal of midwifery, often disparaged by obstetricians, is the pregnant and birthing woman's satisfaction with her care, at least when all goes well. The midwifery approach emphasizes the importance of women's satisfaction and the literature seems to be overwhelming: midwifery care is claimed to be significantly more satisfying to the woman and her family than doctor-centered, medicalized birth care.[12] Moreover, a search of the scientific literature fails to uncover reliable studies demonstrating better outcomes with doctor-led than with midwife-led deliveries for low-risk women.[13–15] The literature, however, is troublingly confused by neglect of the differences between nulliparous and parous labor and focusing on choice of provider or place of birth rather than on labor. Gross but inaccurate generalizations are then easily made.

5.4.2 Bridging the controversies

Ironically, the majority of protraction disorders of labor as well as cases of intrapartum fetal distress occur in completely healthy women giving birth to their first child, and most of these complications arise gradually in the first stage of labor. This makes a clear-cut distinction between the need for primary or secondary care virtually impossible, especially in nulliparous labor. Evidently, quality care requires much closer cooperation and mutual respect among all birth care providers and a redefinition of professional working relations (Chapter 26). In fact, a new balance must be found so that all women in labor will benefit from the complementary skills of both professions. To develop the team spirit that is vital to high-quality care, the professional relations between nurses, midwives and obstetricians must be redefined in a mutually satisfactory manner. This emphasizes the need for a collective plan for the supervision of normal childbirth that stimulates a synthesis of the managerial approach of obstetricians and the individual attention so typical of midwifery care: *proactive support of labor* (Section 3). This is an issue of great practical importance in all childbirth services all over the world. Section 3 of this book will demonstrate how organizational reforms and well-defined mutual responsibilities can improve maternity care immensely. This collective purpose is one of the greatest challenges for obstetricians, midwives, nurses, hospital administrators, and health officials.

> *Maternity care should be woman-centered instead of provider-centered. All pregnant women should benefit from the complementary skills of midwives and obstetricians.*

5.5 Summary

- Modern birth care has surpassed the point at which the benefits of medical technology have reached their limits. Now, the negative effects of excessive medicalization are prevailing.
- A reappraisal of midwifery, focused on personal, supportive care in labor, is urgently needed.
- A return to autonomous midwifery care for low-risk births will not provide the solution, however. This can be deduced from the results of the Dutch midwifery-centered birth system.
- Most labor disorders arise in completely healthy, first-time mothers after a completely uneventful pregnancy. A strict division between autonomous midwifery care and secondary obstetrical care cannot cope with this phenomenon.
- The much-needed improvements in maternity care require structural reforms in current childbirth systems and, above all, in the working relations between obstetricians, midwives, and labor room nurses.
- *Proactive support of labor* represents a system that combines the best of midwifery, personal nursing, and responsible medical care.

REFERENCES

1. Block J. *Pushed: The Painful Truth about Childbirth and Modern Maternity Care.* Cambridge, MA: Da Capo Press; 2007.
2. Wagner M. *Born in the USA: how a broken maternity system must be fixed to put women and children*

first. Berkeley, CA: University of California Press; 2007.

3. Lake R, Epstein E. *The Business of Being Born*. A documentary film (2007) www.thebusinessofbeing-born.com/about.htm.

4. Kaufman KJ. Effective control or effective care. *Birth* 1993; 20(3): 150–61.

5. De Vries R. Midwifery in The Netherlands: vestige or vanguard? *Med Anthropol* 2001; 20: 277–311.

6. http://europe.obgyn.net 2007

7. Stubbs V. Working relations: midwives and obstetricians in The Netherlands. *Midwifery Today Int Midwife* 2003; 67: 52–5.

8. Perinatal care in the Netherlands. 2005 (in Dutch) Stichting Perinatale Registratie Nederland.

9. Rijnders M, Baston H, Schönbeck Y, *et al*. Perinatal factors related to negative or positive recall of birth experience in women 3 years postpartum in The Netherlands. *Birth* 2008; 35(2): 107–16.

10. Drife JO, Künzel W, Ulmsten U, *et al*. The Peristat Project. *Eur J Obstet Gynaecol Reprod Biol* 2003; 111 (Suppl 1): S1–78.

11. Bruinse HW, Evers A. *ATNICID-study (Admission of Term Neonates to Neonatal Intensive Care or Intrauterine Death), interim analysis June 2007*. Utrecht, The Netherlands: University Medical Center Utrecht.

12. Wagner M. Midwifery in the industrialized world. *J Soc Obstet Gynaecol Canada* 1998; 20: 1225–34.

13. Olsen O, Jewell MD. Home versus hospital birth. *Cochrane Database Syst Rev* 2000; (2): CD000352.

14. Brown S, Grimes D. A meta-analysis of nurse practitioners and nurse midwives in primary care. *Nurs Res* 1995, 44. 332–9.

15. MacDorman M, Singh G. Midwifery care, social and medical risk factors, and birth outcomes in the USA. *J Epidemiol Community Health* 1998; 70: 310–17.

6

Self-sustaining mechanisms

Birth professionals – be they doctors, midwives, or nurses – often fail to see the adverse effects their care may have on women's childbirth experiences and the outcomes of labor. "Fish can't see water" as the saying goes. Providers are caught up in complex systems hiding several intrinsic mechanisms that sustain the current methods of childbirth. If the much-needed changes are to be made, these hindering values need to be identified, explored, and overcome.

6.1 The applause phenomenon

Modern intervention possibilities allow even those professionals who lack elementary labor and delivery skills to achieve what appears to be the best result: the birth of a living child. Indeed, there are few problems of labor that cannot be simply resolved by cesarean section. In this way, blasé practitioners may quickly come to feel that they are good care providers and will not recognize the need for proper evaluation of their care. The truth is that labor disorders are much easier to create than to prevent, and although each traumatic birth experience is unintentional, nonetheless it is often the result of unintended mistreatment and violation of a woman in an exceedingly vulnerable position. No matter how empathetic, friendly, and kind the birth professional remains through all this, the end-result is utterly unfriendly to a woman. And yet, there is nearly always applause. . .

> *In the delivery room, even after a mediocre performance, a round of applause typically follows.*

After the cesarean or instrument-assisted delivery of a healthy baby the professional is nearly always regarded as having done a good job, or the "policy" of care is in any case sold in this way. "With the midwife's patience, did the woman not have the best chance of a natural birth?" Because it is she "who could not do it herself," was the vacuum or cesarean delivery not truly inevitable? Did not the patient herself literally plead for the mercy of surgery? After a slow or failed induction, the obstetrician is not recognized as the originator of the woman's protracted ordeal but is thanked as her savior for performing the relieving cesarean. When the fetus that was supposedly "in distress" was operatively delivered and the child was born in good condition, "the intervention was performed adequately in time"; and for the newborn with a poor start "the intervention was well-indicated." What can we professionals possibly do wrong?

Professional satisfaction resulting from a deftly performed operative delivery and the self-image of the heroic, right-on-time obstetrician push the willingness to reflect on the real cause of the problems to the back burner. Performing a surgical intervention is ultimately sexier than attending a spontaneous birth. The negative result of all this is positive reinforcement of the non-management or mismanagement of labor. Moreover, the black cloud phenomenon (Chapter 4) is bolstered by the unmerited applause: the more forcefully an obstetrician stresses the possibility of an unfavorable outcome, the more thankful the parents will be for the operative birth of a healthy baby. Daily affirmation does not inspire self-evaluation and allows for the continuation of this sort of "care." Childbirth services desperately need new quality-control criteria that will make the care providers accountable not only for perinatal morbidity and mortality but also for superfluous interventions, iatrogenic complications, avoidable operative deliveries, physical and emotional trauma, and the (dis)satisfaction of the women subjected to their care (Chapters 27 and 28).

> *Obstetrics needs new quality-control criteria.*

6.2 Patient consumerism

Harmful medicalization of birth is also the result of a change in the attitude of pregnant women themselves. The body is increasingly regarded as something we can control to the extent that discomforts inherent to late pregnancy and birth are no longer acceptable. Women have busy jobs and have children along the way. They regard the free choice of an epidural as their God-given right. Many women give preference to the amenities and supposed safety of the hospital and request an induction of labor or even a cesarean delivery at a time that best suits both their schedule and that of the physician. This is the patient as consumer. Some women go from one doctor to another until they get what they want, and doctor-shopping surely biases obstetricians' responsiveness to the desires of the patient: "If I don't do it, someone else most certainly will."

Sadly, some leading feminists who fight for women's rights have been drawn into believing biased information and as a result have unwittingly promoted the right of women to demand elective obstetric procedures such as labor induction or even a cesarean that are potentially dangerous to themselves and their babies. Ironically, their rightful appeal to self-determination and autonomy is completely nullified through their making themselves totally dependent on the technical skills of physicians. Obstetricians are increasingly confronted with impassioned requests from patients who have been overwhelmed by biased and ill-founded information from the media and the Internet, the sheer volume of which renders the information incoherent. Compelling demands for an induction or cesarean delivery without any identifiable medical indication create a strange excuse for the complications resulting from such superfluous interventions. In the final analysis, however, it is not the clients who are ultimately responsible for this, but the specialist who allows it to happen.

> *Changing expectations and attitudes of pregnant women are no valid excuse for the excessive medicalization of birth. The central problem is that professionals do not have the right answers and, moreover, create most of their patients' insecurities, anxieties, and demands themselves.*

6.2.1 Biased patient information

The issue of potential damage to the pelvic floor in childbirth is attracting more and more attention among laypersons and caregivers alike. Cesarean delivery is often assumed to protect pelvic floor function after childbirth, but this assumption is not supported by evidence. The literature is difficult to interpret owing to multiplicity of study designs, relatively short follow-up, and the lack of randomized studies.[1] Because severe urinary and anal incontinence can follow elective prelabor cesarean delivery, it appears that pregnancy itself can lead to pelvic floor disorders.[2–10]

A large, population-based Australian survey showed that disorders of the pelvic floor are strongly associated with aging, pregnancy, and instrument-assisted delivery, whereas cesarean delivery was not associated with a significant reduction in pelvic-floor disorders over the long term as compared with spontaneous vaginal delivery.[11] Another large Norwegian retrospective study enrolled 15 307 patients and found that women whose deliveries had all been vaginal had a 70% higher risk of urinary incontinence than women whose deliveries had all been by cesarean.[12] The authors cautioned, however, that for an individual woman a decision to deliver all her infants by cesarean would decrease her risk of moderate or severe incontinence only from 10% to 5% overall and that there was no evidence that this effect would persist in the long term. They concluded that their data did not justify an increase in the use of cesarean deliveries. On reviewing the evidence, similar conclusions can be drawn with respect to sexual dysfunction after childbirth.[8,9,13,14]

Real risk factors for relevant pelvic morbidity have repeatedly been defined and include long second stage of labor and operative vaginal delivery.[15–20] Identified prevention strategies include antepartum and postpartum pelvic floor exercises, restricted use of episiotomy, and avoiding instrumental vaginal deliveries, but the preventive role of elective cesarean delivery seems very tenuous.

> *There is no solid evidence to support the widespread assumption that cesarean delivery effectively protects women from long-term sexual and pelvic floor dysfunction.*

Advertisements in women's magazines, offering elective cesarean delivery ("spare your pelvic floor," "keep your honeymoon fresh") serve the bank accounts of private doctors much more than the general health of their potential clients. For now, the stereotypical profile of the primigravida who opts for the knife without any medical indication seems to be a professional woman accustomed to having control over her life and those of others. These suited executive women have even spawned a label seen in medical literature and the lay press: "too posh to push." Also, pop idols and movie stars – role models for many young women – frequently set insidious examples. Each report of a cesarean on celebrity-request in tabloids and magazines encourages thousands more cesareans. Popular magazines never write about disfiguring surgical scars, persisting abdominal pain and/or dyspareunia owing to adhesions and scar tissue, decreased fertility, or life-threatening complications in following pregnancies (Chapter 2).

> *Reduction of surgical consumerism requires provision of honest and factual information to the general public.*

Doctors have a duty not to harm their patients, so they must ensure that any care does more good than harm. As with the introduction of many obstetric procedures, primary elective cesarean delivery may become widely disseminated without proof of benefit and before the potential risks to women have been carefully determined. Moreover, once introduced in routine practice, interventions tend to persist. With more doctors willing to do elective cesarean section and with increasing numbers of young women seeing it as a personal choice, inevitably maternal and neonatal morbidity and mortality will rise proportionally (Chapter 2). Clearly, reduction of inappropriate cesarean rates is as much about education of the general public as about reeducation of knife-loving obstetricians. This is a painful but necessary undertaking for the obstetrical community. It has a chance of success only if childbirth professionals can offer an acceptable alternative ensuring short labor and safe delivery – with the concept of *proactive support of labor* (Section 3).

> *Promoting normal labor and delivery is as much about reeducation of the general public as about reeducation of obstetricians, midwives, and labor room nurses.*

6.3 Liability concerns and control

Clearly, high-quality maternity care is a skilled art, but physicians increasingly circumvent this challenge and take refuge in surgery when labor gets tough. Many doctors feel they regain control with a cesarean, a move that might cut down on malpractice litigation.

6.3.1 Defeatism

Within the spiral of medical excess and intervention, the treacherous waltz of obstetrics with litigation goes on: the more obstetricians intervene in pregnancy and childbirth, the more complications occur, the more obstetricians get sued, and the more they intervene. In many circumstances cesarean birth seems to be safer legally, while it is not so medically. There are even obstetricians who say "the only cesarean I have ever been sued for is the one I didn't do." Such a striking remark not only echoes widespread frustration within medical circles but also reflects the widespread defeatism with regard to the spiraling cesarean rates. Such attitudes, however, seriously call into question whether these physicians operate on the basis of a consistent policy of care for short and safe labor. Structural improvement of labor care is indeed possible (Section 3) if there is the professional will to do so, and this will no doubt coincide with diminishing litigation threats (Chapters 25 and 26).

6.3.2 Convenience

Many women declare their intolerance for long and painful labor by requesting the cesarean solution when labor gets tough. To the doctor a cesarean section is also far more convenient and much more efficient from a time-management perspective than waiting around for natural birth. But the trend goes even further with the avoidance of labor and delivery altogether. Birth is rapidly becoming a 9-to-5 business, circumventing the burden of working at night. What once used to be an emergency intervention is now often a scheduled procedure and parents' biased wishes are a welcome excuse. Patient-choice cesarean delivery already accounts for more than 2% of all births in the USA.[21] Women are more educated and assertive about their healthcare decisions and read magazines that quite often provide unbalanced information provided by biased doctors. As a result, more and more women are demanding a scheduled cesarean section rather than undergoing a natural vaginal birth. They too feel in control knowing in advance the date and time of their delivery, which can be helpful in planning the multitude of activities, from career issues to child care, that surround a birth. Since everyone seems to be content, why bother?

> *It is much easier to comply with parents' biased preferences than to guard the medical necessity of cesarean delivery.*

6.3.3 False information

The crucial question, however, is whether such practical advantages outweigh the risks and whether women are truly informed about the consequences of these practices. The key ethical issue is not the right to choose or demand a major surgical procedure for which there is no medical indication but the right to receive and discuss full, unbiased information prior to any medical or surgical procedure. The rise in cesareans on-demand in low-risk pregnancies is factually a reflection of being told by the medical community that "this is a quick fix without risk, why wouldn't you?" But it is highly unlikely that women would ever consider choosing cesarean delivery if they were given the full scientific evidence on the direct and indirect risks for themselves and their babies (Chapter 2). The obstetrician who promotes or easily decides for a planned cesarean delivery actually remains co-responsible for all uterine scar-related complications in the woman's future pregnancies and childbirths. But by the time women (and lawyers) figure that out, these doctors are going to be long gone. . .

> *Women considering elective cesarean delivery should be counseled on the basis of the evidence: a significantly increased risk of maternal and perinatal morbidity and mortality in the index and future childbirths, and no significant protection from pelvic floor dysfunction (Evidence levels B and C).*

Since severe maternal and neonatal morbidity and even death may occur in association with repeat cesareans or VBACs in future pregnancies, all studies on the short-term effects of a primary cesarean delivery underestimate total morbidity and mortality. Despite this, ACOG has released a formal opinion supporting American obstetricians who honor a patient's request for cesarean delivery in the absence of any medical indication, citing the ethical premise of patient autonomy and informed consent.[22] Strangely, the question of patient choice asks only whether a woman should have the right to choose a cesarean delivery, whereas a woman's right to choose vaginal delivery is not addressed.[23] Paradoxically, the choice of women for VBAC or of a breech-presenting fetus is bluntly overruled in many hospitals, although these options can be relatively safe in selected cases.[24–27]

> *The key ethical issue is not the right to choose a cesarean delivery but the right to receive and discuss full, unbiased information prior to any medical or surgical procedure.*

6.3.4 Remuneration practices

A cesarean not only decreases the chance of being sued but it is also far more lucrative for doctors. And hospitals are more than happy to comply since they get paid as much as $9000 more by insurance companies for a cesarean than for an uncompli-

cated vaginal birth. Besides, new mothers can often get an additional two weeks of paid maternity leave from their employers after a cesarean. These provisions do not stimulate changes in the right direction. Policy makers in governmental health departments, insurance companies, labor unions, and employer organizations should wake up and realize that they are actually promoting improper medical care.

> *Current financing and insurance systems promote improper incentives for cesarean delivery.*

6.3.5 Inflation

Inevitably, the more readily an obstetrician honors a woman's request for a cesarean section without any medical reason, the lower becomes his or her threshold for surgical solutions for minor problems in labor. Such an inflation of indications is especially worrying in teaching hospitals where residents no longer master prevention and appropriate handling of labor disorders and grow permanently malconditioned by the liberal surgical practices of their teachers. The cesarean virus has spread to pandemic proportions as a result (Chapter 2).

6.4 Ignoring the evidence

There is a fundamental difference between the practice of science and the practice of medicine: to generate and test hypotheses scientists must believe they do not know, whereas practicing doctors, to have the confidence to make life and death decisions, must pretend they know. In reality, however, practitioners often do not know the exact risks in individual cases. As a result, adversity odds are generally overestimated whereas normalcy odds are significantly underestimated. The epidemiological impact was epitomized by Woolf and Kamerow: "Preoccupation with the potential benefit to the numerator may make doctors less sensitive to the adverse effects on the population."[28] This partially explains the continuing gap between obstetric practice and the scientific evidence.

> *Doctors usually overestimate adversity odds and underestimate normalcy odds.*

6.4.1 Invalid excuses

Despite a positive movement toward evidence-based obstetrics, still many obstetricians are familiar neither with recent evidence nor with the means of obtaining it, whereas the majority of those who are aware of the concept of evidence-based medicine first consult another obstetrician rather than the literature when faced with a difficult clinical problem.[29] "Some obstetricians simply reject the evidence in their practice using excuses like 'the evidence is out of date; collecting evidence is too slow and prevents progress; evidence erodes physician autonomy; I use clinical judgment and my experience; trust me, I am a doctor, and stop doctor-bashing.'"[30] Other practitioners use anecdotal "horror stories" to try to prove the need for an intervention that the evidence has shown to be unnecessary, or quote evidence of poor and/or inadequate quality. The first response of most obstetricians whose cesarean rates are compared unfavorably with those of their peers is: "My patients are more complicated than average" (is that so?) or "Our women have smaller pelvises" (nonsense), or "Our babies are getting bigger" (not true), and "Our population is not as homogenous" (no evidence). Such uncritical attitudes explain the tenacity of current methods of birth care despite the overwhelming evidence of the adverse and even harmful effects of excessive interventions.

> *The explosion of cesarean delivery rates is the greatest uncontrolled medical experiment in modern medicine.*

Several professional associations, among which are ACOG and RCOG, have published extensive systematic reviews of all the ins and outs of cesarean delivery, mainly focusing on the prevention of surgical complications and only superficially addressing some measures to prevent cesarean section.[31,32] The importance of these guidelines is beyond question, but the sheer volume of stand-alone recommendations obscures or lacks a central strategy for labor care and the prevention of surgery. Such an evidence-based birth-plan will be presented in Section 3: *Proactive Support of Labor.*

6.4.2 Resistance to change

Obstetricians remain human. Past and recent evidence shows that most practitioners tend to stick to the ways of practice they mastered during their training and are highly reluctant to change. Nevertheless, we professionals must redesign birth care services ourselves, and in such a way that we, the front-line caregivers, lead the process of change. Otherwise, health care managers, insurance carriers, and politicians will inevitably take the initiative.

> *If we professionals want to stay in control, we will have to take the lead in the much-needed reforms of childbirth services, rather than being forced to change by health care managers and insurers.*

6.5 Educational flaws

A new generation of obstetrician-perinatologists has now emerged who are highly trained in prenatal diagnosis, fetal medicine, and high-risk obstetrics, but not infrequently devoid of normal labor and delivery skills, as almost any problem can be and is resolved by cesarean delivery.

6.5.1 Deficient training in labor and delivery skills

Residents and fellow obstetricians often fail to gain insight into everyday clinical complexities in the labor ward, because training priorities are set on the detection of maternal disease and fetal compromise instead of the management of normal labor and handling everyday labor problems in the delivery room adequately. Added to this, too much of residents' training time is consumed by research to enhance the publications of their superiors; after all, it is "publish or perish." During the past three decades, most professors in obstetrics, being ultimately responsible for the skills of future practitioners, specifically focused attention on fetal and maternal diseases, while often neglecting the basic education in and evaluation of normal childbirth practice. Other obstetricians working in university and training hospitals have equally become excessively burdened with organizational, instructional, and analytical tasks, such as management participation, educational reforms, and research. As a result, the basic work in the delivery room is mostly delegated to others in positions of lesser authority and training. The unfortunate consequence of this is that those who lead and decide the direction of studies and professional education have cut themselves off from the only true source of obstetrical acumen: the daily observation of pregnant and laboring women. Modern obstetricians seem to be more interested in technical developments and the study of illnesses and relatively rare clinical phenomena than in the evaluation of care for the everyday birth. They spend more time behind the desk than in the labor and delivery rooms. Yet it is precisely a daily presence in the labor ward that would supply the crucial information needed to preserve the wellbeing of the female half of humankind, such as the need for reducing the number of superfluous operative deliveries and preventing physical and emotional trauma.

More than 90% of all women pass their pregnancy uneventfully until the moment of delivery. Accordingly, obstetricians interested in research and science should not focus solely on filling in the holes in knowledge surrounding rare diseases but also on the countless frictions that occur in everyday work in the labor and delivery rooms. Lack of direct involvement in labor management at the consultant level inevitably results in lack of authoritative guidance on the working floor. Given the current high intervention rates in labor and delivery, obstetricians should devote more attention to the prevention of difficult labor than to its cure. In conclusion: they need to return to the delivery room.

> *Obstetricians must return to the labor room – both intellectually and physically – and take on the many challenges it presents.*

On the other hand, most midwives have not been educated in the creation and critical review of scientific studies. This explains the paucity of scientific work originating at the level of midwifery care. Official evidence-based guidelines on the supervision of labor at home or in primary-care birth centers are actually non-existent. In fact, a reappraisal of typical midwifery wisdom will show that much of it is deceptive, as will be demonstrated time and again in the next two sections of this manual.

> **Fundamental problem 11**
>
> *Most gynecologists are not really interested in normal birth, whereas many midwives are insufficiently interested in scientific evidence and objective quality assessments.*

6.5.2 Post-doctoral education and development

To keep pace with developments in professional knowledge, doctors and midwives scan journals and attend symposia. Speakers at conferences are invited to lecture for 10, or at most 20 minutes. Inevitably, information is fragmented and detached from its complex clinical context. All too often, research data are presented in isolation, and suggestions for an approach to specific clinical problems are carelessly offered without taking into account the direct and indirect effects they will have on all other aspects of care. Induction techniques, opioids in labor, epidural block, and routine elec-tronic fetal monitoring are only a few examples of many that will be addressed in Section 3.

> *The contemporary culture of medical education and science is characterized by a preoccupation with details that results in a loss of clinical perspective.*

Scientific literature is like the Internet: pertinent information is nearly impossible to find in the never-ending stream of publications that have no direct clinical relevance. The common solution – not reading at all or simply relying on authoritative "evidence-based" guidelines – is not always in the patient's best interest: meta-analyses of clinical trials on specific clinical questions, and how important these may be, often neglect to account for the complexity of everyday practice. The ten-dency is that patients must comply with "the evidence" of isolated issues rather than the evi-dence fitting a patient's case. Both logic and clin-ical behavior may be seriously warped as a result.

> *Uncritical application of "evidence-based" cook-ery-book measures may seriously harm patients.*

6.6 Evidence-based versus concept-based care

Despite clear medical gains since its introduction, evidence-based medicine may be further criticized for its ideological biases and the shortcomings of the technique. The validity of randomized con-trolled trials may be subject to severe limitations when used for the evaluation of complex phe-nomena and procedures like labor and delivery.[33] "Evidence" rests on clinical practice, which in turn is rooted in structural arrangements and cultural ideas. Devries, for instance, using "the best avail-able evidence" from the debate over home delivery versus hospital birth, pointed out that "the evidence" is actually the product of a researcher's assumptions about the practice in question.[34] Ideological differences give rise to irresolvable disagreements about what constitutes evidence and how that evidence is to be interpreted. In this way "evidence" rather becomes a rhetorical justi-fication for whatever particular groups were going to do anyway.[34] Clearly, for many complex issues "evidence" cannot settle scientific disputes in any simple way. One of the most influential biases in the acquisition of "evidence" is the choice of the question, and the best evidence in answer to the wrong question is useless. Numerous examples of this will be given in the following chapters. What is more, meta-analyses of clinical trials only describe *what* happens, but not *why*. Therefore, generally speaking, "evidence-based" policies without a leading concept are usually meaningless. Con-versely, a logical concept-based approach unsup-ported by evidence is equally useless. Clearly, a synthesis of both approaches is needed and that is precisely the foundation of *proactive support of labor* (Section 3). So before this method of care and the clinical evidence can be explained, its conceptual, biological basis needs to be addressed as well as some pervading misconceptions about the physiology of normal birth that still dominate the various types of childbirth services (Section 2).

> *Childbirth practices should be based on a logical, integral concept of childbirth supported by clinical evidence. Isolated research "evidence" without a clinical concept of birth is pointless.*

6.7 Summary

- Numerous factors sustain the excessive medica-lization of childbirth, such as liability concerns, convenience, remuneration factors, educational flaws, basic reluctance to change, biased wishes of ill-informed patients, and the applause phe-nomenon.

- Breaking these cycles is possible only through professional, open-minded introspection and the willingness to implement fundamental and structural improvements.
- We need new quality criteria of birth care, whereby birth professionals must account not only for perinatal morbidity and mortality but also for superfluous interventions, iatrogenic complications, avoidable operative deliveries, physical and emotional trauma, and the (dis) satisfaction of the women subjected to our care.
- Much-needed reforms are as much about medical reeducation and changing practice patterns of birth professionals, as about changing patients' childbirth expectations.
- Improvement of childbirth services requires an overall, integrated, and conceptual plan for normal childbirth, supported by solid clinical evidence: *proactive support of labor.*

REFERENCES

1. Minkoff H, Frank A, Chervenac A. Elective primary cesarean delivery. *N Engl J Med* 2003; 348: 946–50.
2. Farral SA, Allen VM, Basket TF. Parturition and urinary incontinence in primiparas. *Obstet Gynecol* 2001; 97: 350–6.
3. Lal M, Mann C, Callender R, Radley S. Does cesarean section delivery prevent anal incontinence? *Obstet Gynecol* 2003; 101(2): 305–12.
4. Wijma J, Potters AE, Wolf BT, *et al.* Anatomical and functional changes in the lower urinary tract following spontaneous vaginal delivery. *Br J Obstet Gynaecol* 2003; 110: 658–63.
5. Wilson PD, Herbison RM, Herbison GP. Obstetric practice and the prevalence of urinary incontinence three month after delivery. *Br J Obstet Gynaecol* 1996; 103: 154–61.
6. Klein MC, Kaczorowski J, Firoz T, *et al.* A comparison of urinary and sexual outcomes in women experiencing vaginal and cesarean births. *J Obstet Gynaecol Can* 2005; 27(4): 332–9.
7. Wang A, Guess M, Connell K, *et al.* Fecal incontinence: a review of prevalence and obstetric risk

factors. *Int Urogynecol J Pelvic Floor Dysfunct* 2006; 17(3): 253–60.
8. Connolly A, Thorp J, Pahel L. Effects of pregnancy and childbirth on postpartum sexual function: a longitudinal prospective study. *Int Urogynecol J Pelvic Floor Dysfunct* 2005; 16(4): 263–7.
9. Hicks TL, Goodall SF, Quattrone EM, Lydon-Rochelle MT. Postpartum sexual functioning and mode of delivery: summary of the evidence. *J Midwifery Women's Health* 2004; 49: 430–6.
10. Viktrup L, Lose G. Epidural anesthesia during labor and stress incontinence after delivery. *Obstet Gynecol* 1993; 82: 984–6.
11. MacLennan AH, Taylor AW, Wilson DH, Wilson D. The prevalence of pelvic floor disorders and their relationship to gender, age, parity and mode of delivery. *Br J Obstet Gynaecol* 2000; 107: 1460–70.
12. Rortveit G, Kjersti Daltveit A, Hannestad YS, Hunskaar S. Urinary incontinence after vaginal delivery or cesarean section. *N Engl J Med* 2003; 348: 900–7.
13. Buhling KJ, Schmidt S, Robinson JN, *et al.* Rate of dyspareunia after delivery in primiparae according to mode of delivery. *Eur J Obstet Gynecol Reprod Biol* 2006; 124(1): 42–6.
14. Barret G, Peacock J, Victor CR, Manyonda I. Cesarean section and postnatal sexual health. *Birth* 2005; 32(4): 306–11.
15. Groutz A, Fait G, Lessing JB, *et al.* Incidence and obstetric risk factors of postpartum anal incontinence. *Scand J Gastroenterol* 1999; 34(3): 315–18.
16. Casey BM, Schaffer JI, Bloom SL, *et al.* Obstetric antecedents for postpartum pelvic floor dysfunction. *Am J Obstet Gynecol* 2005; 192(5): 1655–62.
17. Andrews V, Sultan AH, Thakar R, Jones PW. Risk factors for obstetric anal sphincter injury: a prospective study. *Birth* 2006; 33(2): 117–22.
18. Kearney R, Miller JM, Ashton-Miller JA, DeLancey JO. Obstetric factors associated with levator ani muscle injury after vaginal birth. *Obstet Gynecol* 2006; 107(1): 144–9.
19. Dietz HP, Wilson PD. Childbirth and pelvic floor trauma. *Best Pract Res Clin Obstet Gynaecol* 2005; 19(6): 913–24.
20. Bahl R, Strachan B, Murphy DJ. Pelvic floor morbidity at 3 years after instrumental delivery and cesarean delivery in the second stage of labor and the impact of a subsequent delivery. *Am J Obstet Gynecol* 2005; 192 (3): 789–94.

21. Health Grades Quality Study. 3rd annual report on "Patient choice" cesarean rates in the United States. 2005. www.healthgrades.com/media/dms/pdf/PatientChoiceSectionStudy-2005sept12pdf. Accessed November 20, 2005.

22. American College of Obstetricians and Gynecologists. Committee Opinion. Surgery and patient choice: the ethics of decision making. *Obstet Gynecol* 2003; 102: 1101–6.

23. Leeman LM, Plante LA. Patient-choice vaginal delivery? *Ann Fam Med* 2006; 4: 265–8.

24. Alarab M, Regan C, O'Connel MP, *et al.* Singleton vaginal breech delivery at term: still a safe option. *Obstet Gynecol* 2004; 103: 407–12.

25. Yamamura Y, Ramin KD, Ramin SM. Trial of vaginal breech delivery: current role. *Clin Obstet Gynecol* 2007; 50(2): 526–36.

26. Landon MB, Hauth JC, Leveno KJ, *et al.* Maternal and perinatal outcomes associated with a trial of labor after prior cesarean delivery. *N Engl J Med* 2004; 351: 2581–9.

27. American Academy of Family Physicians. Trial of labor after cesarean (TOLAC), formerly trial of labor versus elective repeat cesarean section for the woman with a previous cesarean section. 2005. www.annfam med.org/cgi/content/full/3/4/378/DC1. Accessed September 2, 2005.

28. Woolf SH, Kamerow DB. Testing for uncommon conditions: the heroic search for positive results. *Arch Int Med* 1990; 150: 2451–8.

29. Olatunbosun OA, Edouard L, Pierson RA. Physicians' attitudes toward evidence based obstetric practice: a questionnaire survey. *BMJ* 1998; 316: 365–6.

30. Wagner M. Fish can't see water: the need to humanize birth. *Int J Gynaecol Obstet* 2001; 75: S25–37.

31. American College of Obstetricians and Gynecologists/Task Force on Cesarean Delivery Rates. Evaluation of Cesarean Delivery. Systematic Review and Evidence Based Guidelines. 2000.

32. Royal College of Obstetricians and Gynaecologists/National Collaborating Centre for Women's and Children's Health. Caesarean Section. Systematic Review and Clinical Guideline. RCOG Press; 2004.

33. Kotaska A. Inappropriate use of randomised trials to evaluate complex phenomena: case study of vaginal breech delivery. *BMJ* 2004; 329:1039–42.

34. Devries RG. The warp of evidence-based medicine: lessons from Dutch maternity care. *Int J Health Serv* 2004; 34(4): 595–623.

Back to basics

"The real act of discovery is not in finding new lands, but in seeing with new eyes."

–Marcel Proust

7

Lessons from nature

"Our cultures, ways of life, judicial systems, and religions are parts of the ecological niche in which we human beings live."[1] There is no doubt that each person is conditioned by his or her cultural and social background. In biological terms, however, every human being is a product of millions of years of evolution. Accordingly, the basic biological processes of parturition are essentially the same in different mammalian species.

7.1 Comparative biology

Comparative studies have shown that most mammals, including *Homo sapiens*, exhibit increased activity prior to the onset of labor; they are busy gathering nesting materials. Apparently, the hormonal changes in late pregnancy that prepare the uterus for the forthcoming labor (Chapter 8) also set the behavioral nesting impulse in motion. The biological purpose speaks for itself in that safety and protection during birth are essential requirements for the preservation of the species. By the same basic principle, it follows that the preparation of the female body for birth is normally not unduly taxing. Despite prelabor bodily changes and latent uterine contractility, the expectant mother takes and gets sufficient rest to be fit enough to begin the real exertion of birthing.

7.1.1 Duration of natural birth

Parturition is a tremendous physical challenge for all mammalian species. That is why the process of natural birth is short. Most observers of domesticated mammals estimate a duration of total parturition of a couple of hours and at the most half a day, even for the first offspring.[1–6] Although observations of primates giving birth in the wild are rare, we know that diurnal monkeys generally give birth within the confines of one night, whereas nocturnal species such as prosimians usually give birth during the restricted hours of daylight – so within the timeframe of half a day at the most.[7] There is no precedent in the animal world to indicate that the fetus benefits from striving overlong to escape from the womb, and there is no evidence that the time required for human childbirth must necessarily be substantially different from that required for the birth process in other higher mammals: less than half a day.

Advocates of "natural childbirth" should know the true nature of physiological or biological birth: the whole process of actual labor and delivery in the animal world normally takes only a few hours and at the most half a day. Procreation in the wild is above all a selection process and nature is a bad obstetrician indeed. As a renowned scientist in comparative biology pointed out: "The only obstetric help in nature is that offered by predators who will shorten the period of pain by killing the laboring female and eating her."[1] Nature is cruel.

> *The natural process of birth is short. In nature, mammalian labor and delivery normally take only a couple of hours.*

7.2 The biological functions of labor pain

In the western world, human procreation has long ceased to present a serious threat to the lives of healthy women, but the emotional impact of labor remains a matter of common concern. As a human female physiological process, natural childbirth is intensely physical, immensely emotional, and surely painful. No good purpose is served by pretending otherwise. "Labor pain is a phenomenon embedded in the very nature of human female existence. Unlike other acute and chronic pain experiences, labor pain is not associated with pathology but with the most basic and fundamental of life's experiences: the bringing forth of new life."[8]

> Giving birth is the only physiological process in nature that causes pain. As with everything in biology, this has specific functions.

Pain in childbirth is a ubiquitous biological phenomenon: all mammals deliver their young with great effort and most species show signs of discomfort and even severe pain.[1] "Why the physiologic process of birth should cause pain has been the subject of philosophic and religious debate, but the biological explanation is simple: labor 'hurts' so that the expectant mother has sufficient warning to get to a place of safety in which to birth her infant."[8] In addition, the pain-related production of endorphins strongly promotes maternal behavior. Both effects are critical for survival of the helpless newborn in nature and the preservation of the species.

7.2.1 Warning sign

The pain of contractions warns laboring animals to go and find a place where predators are least likely to be around. They instinctively seek the isolation and protection of their den and stay there, whereas humans call for professional help. Women will also instinctively seek surroundings in which they feel safe. For some this is the sanctity of their own home

and for others it is a hospital. Nearly all mammals that live in groups are protected during labor and delivery by their group members. Unrest, a change in the environment, or simply being left alone can so disturb the autonomic vegetative balance that labor stalls. This is no different in humans.

7.2.2 The role of endorphins

Females of all mammalian species show maternal behavior immediately after birth, which is vital to the survival chances of the cub and thus for the preservation of the species. Maternal nursing behavior is a critical biological effect promoted through the natural pain of labor. Labor pain induces the production of large amounts of endorphins in the mother's brain and these play a crucial role in the instant establishment and maintenance of maternal nursing behavior. Moreover, maternal endorphins cross the placenta and promote suckling behavior in the newborn.[1] In wildlife, endorphins are critical for effective mother–child bonding. Again, there is no reason to assume that this should be any different in the human species. In fact, human studies show that after analgesic medication during labor, the neonates exhibit decreased alertness,[9] inhibition of suckling,[10] lower neurobehavioral scores,[11] and a delay in effective feeding.[12–15]

> The natural pain of labor has important biological functions, especially for mother–child bonding. Endorphins encourage the natural establishment of a bilateral nursing–suckling relationship.

7.3 Psychovegetative regulation

Whenever an animal in labor is disturbed, uterine contractions are inhibited so that the female is able to leave the spot and find another safe place before she actually gives birth. This adaptive mechanism clearly shows the importance of a perception of safety and avoidance of disturbance during labor and delivery.

7.3.1 The parasympathetic system

From the biological point of view, labor is a parasympathetic process, a physiological condition that requires rest, ease, comfort, and a feeling of confidence and security. Our own species is not an exception, and for this reason home birth is in greater accord with people's basic instincts than is going out in the dark to a hospital, unless faith in medicine so exceeds trust in nature that the hospital is perceived to be safer. For many women, however, leaving home is the greatest stress of the whole process of parturition.[16] The change of environment is actually the reason why ineffective labor occurs more frequently since hospitals have replaced the home as the place for birth, although this is not always recognized or admitted by clinicians. Birth attendants should make more allowances for the basic conditions of natural birth and instinctive behavior. Doing so would create an intimate, safe, and private atmosphere. The serious lack of this in many hospitals was documented in Chapter 4.

> *Giving birth is a parasympathetic process: labor is easiest during parasympathetic dominance, whereas sympathetic stimuli inhibit labor.*

7.3.2 Biological effects of stress

In all mammalian species the course and outcome of labor and delivery are strongly influenced by environmental disturbances. Anxiety and fear invariably lead to prolongation of labor.[1] A laboring wild mare, for instance, is capable of stopping labor and running for her life when she observes wolves. As soon as the cause of anxiety has disappeared, she resumes her discontinued activity. If the disturbance is too long, she loses her unborn foal and sometimes even her own life.

> *Anxiety and stress invariably lead to prolongation of labor.*

An epinephrine (adrenalin) surge from fear or anxiety has the biological effect of weakening and even stopping contractions. Stress hormones suppress the oxytocin receptor's activity and lower the concentration of free calcium ions in the myometrial cells so that the frequency and force of contractions decrease and contractions may eventually stop completely.[17] Suppression of uterine activity is a life-saving adaptation for the laboring animal developed through evolution – *fright: fight or flight* – in which mammals halt birth when they feel threatened so that they can flee to safety. The sympathetic control system is primarily activated by fear. What was originally a protective mechanism has in the human situation, where it is not necessary to flee to protect one's life, turned against the parturient. A recent prospective human study of 908 term low-risk women showed that the prelabor level of anxiety, assessed at 36 weeks' gestation, is an independent predictor of long dilatation time during labor.[18]

> *Stimulation of the stress response is one of the most important causes of (iatrogenic) dynamic birth disorders.*

After many millions of years of evolution, human biology cannot change as quickly as can civilization and patterns of culture, and the biological stress response is, without a doubt, a factor of major importance in the currently high incidence of iatrogenic birth disorders. A strange environment, discontinuity of care, negative psychological conditioning, crippling uncertainty, and indecisive conduct and care not infrequently play a pivotal role in dysfunctional, protracted labor (Chapter 4). All the standards of care for *proactive support of labor* are focused on preventing, overcoming, and ending this vicious circle of undue stress (Section 3).

7.4 Summary

- Giving birth is the only physiological process that causes pain.
- Endorphins play an important biological role in the establishment of a natural bilateral nursing–suckling relationship between mother and child.
- Care providers advocating "natural birth" should be aware of the characteristics of birth in nature.
- Physiological labor is short: birth in nature of any mammalian species takes less than half a day.
- Birth is a parasympathetic process requiring calmness, confidence, comfort, and a feeling of safety.
- Stimulation of sympathetic stress responses strongly undermines the effectiveness of labor, which invariably leads to long labors and related complications.
- A sympathetic response to (iatrogenic) stress and anxiety is a major contributor to dystocia and high cesarean delivery rates.
- Avoidance of undue stress requires a comforting and reassuring birth environment and an overall plan governing the reassuring attitude of all birth attendants: *proactive support of labor.*

REFERENCES

1. Naaktgeboren C. The biology of childbirth. In: Chalmers I, Keirse MJNC, Enkin M, eds. *Effective Care in Pregnancy and Childbirth*, vol. 2: Childbirth. Oxford: Oxford University Press; 1998.
2. Parkes AS. *Marshall's Physiology of Reproduction*, 4th edn. vol. 2. London: Longmans, Green; 1958: 504–5.
3. Young IR. The comparative physiology of parturition in mammals. *Front Horm Res* 2001; 27: 10–30.
4. Fortman JD, Hewett TA, Bennet BT. *The Laboratory Non-Human Primates.* Boca Raton, FL: CRC Press; 2000.
5. Jensen P. *The Ethology of Domestic Animals: An Introductory Text.* New York: CABI Publishing; 2002.
6. Waring HG. *Horse Behavior*, 2nd edn. Norwich, NY: William Andrew Publishing; 2002.
7. Jolly A. Primate birth hour. *Int Zoo Yearb* 1973; 13: 391–7.
8. Lowe NK. The nature of labor pain. *Am J Obstet Gynecol* 2002; 186: S16–24.
9. Belsey EM, Rosenblatt DB, Lieberman BA, *et al.* The influence of maternal analgesia on neonatal behaviour: I. Pethidine. *Br J Obstet Gynaecol* 1981; 88(4): 398–406.
10. Kron RE, Stein M, Goddard KE. Newborn sucking behavior affected by obstetric sedation. *Pediatrics* 1966; 37: 1012–16.
11. Hodgkinson R, Bhatt M, Wang CN. Double-blind comparison of the neurobehaviour of neonates following the administration of different doses of meperidine to the mother. *Can Anaesth Soc J* 1978; 25(5): 405–11.
12. Righard L, Alade MO. Effect of delivery room routines on success of first breast-feed. *Lancet* 1990; 336(8723): 1105–7.
13. Nissen E, Lilja G, Matthiesen AS, *et al.* Effects of maternal pethidine on infants' developing breast feeding behaviour. *Acta Paediatr* 1995; 84(2): 140–5.
14. Matthews MK. The relationship between maternal labour analgesia and delay in the initiation of breastfeeding in healthy neonates in the early neonatal period. *Midwifery* 1989; 5: 3–10.
15. Crowell MK, Hill PD, Humenick SS. Relationship between obstetric analgesia and time of effective breast feeding. *J Nurse Midwifery* 1994; 39(3): 150–6.
16. Friedman DD. Conflict behavior in the parturient. In: Hirsh H, ed. *The Family. Proceedings of the 4th International Congress of Psychosomatic Obstetrics and Gynecology.* Basel: Karger; 1975: 373–6.
17. Lopez Bernal A. Overview of current research in parturition (Uterine Contractility Symposium of the Physiological Society). *Exp Physiol* 2001; 86(2): 213–22.
18. Wijnen HA, Denollet J, Essed GG, *et al.* High maternal anxiety during late gestation predicts protraction of labor. In: Wijnen HA, ed. *The Kempen Study.* Academic Thesis 2005, University of Tilburg, The Netherlands.

8

Elementary biophysics of birth

Although the basic physiology of parturition is a permanent design of nature, the professional conduct and care of normal childbirth vary significantly (Chapter 5). This diversity in approaches to labor and delivery reflects differences in appreciation or knowledge of the elementary processes that control normal birth. By and large, interventionist obstetricians tend to override biology, whereas conservative caregivers often allow labor to derail from the physiological track for too long. If scrutinized, both dogmatic approaches allow professionals to attend birth with neglect or even ignorance of the basic natural science of normal parturition.

Rational birth care must be based on a solid understanding of the biology of birth and this is precisely the hallmark of *proactive support of labor* (Section 3). For comprehension of the physiological basis of this method of care, this chapter is of critical importance to all professionals involved in childbirth: physicians, midwives, and nurses. Laypersons without a medical background, however, might be discouraged from further reading by the bio-technical aspects of birth in this chapter, and may wish to scan only the boxed key points and summary and proceed directly to Chapter 9.

8.1 The prelabor preparation of the uterus

The function of the uterus changes radically at the end of pregnancy. For nine months the uterus maintains a state of functional quiescence in which the natural contractility of the myometrium is effectively suppressed and the resistance of the cervix is kept high enough to ensure that the fetus remains safely inside the womb. At the end of nine months, however, the uterus must suddenly recover its contractile competence and effectively expel the fetus.

> The biological transformation
>
> *At term, the uterus changes radically from being a safe, inert cocoon to a powerful expulsive organ.*

Slow progress in our understanding of prelabor uterine transformation reflects the difficulty in extrapolating from the control mechanisms in various animal models to human parturition, a process that in humans precludes direct investigation. Although the precise starting signal of parturition seems to vary, the final common pathway from the decline in functional progesterone at tissue level is probably common in all mammalian species, including humans. Comprehensive analyses of the complex paracrine/autocrine pathways involved have been reviewed by several distinguished researchers in this field.[1–13] We briefly summarize only those essentials that are needed for an appropriate clinical understanding of the physiological process of human birth.

8.1.1 The fetal trigger

Considerable evidence suggests that the fetus is in control of the uterine preparation for labor and the timing of birth. The signals that initiate the functional transformation of the uterus represent the expression of the fetal genome acting through endocrine pathways involving the fetal brain, adrenal glands, and placenta, as well as mechanical signals acting directly on the myometrium (distension and stretch) as a result of the growth of the fetus. Together, these fetal signals contribute to the timely, safe, and effective birth at term.

> *During the weeks preceding birth, it is the fetus itself that triggers the uterine preparation for birth.*

8.1.2 Biochemistry

Weeks before there is any indication of labor onset, the maturation and activation of the fetal endocrine system cause the fetal hypothalamus to produce and release corticotropin-releasing hormone. This neuropeptide stimulates the fetal pituitary gland to produce adrenocorticotropin hormone, or corticotropin, which activates the fetal adrenal glands to produce and release DHEAS (dehydroepiandrosterone sulfate). The placenta and fetal membranes convert DHEAS into estrogens, which are transferred to the mother. The conversion of DHEAS to estrogen at the level of the fetoplacental unit is critical for the preparation of the uterus for labor; as a result, the ratio of progesterone to estrogen begins to decline at the level of the uterine tissues. In addition, progesterone withdrawal may be effected functionally through blockade of progesterone receptor action at the level of the genome. The decrease in functional progesterone and the declining progesterone to estrogen ratio induce intricate biochemical changes in both the cervix and the myometrium.

8.1.3 Functional transformation at two distinct levels

To achieve a proper understanding of the physics of birth, we must first of all distinguish between the prelabor transformation of the myometrium and that of the cervix, because normal labor relies on the balance between myometrial force and the resistance of the cervix. This balance is orchestrated physiologically, but the two events are not necessarily synchronous.

> Prelabor biophysical transformation
>
> *The cervical transformation determines how much resistance must be overcome to open the womb. The myometrial transformation determines how much force can be exerted to achieve this.*

8.2 Prelabor transformation of the cervix

The process of prelabor cervical maturation is a complex enzymatically controlled process with substantial remodeling of the cervical extracellular matrix. In brief: the decrease in inhibitory progesterone activity triggers the production of inflammatory cytokines particularly in the area of the internal os of the cervix. These cytokines (especially interleukin-8 [IL-8]) stimulate fibroblasts to produce hyaluronic acid, which promotes cervical ripening. Cytokines may also play a direct role: through chemotaxis IL-8 attracts granulocytes that release collagenases and elastases in the proximal part of the cervix. These proteins act to break down the mucopolysaccharide bonds and allow the collagen fibers to shift in relation to one another, with a resultant softening (ripening) and shortening (effacement) of the cervix. Nitric oxide may be a mediator of cervical competence during pregnancy, whereas this same agent, acting through the cyclic guanosine-monophosphate (cGMP) signal transduction pathway, may paradoxically promote cervical ripening in late pregnancy.[14–16]

8.2.1 Cervical ripening

The term effacement refers to the upward incorporation of the cervix into the lower segment of the uterus. This process begins at the internal os of the cervix and proceeds gradually downward to the external os, at which point the cervical body has disappeared and effacement is complete. Effacement begins several days to weeks before the end of pregnancy and progresses slowly to the time of labor. Effacement is mostly, but not always, complete before the clinical onset of labor.[17] In this context it should be noted that complete effacement and beginning of dilatation of the cervix are not requirements for a clinical diagnosis of labor (Chapter 14). However, labor is likely to be prolonged if effacement has not taken place to a substantial extent beforehand. These are usually the troublesome cases. When the cervix is fully effaced at the start, labor can be expected to proceed smoothly and without any intervention. In this situation, progress is usually rapid, and the woman is likely to deliver spontaneously within a matter of hours.[18]

> *Optimal prelabor cervical transformation is essential for a smooth first stage of labor.*

8.3 The prelabor transformation of the myometrium

Labor may best be regarded as an event initiated by the removal of the inhibitory effects of pregnancy on the myometrium rather than as an active process governed by uterine stimulants.[5] The maintenance of the state of uterine quiescence during pregnancy involves active blockade of the expression of genes that increase myometrial contractility. In particular, progesterone inhibits myometrial contractility, cell–cell coupling, and responsiveness to endogenous stimulants such as oxytocin and stimulatory prostaglandins. The myometrial preparation for labor involves a remarkable change in the phenotype of the myometrium near term, restoring uterine contractile competence. The relative rise in estrogens stimulates hypertrophy of the myometrial cells and induces the production

of prostaglandin E_2 (PGE_2) in the myometrium, enhancing the myotropic effect.

8.3.1 Braxton Hicks contractions

The beginning of myometrial transformation often becomes clinically apparent when the pregnant woman experiences intermittent periods of discomfort from contractions at irregular intervals – often 10–30 minutes apart. Such periods of Braxton Hicks contractions that come and go may be noticed for several weeks before true labor begins. Every myometrial cell can act as a local pacemaker and stimulate nearby muscle cells to contract, but there is still no coordination, and therefore Braxton Hicks contractions have no substantial effect on the cervix.

> *The myometrial preparation for labor involves a remarkable change in the phenotype of the myometrium near term.*

8.3.2 The activation of the myometrium

During labor, the uterus must produce forceful contractions to overpower the resistance of the cervix. To this end, radical changes take place in the myometrium during the final days of pregnancy. This process is called the activation of the myometrium. The rise of myometrial estrogen levels and the relative decrease of progesterone activate the expression of a cassette of genes encoding contraction-associated proteins (CAPs), including connexin-43, oxytocin receptors, and prostaglandin receptors. Oxytocin levels do not rise prior to or during labor, but the effect of endogenous (and exogenous) oxytocin on uterine contractility becomes greater as the number of oxytocin receptors increases.[19,20] The binding of oxytocin to its receptors initiates the local production of PGE_2 at the precise location where it must act: in the myometrium. PGE_2 enhances the formation of mRNA which codes for specific intercellular proteins (*connexons*)[21] that are quickly capable of creating large-scale stimulus-conducting connections between the myometrial cells, known as *myometrial gap junctions*. These are small, intercellular channels that have a low resistance to ions and a high electrical conductivity for action potentials. This cell–cell conduction system develops suddenly (normally within a few hours) and is essential for the coordination of myometrial cell contractions and thus for the achievement of forceful contractions and effective labor.

> *Optimal myometrial transformation is essential for a smooth birth.*

8.4 The onset of labor

The final step of myometrial transformation – the sudden formation of the myometrial gap junctions – takes only a few hours. Prior to labor, gap junctions are scarcely present, if at all. In fact, it is precisely the sudden and widespread formation of gap junctions that triggers the onset of clinical labor. The orchestration of myometrial cell contractions occurs in a very short time, resulting in propagated contraction waves, and the newly coordinated contractions begin to have an impact on the softened cervix. In this way, the physical connection between the fetal membranes and the lower decidua is disrupted and the production of PGE$_2$ further increases. The formation of gap junctions accelerates rapidly, and the process reinforces itself through positive feedback: labor has begun.

> *The sudden formation of the myometrial gap junctions triggers the onset of labor.*

8.4.1 Electromechanical coupling

As with other types of muscle contractions, uterine action potentials must be generated and propagated to yield effective contractions in a process known as electromechanical coupling. Uterine action potentials during labor occur in bursts originating in one of the fundal corners of the uterus where cells have a higher resting potential than other myometrial cells. These cells act as "pacemakers." Contraction waves are propagated through the conduction system of myometrial gap junctions, and the electrical activity is translated into uterine force exerted on the contents of the uterus. The electrical orchestration determines the number of myometrial cells recruited for action, which in turn determines the strength of each contraction. Uterine relaxation between contractions is secured by a refractory period of the myometrial cells for at least one minute after each excitation wave.

> *The efficiency of labor contractions relies on the degree and quality of the myometrial transformation.*

8.5 The physics of effective labor

For labor to be effective the uterine force must overpower the resistance of the cervix. In terms of physics, force is a vector, meaning it has direction. This elementary principle is too often forgotten in obstetrics. From a physics point of view, uterine force is a fundamentally different parameter from uterine tone assessed by manual palpation and from intrauterine pressure measured with intrauterine catheters.

8.5.1 Uterine coordination

To gather effective, directional force, uterine contractions must propagate in a coordinated fashion. This, in turn, requires a functional electrical conduction system and thus a fully and adequately transformed myometrium. Pacemaker cells in the right cornu usually predominate over those in the left cornu and start the great majority of contractions. The excitation wave first propagates laterally and subsequently downward toward the cervix at 2 cm/s, depolarizing the whole organ within 15 seconds. In this way, the uterine tube first stiffens and then shortens, producing effective traction on the dilatation ring and thrusting force on the cervix via the fetal head or the bulging amniotic sac (wedging action). Only coordinated contractions are efficient contractions, and only efficient contractions can be effective. The overall effectiveness of labor depends on the frequency and efficiency of the contractions versus the cervical resistance.

Propagation of contractions

An efficient contraction first stiffens and then shortens the uterus, thus creating effective, directional force on the cervix. Essential myometrial orchestration requires a fully transformed myometrium.

8.5.2 Uterine force

Uterine force comprises two components: pulling and pushing forces.[22] In a physical sense, the combination of pulling and pushing is comparable to what happens when one pulls on a sock: there is traction on the cervix and in addition a pushing force is applied to the cervix by the presenting part (wedging action). In other words, cervical dilatation is achieved by traction combined with hydrostatic action of the unruptured membranes or, after their rupture, by direct application of the descending fetal head against the cervix. The presenting fetal part functions as a wedge. As in pulling on socks, in labor the initial force is predominantly traction, whereas the contribution of the pushing (descending) component gradually increases in importance later in time. Descent is needed to maintain wedging action and to complete the last centimeters to full dilatation.

Uterine force comprises two components: pulling and pushing forces.

In a laborious experimental setting, the "head-to-cervix force" (HCF) can be measured with a sensor between the caput and the cervix.[23] HCF can be regarded as the approximate uterine force. Studies analyzing the time relationship between HCF and intrauterine pressure show that HCF increases before pressure does and that HCF is lower in labor that requires augmentation. An increase in the frequency of contractions also increases HCF.[24] Most importantly, HCF is a better predictor of the successful achievement of vaginal birth than is intrauterine pressure or even dilatation rate.[25] These findings support the assertion that force and not pressure is the most important factor for a successful birth and, by extension, that efficient coordination of contractions is the deciding factor in the effectiveness of labor.

Force is a vector and therefore has direction. Uterine force is a fundamentally different parameter from the clinical measures of uterine tone or intrauterine pressure.

8.5.3 Cervical resistance

The resistance of the cervix determines how much cumulative force the uterus must generate to accomplish full dilatation. Direct measurement of the cervical resistance is not possible. Clinical assessment of cervical softness provides only an indirect and subjective impression. This is true both prior to and during labor. One way to overcome slow progress in labor is to enhance uterine force by rupturing the membranes (amniotomy) and by the use of oxytocin. Another approach would be to reduce cervical resistance. In fact, several methods for influencing cervical resistance to accelerate slow labor have been tested.[26] These techniques include parenteral administration of porcine relaxin, local cervical injections of hyaluronidase, electrical vibration of the cervix, and local application of prostaglandins. To date, however, controlled trials have not demonstrated any significant advantage in the use of these methods, whereas the safety of these measures requires further assessment.[26]

> *There are no effective and safe measures to reduce cervical resistance in labor.*

8.5.4 A clinical measure for effective labor

In daily practice, the vector force of a contraction cannot be measured directly. For this reason, nurse-midwives manually assess uterine action on the basis of frequency, intensity (tone), and duration of the contractions. However, such clinical assessment of the uterine tone gives no real information about the direction of the uterine force. Indeed, the assessment of uterine activity by palpation is highly inaccurate and its correlation with the speed of dilatation is rather poor.[27]

Obstetricians often use intrauterine pressure measurements to evaluate uterine action. However, these practitioners should realize that in doing so they are measuring an entirely different physical variable from force. Intrauterine pressure is only indirectly related to uterine force and relays little to nothing about the pulling and pushing direction of uterine force. In fact, poorly coordinated contractions can surely build up pressure without causing an effective thrusting force onto the cervix. In conclusion, intrauterine pressure monitoring is not as useful in evaluating the efficiency of uterine contractions as it is typically believed to be. Pressure is not the measure. Force is the course.

Since neither uterine force nor cervical resistance are truly measurable, the only real and clinically relevant parameter for evaluating labor is the net effect that results from the interaction of both: i.e., progression of dilatation. Since resistance cannot be influenced safely, augmentation of uterine force through amniotomy and oxytocin is the only possible procedure for improving the effectiveness of labor, if necessary.

> *The clinical characteristics of uterine contractions (frequency, intensity or tone, and duration) or intrauterine pressure readings cannot be relied on as measures of effective labor or as indices of normality. The only relevant parameter is progression in dilatation (Evidence level B).*

8.6 Exhaustion of the uterus

Prolonged labor leads to accumulation of lactic acid in the myometrium.[28] In addition, long labor and belated and prolonged augmentation result in myometrial desensitization through a significant reduction in both oxytocin-binding sites and oxytocin receptor mRNA.[29,30] Consequently, the uterus gradually loses its ability to respond to oxytocin stimulation – the result is sometimes described as oxytocin-resistant dystocia – or the uterus reacts like any overburdened muscle with disorganized hypertonia (tetanic spasms), leading to fetal distress. This is the exhausted, refractory uterus, a common but mostly unrecognized complication in conventional obstetrics, when the decision to accelerate slow labor is generally postponed far too long (Chapters 17 and 21).

> **The refractory uterus**
>
> *In abnormally slow labor the uterus gradually loses its ability to respond to oxytocin stimulation.*

8.7 First labor compared with subsequent labors

The most significant difference between nulliparous and parous labor is the relatively long duration of first births. This is largely accounted for by the slower evolution of the nulliparous cervical changes in early labor. Beyond 3 cm dilatation the mean rate of cervical dilatation for nulliparas nearly equals that of multiparas,[17] and from that point 95% of all nulliparous and parous women reach full dilatation in eight hours or less (Chapter 15).

8.7.1 The fundamental parity difference

The difference in speed in accomplishing the early process of completing full effacement and establishing the first 3 cm dilation is the result of the relatively higher resistance-to-force ratio in first labors. There are two sides to this equation:

1. The average resistance of the nulliparous cervix is likely higher because it has never before been stretched and opened.
2. There are strong indications that the absolute force that the nulliparous uterus is initially able to generate is usually less because the contractions are often less efficiently coordinated.[23,31]

Both factors explain why early dynamic dystocia is a frequent disorder in first labors. The main factor seems to be less-efficient contractions because, even after correcting for cervical ripeness at the onset of labor, the nulliparous uterus requires twice as much effort to effect normal vaginal delivery as its multiparous counterpart (measured by intra-uterine pressure measurements).[32] It appears that myometrial activation – like so many other complex biological processes – is not always executed as swiftly and as well on the first attempt as it is on subsequent occasions. One could say that the nulliparous uterus still has to learn how to birth and that in the experienced parous labor the blueprint is already present and, therefore, the activation of the parous myometrium commonly proceeds more rapidly and more successfully. While for some scientists it may still be open for debate whether the longer duration of early nulliparous labor is predominantly a result of higher cervical resistance or mainly the result of less force per contraction, the clinical fact remains that ineffective early labor is a problem specific to first labors. Parous women do not suffer from dynamic dystocia to any significant extent, unless their labor is induced.

> *Ineffective uterine contractions are a problem specific to first-time labor.*

8.8 Fetal oxygenation during labor

The importance of the myometrial gap junction system is electrical orchestration of the myometrium, establishing forceful contractions and regulating interval uterine relaxation. Adequate inter-contraction relaxation is a prerequisite for adequate fetal oxygenation during labor and delivery.

8.8.1 The placental reserve capacity

A healthy fetus is exceptionally well equipped to endure the stress and pressures of normal labor. Fetal blood flow through the placenta remains unimpeded during contractions, unless the umbilical cord is compressed by accident. In contrast, the maternal blood supply to the placenta is blocked during each normal contraction owing to external compression of the spiral arteries in the myometrium. The normal, healthy fetus is perfectly able to tolerate this potentially stressful situation because the placental circulatory system has a functional reserve capacity. The maternal blood pool within the placenta is sufficiently large and saturated to maintain a positive maternal–fetal oxygen gradient throughout a normal contraction, thereby ensuring normal fetal oxygenation. During the intervals between contractions, the spiral arteries open again and maternal–placental blood is refreshed. In other words: both adequate placental reserve capacity and adequate uterine relaxation in the intervals between contractions are essential preconditions for the fetus to survive labor. These obligatory intervals are secured by a physiological refractory period of the myometrium for at least one minute after each excitation wave.

> Reserve capacity of the placental circulation
>
> *The healthy fetus is well equipped to tolerate the arrest of maternal blood flow to the placenta during each contraction.*

8.8.2 Interval uterine relaxation

The force of contractions poses no threat to a healthy fetus, but insufficient uterine relaxation between contractions certainly does. Good uterine relaxation depends on coordination and electrical orchestration, which means that safe and effective contractions require a completely transformed myometrium. Even in a healthy fetus with a completely normal placenta, insufficient uterine relaxation between contractions (uterine hypertonia) invariably leads to fetal hypoxia. Uterine hypertonia is a frequent complication particular to induction and is attributable to the attempt to force a non-transformed or incompletely transformed myometrium into contractions. The clinical implication is clear: a safe labor involves waiting for the spontaneous onset of labor and refraining from induction. Inter-contraction uterine hypertonia may also result from accumulation of lactic acid. In order to avoid this fetal predicament, dysfunctional labor is best corrected in time (Chapters 15, 17, 21).

Adequate uterine relaxation between contractions is vital to fetal oxygenation.

8.8.3 Disorganized uterine action and fetal distress

In other non-physiological conditions, uterine relaxation may be compromised through random excitation of myometrial cells by intrauterine infection, meconium, or free blood, leading to dysfunctional labor and fetal distress. The fetal bowels contain bile acids and salts that render meconium very corrosive. This may, as in cases of intrauterine infection, result in cytokine production in the fetal membranes and the decidua.[33,34] Inflammatory cytokines may disorganize myometrial coordination and consequently lead to dystocia in conjunction with hypertonia in the contraction intervals.[33–38] A vicious circle of fetal distress and dysfunctional labor may ensue

(Chapters 21 and 24). Free blood in utero due to (partial) placental abruption may act similarly.

Hypertonic dystocia

Intrauterine bacteria, meconium, or free blood may lead to a vicious circle of fetal compromise and dysfunctional labor through inflammatory cytokines provoking disorganized uterine hypertonia.

8.9 Important clinical implications

Obstetricians who advocate daytime obstetrics with liberal induction policies override biology and tend to ignore the fundamental physiological preconditions for a smooth birth. On the other hand, conservative childbirth attendants who advocate expectancy and the maxim "let nature take its course with the least possible intervention" tend to forget that first childbirth is – in terms of evolution – a selection process that often fails. This is an observable fact in all mammalian species, including humans. The current cesarean rates for failed first labors speak for themselves (Chapter 2).

Only coordinated uterine contractions are efficient contractions, and only efficient uterine contractions can be effective.

8.9.1 Induction of labor

Complete transformation of both the cervix and the myometrium is essential for a smooth and safe birth. Since neither of these two physiological processes has had a chance to achieve full completion when labor is induced, every pregnant woman who undergoes induction of labor is put at a disadvantage from the outset. The cervix is always more resistant than it would be if labor had started spontaneously, and the myometrium is much less efficient at exerting force. While it is true that locally applied exogenous prostaglandins may sometimes soften an unripe cervix, this so-called cervical priming is generally ineffective in achieving the activation of the myometrium. Quite often the relevant proteins (*connexons*) needed for the crucial formation of gap junctions are simply not yet present. This explains why priming/induction with prostaglandins or induction with amniotomy and oxytocin often leads to ineffective labor despite "cervical ripeness." The cesarean delivery rate in low-risk women with a Bishop score of 7 or greater is significantly increased after elective induction compared with women with spontaneous labor onset.[39,40] Furthermore, oxytocin is much less safe and effective when used to induce labor than when used to augment spontaneous but slow labor. There are fewer oxytocin receptors present in an induced labor and the uterus lacks a functional stimulus conduction system. It is for this reason that oxytocin administered for induction often either has little effect or leads to hypertonic uterine dysfunction, the latter being characterized by ineffective labor and a high incidence of fetal distress (Chapters 21, 24).

> *"Oxytocin is not nearly so predictably effective and safe in initiating the process of labor as it is in accelerating progress after labor has already started spontaneously."*[18]

8.9.2 Augmentation of labor

In contrast, early augmentation of spontaneous labor is generally safe and usually extremely effective. Connexons and oxytocin receptors are widespread and the binding of oxytocin to these receptors enhances the formation of PGE_2 in the myometrium – the precise location where it must act. When the formation of the gap junctions is not yet complete, oxytocin quickly overcomes this. Spontaneous but initially ineffective labor is greatly improved by early stimulation with amniotomy and oxytocin. Failure of the cervix to dilate in response to oxytocin constitutes an indication to

review the diagnosis of labor (Chapter 14). Other explanations are an inordinate delay before commencement of oxytocin (resulting in a refractory uterus) or intact membranes (Chapter 17).

> *Timely augmentation normalizes slow labor, whereas induction creates a slow and difficult labor.*

8.9.3 Only progress counts

A postponed decision to accelerate slow labor frequently originates in the false assumption that the quality of labor can be judged on the basis of the external appearance of the parturient, in particular the painfulness, the frequency, and the tone of the contractions. If contractions appear to be strong, the traditional policy is to refrain from vaginal examinations – often regarded as a burdensome interference – and to wait four hours or more. This is a common and widespread mistake. Four hours is much too long to discover that labor has hardly progressed (Chapters 15, 21). The efficacy of labor can only be measured in terms of dilatation, and dilatational progress correlates poorly with both the subjective element of pain, as felt by the mother, and the pseudo-objective tone of the contractions, as assessed by palpation.[27] The same holds true for intrauterine pressure readings. Labor must not be evaluated by these methods. Only progress counts (Chapter 15).

> *The only possibility for assessing uterine force and resistance is the net effect: progress in dilatation. The only safe and effective way to accelerate slow labor is to intensify the uterine force.*

8.10 Summary

- Rational and responsible birth care must be based on a solid understanding of the physiology of natural parturition.

- At term, the uterus transforms from an inert cocoon into a powerful, expulsive organ.
- The biophysical transformations of the cervix and the myometrium must be distinguished from one another. The degree of prelabor cervical transformation determines how much resistance must be overcome for dilatation, whereas the prelabor myometrial transformation determines how much force can be exerted to accomplish this.
- The ratio of force to resistance decides the effectiveness of labor. A fully transformed cervix with low resistance and a fully transformed myometrium enabling forceful contractions are both crucial for an easy birth.
- The biophysical trigger for the onset of labor is the sudden appearance of a stimulus-conducting system of myometrial gap junctions, coordinating myometrial cell contractions. The appearance of this electrical conduction system is a prerequisite for efficient contractions and effective labor.
- Uterine force is a vector and therefore has direction. Effective contractions require efficient coordination in which the uterus first stiffens and then shortens so that uterine force is effectively directed upon the cervix. This requires an optimally transformed myometrium.
- Only coordinated contractions are efficient contractions, and only efficient contractions can be effective. The overall effectiveness of labor depends on both the efficiency of the contractions and the cervical resistance.
- Uterine force is the deciding factor for a successful birth, but the clinical features of uterine contractions – frequency, intensity, and duration – cannot be relied on as measures of effective force or as indices of labor normality. The same goes for intrauterine pressure monitoring.
- The only relevant parameter is progression of labor. Inadequate progression is an indication for augmentation of uterine force, and a restoration of progression is the only means of evaluating the efficacy of this procedure.
- Uterine force poses no risk to the fetus, but insufficient uterine relaxation between contractions surely does. The uterus's ability to relax depends on coordination, which is why effective

and safe contractions require a fully transformed myometrium.
- *Proactive support of labor* means exhibiting the utmost restraint with induction and thus patiently waiting for the complete prelabor transformation of both the cervix and the myometrium, i.e., waiting for the spontaneous onset of labor.
- Induction of labor creates long and unsafe labor, whereas augmentation promotes short and safe labor.
- Whenever spontaneous labor is slow, prompt acceleration by amniotomy and oxytocin is warranted, because after an extended period the uterus gradually loses its ability to respond to oxytocin properly, or reacts like any overburdened muscle with continual spasms, leading to fetal distress.

REFERENCES

1. Smith R. Parturition. *N Engl J Med* 2007; 356: 271–83.
2. Liao JB, Buhimshi CS, Norwitz ER. Normal labor: Mechanism and duration. *Obstet Gynecol Clin N Am* 2005; 32: 145–64.
3. Lye SJ, Challis JRG. Parturition. In: Harding R, Bocking AD, eds. *Fetal Growth and Development*. Cambridge University Press; 2001: 241–266.
4. Challis JGR, Matthews SG, Gibb W, *et al*. Endocrine and paracrine regulation of birth at term and preterm. *Endocr Rev* 2000; 21: 514–20.
5. Norwitz ER, Robinson JN, Challis JRG. The control of labor (review articles). *N Engl J Med* 1999; 341(9): 660–6.
6. Norwitz ER, Robinson JN, Repke JT. *The Initiation Of Parturition: A Comparative Analysis across the Species*. New York: Mosby; 1999.
7. Majzoub JA, McGregor JA, Lockwood CJ, *et al*. A central theory of preterm and term labor: putative role for corticotropin-releasing hormone. *Am J Obstet Gynecol* 1999; 180: S232–41.
8. Goodwin TM. A role for estriol in human labor, term and preterm. *Am J Obstet Gynecol* 1999; 180: S208–13.
9. Garfield RE, Saade G, Buhimschi C, *et al*. Control and assessment of the uterus and cervix during pregnancy and labour. *Hum Reprod Update* 1998; 4(5): 673–95.
10. Nathanielsz PW. Comparative studies on the initiation of labor. *Eur J Obstet Gynecol Reprod Biol* 1998; 78(2): 127–32.

11. Challis JR. Characteristics of parturition. In: Creasy RKRR, ed. *Maternal-Fetal Medicine: Principles and Practice.* Philadelphia: WB Saunders; 1994: 482.

12. Cunningham FG, Leveno KJ, Bloom SL, *et al.* Chapter 6: Parturition. In: *Williams Obstetrics,* 22nd edn. New York: McGraw-Hill; 2005: 161–86.

13. Lopez Bernal A. Overview of current research in parturition (Uterine Contractility Symposium of the Physiological Society). *Exp Physiol* 2001; 86(2): 213–22.

14. Vaisanen-Tommiska M, Nuutila M, Ylikorkala O. Cervical nitric oxide release in women post term. *Obstet Gynecol* 2004; 103(4): 657–62.

15. Okawa T, Vedernikov YP, Saade GR, *et al.* Effect of nitric oxide on contractions and cervical tissues from rats. *Gynecol Endocrinol* 2004; 18(4): 186–93.

16. Chen DC, Ku CH, Huang YC, *et al.* Urinary nitric oxide metabolite changes in spontaneous and induced onset active labor. *Acta Obstet Gynecol Scand* 2004; 83(7): 641–64.

17. Hendricks CH, Brenner WE, Kraus G. Normal cervical dilatation pattern in late pregnancy and labor. *Am J Obstet Gynecol* 1970; 106: 1065–82.

18. O'Driscoll K, Meagher D, Robson M. *Active Management of Labour,* 4th edn. Mosby; 2003.

19. Shojo H, Kaneko Y. Characterization and expression of oxytocin and the oxytocin receptor. *Mol Genet Metab* 2000; 71(4): 552–8.

20. Blanks AM, Thornton S. The role of oxytocin in parturition. *Br J Obstet Gynaecol* 2003; 110 (Suppl 20): 46–51.

21. Chow L, Lye SJ. Expression of the gap junction protein connexin-43 is increased in the human myometrium toward term and with the onset of labor. *Am J Obstet Gynecol* 1994; 170(3): 788–95.

22. Buhimschi C, Buhimschi IA, Malinov AM, *et al.* The forces of labour. *Fetal and Maternal Medicine Review* 2003; 14(4): 273–307.

23. Gough GW, Randall NJ, Genevier ES, *et al.* Head-to-cervix forces and their relationship to the outcome of labor. *Obstet Gynecol* 1990; 75: 613–18.

24. Allman AC, Genevier ES, Johnson MR, *et al.* Head-to-cervix force: an important physiological variable in labour. 1. The temporal relation between head-to-cervix force and uterine pressure during labour. *Br J Obstet Gynaecol* 1996; 103: 763–8.

25. Allman AC, Genevier ES, Johnson MR, *et al.* Head-to-cervix force: an important physiological variable in labour. 2. Peak active force, peak active pressure and mode of delivery. *Br J Obstet Gynaecol* 1996; 103: 769–75.

26. Enkin M, Keirse MJNC, Neilson J, *et al. A Guide to Effective Care in Pregnancy and Childbirth,* 3rd edn. Oxford: Oxford University Press; 2000: 332–40.

27. Arrabal PP, Nagey DA. Is manual palpation of uterine contractions accurate? *Am J Obstet Gynecol* 1996; 174: 217–19.

28. Quenby S, Pierce SJ, Brigham S, Wray S. Dysfunctional labor and myometrial lactic acidosis. *Obstet Gynecol* 2004; 103(4): 718–23.

29. Phaneuf S, Aboth G, Carasco MP, *et al.* Desensitization of oxytocin receptors in human myometrium. *Hum Reprod Update* 1998; 4(5): 625–33.

30. Phaneuf S, Rodriguez Linares B, Tamby Raya RL, *et al.* Loss of oxytocin receptors during oxytocin-induced and oxytocin-augmented labour. *J Reprod Fertil* 2000; 120: 91–7.

31. Fairlie FM, Phillips GF, Andrews BJ, Calder AA. An analysis of uterine activity in spontaneous labour using a microcomputer. *Br J Obstet Gynaecol* 1988; 95(1): 57–64.

32. Arulkumaran S, Gibb DM, Lun KC, *et al.* The effect of parity on uterine activity in labour. *Br J Obstet Gynaecol* 1984; 91(9): 843–8.

33. Matsubara S, Yamada T, Minakama H, *et al.* Meconium-stained fluid activates polymorphonuclear leucocytes; ultrastructural and enzyme cytochemical evidence. *Eur J Histochem* 1999; 43: 205–10.

34. Anahya SN, Kakshmanan J, Morgan BL, Ross MG. Meconium passage in utero: mechanisms, consequences, and management. *Obstet Gynecol Surv* 2005; 60(1): 45–56.

35. Mark SP, Croughan-Minihane MS, Kilpatrick SJ. Chorioamnionitis and uterine function. *Obstet Gynecol* 2000; 95(6): 909–12.

36. Edwards RK. Chorioamnionitis and labor. *Obstet Gynecol Clin N Am* 2005; 32: 287–96.

37. Rauk PN, Chiao JP. Oxytocin signaling in human myometrium is impaired by prolonged exposure to interleukin-1. *Biol Reprod* 2000; 63: 846–50.

38. Rauk PN, Friebe-Hoffman U. Interleukin 1-beta down regulates the oxytocin receptor in cultured uterine smooth muscle cells. *Am J Reprod Immunol* 2000; 43: 83–9.

39. Yeast JD, Jones A, Poskin M. Induction of labor and the relationship to cesarean delivery; a review of 7001 consecutive inductions. *Am J Obstet Gynecol* 1999; 180: 628–33.

40. Hamar B, Mann S, Greenberg P, *et al.* Low-risk inductions of labor and cesarean delivery for nulliparous and parous women at term. *Am J Obstet Gynecol* 2001; 185: S215.

9

First-stage labor revisited

To allow the passage of the fetus, the cervix must vanish completely, accomplished by effacement and dilatation. These clinical phenomena are consecutive manifestations of one and the same process: the incorporation of the cervix into the lower segment of the uterus. In effective labor, the previously softened cervix first effaces completely (full effacement), followed by progressive dilatation until it has disappeared completely (full dilatation). From this point the uterus, its lower segment, and the vagina form a single open tube through which the baby can be born.

9.1 Normal pattern of dilatation

Current teaching and theoretical understanding of normal dilatation rates is still dominated by the work of Friedman,[1] who deserves credit for being the pioneer in this field of research more than 50 years ago, but whose conclusions were actually incorrect. Friedman arbitrarily divided first-stage labor into three artificial sections – from 0 to 3 cm, from 3 to 8 cm, and from 8 cm to full dilatation – and subsequently analyzed these sections statistically, a novelty in those days. As a result he described a characteristic pattern for labor when cervical dilatation is graphed against time: "[The average dilatation curve] takes on the shape of a sigmoid curve: a relatively flat latent phase, followed by the acceleration phase, a steep phase of maximum slope, and ending in a deceleration phase."[2]

9.1.1 The Friedman doctrine defeated

Unfortunately, this classic Friedman curve is still reproduced today in most textbooks as the reference curve of "normal labor" in spite of its invalidity. Firstly, Friedman's study population included patients with breech presentation, twins, oxytocin, heavy sedation, and a high rate of forceps delivery, and thus did not represent a "normal labor and delivery" population. Secondly, labor and delivery times do not follow a normal distribution, indicating that the use of parametric statistics (means) – as Friedman did – is not correct; it falsely lengthens the duration of labor, and the separate analysis of artificial sections gives the illusion of a sigmoid dilatation curve.[3]

> *The sigmoid curve for normal dilatation is one of the many mistaken but persistent sacred concepts of conventional obstetrics and midwifery.*

9.1.2 Fundamental reassessment

It was Charles Hendricks and co-workers who demonstrated significant differences between labors in practice and the description of labor found in most textbooks, dividing first-stage labor into a latent phase and an active phase.[4] They also noted a large body of evidence in the obstetric literature on normal progression in dilatation which was at wide variance with the standard textbook teaching. They boldly challenged and successfully disproved one of the sacred concepts of conventional obstetrics: Friedman's sigmoid reference curve for normal dilatation. Their principal differences include:

1. Absence of a latent phase
2. Brevity of normal labor
3. No deceleration phase in normal labor

Hendricks and co-workers justifiably disputed the methodology of Friedman's classic study: Friedman had divided each labor artificially into sections and extrapolated the onset of labor back to zero dilatation at time zero and subsequently the means of each section were derived. By arbitrarily dividing the data, extrapolating back, and obtaining means, a sigmoid curve was derived that does not represent the mean course of normal cervical dilatation time. It masks the true nature of normal dilatation – which is actually linear – and tends to be far too long in the initial part (the so-called "latent phase"). As Hendricks convincingly demonstrated, most women go into labor with an already effaced cervix, and the average dilatation of nulliparas at the onset of labor is actually 2.5 cm, while that of multiparas is 3.5 cm.[4] He rightly disputed the very existence of a latent phase, because he carefully observed in his study that contractions in late pregnancy may come and go, and that effacement and incipient dilatation – presumed to be typical of the latent phase of labor – actually occur during the final four weeks before women go into clinical labor. In fact, labor is considerably longer when a latent phase is included. Even worse, primary dysfunctional labor is often misconstrued as "latent labor," preventing adequate treatment of early labor disorders (Chapters 15, 17, 21).

> *The classic sigmoid reference curve for normal dilatation, assessed by Friedman, was actually based on hypothetical extrapolations with regard to dilatation in early labor. In addition to this, erroneous statistics were used. The Friedman curve is therefore incorrect (Evidence level B).*

9.1.3 The fallacy of the latent phase

Clearly, the so-called latent phase of first-stage labor is poorly understood and differentiating between a prolonged latent phase and false labor is difficult, if possible at all. In fact, such a distinction is only possible in retrospect. The mean duration of the latent phase – defined by Friedman to begin at the moment regular contractions occur and to end at 3 cm dilatation, at which point an acceleration of cervical dilatation is noted – was 8.6 hours (+2 SD 20.6 hours) for first labor and the range was 1–44 hours with a maximum of 20 hours still accepted as statically normal (sic!). Little wonder that a long "latent phase" of labor is strongly associated with poor labor outcomes: more fetal distress, undue maternal exhaustion, more interventions, and more surgical deliveries.[5,6]

> *Dividing first-stage labor into a latent and an active phase constitutes a persistent fallacy and one of the most pervasive impediments to appropriate labor management.*

9.1.4 Defining the beginning of labor

Most caregivers diagnose the beginning of labor – in accordance with Friedman's vague definition – on the degree of discomfort associated with regular and painful contractions, while the significance of complete effacement for the diagnosis of labor is generally overlooked (Chapter 14). *Williams Obstetrics*[7] states that with intact membranes and painful contractions, a cervical dilatation of at least 3–4 cm should be used to confirm labor and should serve as a convenient starting point of labor management. Such an approach would mean that labor cannot be reliably determined until most if not all the alleged "latent phase" has been completed. This sentiment is echoed in the ACOG bulletin on dystocia (2003), which avoids discussing the "latent phase" entirely and "focuses on labor subsequent to entering the active phase. . .."[8] These contentions leave the care provider with no current guidelines for the approach of the alleged latent phase. As a result, most providers continue to use Friedman's original classification system with all the associated vagueness and clinical indecisiveness during "latent labor." For years, and even still today, the arbitrary concept of the latent phase provided the vague theoretical basis and false justification for the expectant attitude in early labor and the reluctance to perform amniotomy if early ("latent") labor is slow. Clearly, the greatest challenge in the supervision of labor is recognizing its start (Chapter 14), and the concept of the "latent phase" of labor in particular has prevented progress in the conduct of labor for a very long time (see also Chapter 11).

9.1.5 Duration of normal labor

Our perception of the normal duration of first-stage labor may be clouded not only by the fallacious concept of the latent phase but also by the many clinical variables that affect the conduct of labor and the many routine measures and interventions that interrupt the natural course of labor in modern maternity units, such as induction, augmentation, sedation, and epidural analgesia.

Hendricks was the first to suggest that the duration of labor be measured from the time of admission to a delivery unit. Since then most studies on the timing of providing labor care and timing of labor interventions accordingly define the onset of labor as the time when the patient is admitted to the labor ward. This works extremely well, provided that strict criteria for admission are used, such as those promulgated by O'Driscoll and co-workers.[9] Their criteria include painful contractions associated with any one of the following: ruptured membranes, bloody show, or complete effacement. These criteria for the diagnosis of labor will be addressed extensively in Chapter 14.

> *The greatest impediment to understanding labor is recognizing its start.*

In nature, normal labor and delivery take any female of any mammalian species less than half a day (Chapter 7) and the human species is no exception: normal labor is short. In the 1970 study of Hendricks *et al.*, the average time from admission to full dilatation was shown to be 4.8 hours for nulliparas and 3.2 hours for multiparas.[4] Moreover, cervical dilatation progressed in a straight line. These findings were similar in all other studies on normal labor. For example, spontaneous labor was analyzed in 25 000 women who delivered at term in the Parkland Hospital in Dallas, Texas, in the early 1990s.[3] Labor and delivery times did not follow a normal distribution. Parity (nulliparous or multiparous) and cervical dilatation on admission were significant determinants of the length of spontaneous labor. The median time from admission to spontaneous delivery was 3.5 hours and 95% of all women delivered within 10.1 hours. These results provide the ironclad evidence that normal human labor is relatively short for both nulliparas and multiparas, despite contradicting views by traditional midwives and conventional obstetricians. *Proactive support of labor* adheres to the strong evidence that normal dilatation progresses at least 1 cm/h from the very onset and most often much faster (Chapter 15). Expert labor care rests on the anticipation and proactive assurance of this normal dilatation rate (Section 3).

> *Normal labor is short: 95% of all women who deliver their babies spontaneously complete their labor and delivery within 10 hours (Evidence level B).*

9.1.6 No deceleration phase

The Friedman curve is incorrect at both ends. When patients with dysfunctional labor are included in the computation of a reference dilatation curve, that graph inevitably tends to flatten out in its final proportion. The Friedman curve thus computed, while indeed being the mean dilatation curve, is *not* representative of the mean *normal* cervical dilatation curve. In actual practice, a sigmoid pattern of dilatation is hardly ever seen in normal labor. Proper non-parametric statistical analysis reveals a continuously accelerating dilatation rate without a final decelerative phase in normal labor. Normal dilatation proceeds at least in a straight line.[4] Several reference labor graphs have been published since the work of Friedman, and the principal difference between these graphs is contingent on when labor is determined to begin.[3] When labor is diagnosed at admission on the basis of strict criteria, rather than with onset of regular contractions, a remarkable similarity of individual labor curves becomes apparent.[3] When a latent phase is excluded, dilatation proceeds in a straight line to full dilatation. The ACOG Task Force on Cesarean Delivery respectfully concluded a systematic review of the relevant literature with the understatement that "the Friedman curve may not be as applicable today as it once was thought to be."[10]

> When graphed against time, normal dilatation proceeds in a straight line (Evidence level B).

9.2 Dynamics and mechanics of first-stage labor

While there may be many questions regarding the clinical definition, the relevance, and the very existence of the latent phase of labor, and while the rate of dilatation usually accelerates rather than decelerates when approaching full dilatation, an astute understanding of the classical distinction between the maximum slope and the deceleration phase of dilatation remains of critical importance for comprehension of the dynamics and mechanics of *difficult* labor.

9.2.1 Wedging action through descent

In order for first-stage labor to be successful, uterine force must be effectively transmitted to the cervix, for which the presenting fetal part – functioning as a blunt wedge – must be adequately applied to the cervical dilatation ring (Chapter 8). The pushing force is transmitted through the bulging amniotic sac or, in the case of ruptured membranes, directly by the fetal head. In order to maintain functional wedging action once dilatation has reached about 7–8 cm, the presenting fetal part must descend. Molding and formation of caput succedaneum additionally encourage adequate lock and impact on the dilatation ring, facilitating further dilatation. Descent and adequate impact of the fetal head are needed for proper wedging action to complete the last centimeters of dilatation.

> Initially, descent of the fetal head is not a factor for the progress of dilatation. However, progress of the last centimeters to full dilatation surely requires descent of the presenting part.

9.2.2 Retraction phase and wedging (descent) phase of first-stage labor

On these physical grounds the first stage of labor is best subdivided into two phases with its transition at about 7 cm (Fig. 9.1). The defining nomenclature is open to debate. We prefer the terms retraction phase and wedging phase because the former emphasizes the explicit role of uterine force at that point, and the latter emphasizes the combined roles of force and mechanical cephalopelvic proportions in that phase. Other options could be the initial dynamic phase followed at about 7 cm by the mechanical phase, or descent phase, or pelvic phase of first-stage labor. What label one prefers is not really important. The crucial point is that in the context of the dynamics and mechanics of birth, two distinct phases can and must be distinguished in the first stage of labor, with transition at about 7 cm and its completion at the onset of the irresistible reflex to bear down (Fig. 9.1).

The physical distinction between the retraction phase and the wedging phase in first-stage labor has significant clinical relevance in *difficult labor only*. While in normal labor the transition from retraction phase into wedging phase typically goes unnoticed, the existence of the wedging phase becomes clinically manifest in abnormal labor, when dilatation has been satisfactory in the retraction phase up to about 7–8 cm but starts to decelerate or even stagnates after that point. This is called secondary protraction, or secondary failure to progress, and eventually secondary arrest (Chapter 21).

> *The first stage of labor is subdivided into the "retraction phase" and the "wedging phase." The transition at 7–8 cm becomes apparent in abnormal labor only through a deceleration in dilatation rate.*

9.2.3 Relationship between dilatation and descent

Lessons should be learned from observations in the nineteenth century, when pelvic deformations caused by rickets were endemic and hydrocephaly remained undetected until birth. In instances when the fetal head could not possibly descend because of an absolute anatomical obstruction, dilatation actually progressed readily to about 7–8 cm, but at that point progress of labor definitively arrested.[12,13] It follows that in the retraction phase, it is uterine force and cervical resistance that are the key factors for labor progress. There is still no relationship between the degree of descent and the speed of the first 7 cm of dilatation (Fig. 9.1). The conclusion must be that slow progress in the retraction phase is not at all indicative of fetopelvic disproportion; slow progress of the first 7–8 cm is the result of ineffective uterine force and must be treated accordingly. However, the achievement of the last centimeters of dilatation requires the continuation of adequate wedging, which requires descent (and compliance) of the presenting fetal part, which in turn requires force. The clinical significance of this is that a genuine cephalopelvic disproportion will manifest itself only in the

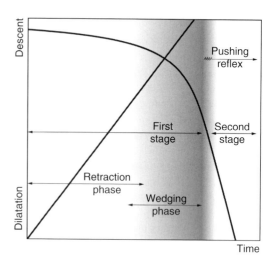

Figure 9.1. Relationship between dilatation and descent of the fetal head. Dilatation proceeds in a straight line. Fetopelvic proportions play a role in the (shaded) wedging phase of the first stage only. This proposition differs fundamentally from the classic contentions still reproduced in most textbooks,[11] which erroneously recognize a deceleration phase in normal labor and regard, in error, the second stage of labor as a part of the mechanical (pelvic) phase of birth.

wedging phase in the form of a secondary arrest of dilatation at about 7–8 cm. Labor arrest due to cephalopelvic disproportion (CPD) will never occur prior to the wedging phase and rarely later. Nonetheless, nowadays insufficient uterine force is still the most likely cause of secondary protraction in first labors – even at this late juncture – and must therefore be treated accordingly (Chapter 21). A reliable diagnosis of CPD cannot be established before the wedging phase of labor and never without forceful contractions (Chapter 22). In first labors, this diagnosis usually requires the use of oxytocin (Chapters 15, 17).

> *The only phase in which the mechanical cephalopelvic relationships play a role in the progression of birth is the wedging phase of the first stage of labor: from 7–8 cm dilatation to the natural start of expulsion when the head is fully engaged; never earlier and rarely later.*

9.2.4 Fetal adaptations to negotiate the birth canal

While descent requires force, the ability of the fetal head to descend also depends upon cephalopelvic proportions. While the pelvic dimensions are essentially static, those of the fetal head are not. The largest diameter entering the pelvis is determined by the head's absolute size, its ability to mold, and the fetus's ability to bend its neck (flexion). In case of relatively unfavorable cephalopelvic proportions even extreme hyperflexion occurs so that the fetus presents the smallest diameter of its head (suboccipito-bregmatic diameter) and the smaller posterior fontanel is presented centrally in the pelvic axis (*extreme hyperflexion*). The largest head diameter to enter the pelvis is made as small as necessary by flexion or as possible by extreme hyperflexion. Adaptation of the fetal head to negotiate the birth canal requires uterine force. This is a reciprocal phenomenon: substantial caput succedaneum formation, molding, and extreme hyperflexion offer clinical proof that uterine contractions are (or have been) forceful during the wedging phase. The reverse is also true: failure to descend and to achieve complete dilatation in the absence of these clinical signs indicates that uterine force is insufficient and must be treated accordingly (Chapter 21).

> *Caput succedaneum, molding, and extreme hyperflexion of the fetal head are manifestations of uterine force.*

9.3 Natural threshold between first- and second-stage labor

At the beginning of the wedging phase (at about 7 cm) the head is still relatively high in the pelvis (Fig. 9.1) and the occiput is in the transverse or diagonal position (Fig. 10.2 in the next chapter). The vagina is not yet stretched. Normally, the fetal head only then begins to descend, facilitating progression of dilatation until completion. Neither the laboring woman nor her attendants are aware of any significant change at that point. Indeed, the fact that the cervix has reached full dilatation would pass entirely unnoticed unless a chance vaginal examination is performed at this juncture.

9.3.1 Misleading and obsolete definition

Unfortunately, leading textbooks still mark full dilatation as the beginning of the second stage of labor.[7,14] This persistent fallacy is based on the obsolete mechanistic view of birth that goes back to the nineteenth century when nothing could be done to improve uterine performance and cesarean section was life-threatening to the mother. For these reasons the approach to slow labor was expectant by default and, eventually, full dilatation marked the point from which difficult labor could be resolved by instrumental vaginal delivery.

9.3.2 Natural demarcation point

Full dilatation is not an end in itself nor is it a natural demarcation line between the first and the second stages of labor. In nature, no laboring mammal knows when she is fully dilated and neither do women who deliver their babies spontaneously without professional attendance (in global perspective, the great majority until recently). Every parturient does, however, invariably notice the often cataclysmic sensation provoked by the descending fetal head the moment it applies pressure to her pelvic floor. This arouses an uncontrollable reflex that compels her to bear down. Evidently, the second stage of labor naturally begins at the moment the irresistible pushing reflex is activated, not earlier. This occurs when the fetal head reaches at least the level of the ischial spines to which the levator muscle is attached (0-station). True reflexive expulsion action is mostly stimulated when the fetal head reaches the pelvic floor, applying pressure on the lower rectum. An inclination to push when the head is still above 0-station should always be regarded with suspicion (Chapter 21).

> *It is* not *full dilatation that is the natural demarcation line between the first and second stages of labor, but the occurrence of the reflexive, irresistible urge to push after full dilatation has been reached.*

An adequate pelvic inlet almost invariably implies an adequate midpelvis and a normal pelvic outlet.[15] As soon as the true expulsion reflex occurs, the fetal head is fully engaged, meaning that its largest diameter has already well passed the pelvic inlet and the entire fetal skull is in the pelvis, making the rest of the birth a matter of pure expulsive force and resistance of the pelvic soft tissues (Chapter 10). This is the true second stage of labor. The natural threshold is the occurrence of the irresistible pushing reflex after full dilatation has been reached and not earlier. As isolated pelvic outlet contraction is exceedingly rare, cephalo-pelvic proportions no longer play a decisive role in the true expulsion stage for the successful conclusion of birth (Chapter 10); a safe vaginal delivery is a near-certain possibility. Thus, the mechanical or pelvic phase of labor, in which passenger-to-passage relationships are decisive factors for progress of labor, represents the last phase of the first stage (wedging phase) and does not transgress into the (properly defined) second stage of labor (Fig. 9.1).

9.3.3 Clinical implications

Although complete dilatation often coincides with the initiation of the woman's reflex to bear down, this is not always the case. If the woman still feels no urge to push after reaching full dilatation, she is still in the first stage of her labor. She should not be encouraged to bear down at this point, because pushing in the first stage of labor results in an unnecessarily long expulsion effort, leading to exhaustion of the mother and instrument-assisted delivery. Continued absence of the pushing reflex at full dilatation is a problem in the first stage of labor and must be treated accordingly. The first step in nulliparous labor is augmentation of labor

using oxytocin, and when this fails to give the desired effect, a cesarean section is the only safe option (Chapters 17, 21, 22).

> *Any interval between a chance assessment of full dilatation and the onset of the irresistible pushing reflex still belongs to the first stage of labor.*

The traditional tenet that marks full dilatation as the beginning of the second stage may have rather unfortunate consequences for women. Too many obstetricians still regard full dilatation as the demarcation line between an abdominal and a vaginal delivery. Whenever there is a need for intervention at this juncture, an instrument-assisted delivery is all too often viewed as a permissible procedure, not to mention a challenge to the obstetrician's manual dexterity. This approach must change. Traction with forceps or vacuum extractor before the natural and true second phase of labor has begun can be genuinely traumatic for both child and mother, because the head is still high, with its largest diameter at or above the pelvic inlet, and the vaginal wall and pelvic floor are yet to be stretched. For this reason, one should never attempt to force a vaginal delivery by instrumental traction in first-stage labor, even if the cervix is fully dilated. Whenever the need for an urgent delivery arises with a fetal head at high station, it should be done by a cesarean.

> *Attempts at vacuum or forceps delivery late in the first stage of labor are evidence of an archaic mechanistic view of birth. This practice must be renounced.*

9.3.4 The evidence

Strong clinical evidence supports our redefinition for the onset of second-stage labor. A large randomized, multicenter study ($n = 1862$) documented that delayed pushing is an effective means of reducing "difficult deliveries" in nulliparous women. The relative risk (RR) was 0.79 with a 95% confidence interval (CI) between 0.66 and 0.95.[16]

The greatest effect was on midpelvic operative vaginal deliveries (RR = 0.72; 95% CI 0.55–0.93).

> *Waiting for deep descent and the natural expulsion reflex to occur before commencement of active pushing reduces instrumental deliveries (Evidence level A).*

9.4 Labor dynamics versus labor mechanics

Since the social conditions that gave rise to rickets were eradicated almost a century ago, nearly all women in the post-industrialized world now have a normally shaped pelvis. For this reason, failure to progress is nearly always a result of insufficient uterine force and/or a lack of remaining expulsive force. Today, true CPD is exceedingly rare (much less than 1%, Chapters 22 and 29). This fact is demonstrated on a daily basis when a fetus is born vaginally with the aid of traction or when the mother – given the chance – spontaneously delivers an equally large or even larger child on a subsequent birth. If a baby can be safely delivered by instrumental traction, then it also, in principle, should have been possible by propulsion, provided the woman had enough strength left.

> *If a woman's pelvis is truly too small, she will not even reach the expulsion stage.*

From what has been discussed thus far, it is clear that it is not so much the mechanical cephalopelvic proportions that determine whether or not spontaneous delivery will occur, but rather the dynamic factors, i.e., effective force. In addition, the relationship between the physical and emotional exertion of the woman and her endurance determines the remaining power available for the successful conclusion of birth by expulsion. This epitomizes the importance of a tolerable and therefore short first stage of labor.

In conclusion: the most important physical factor in labor is the ratio of force to resistance

that must be overcome at the various phases and stages of labor and delivery. This holds for both stages of the birthing process. The mechanical proportions between the size of the fetal head and the bony pelvis play a role in the wedging phase of first-stage labor only. The resistance in the correctly defined second stage of labor consists only of soft pelvic tissues (Chapter 10). In summary:

Physical factors determining the progression of labor		
FIRST STAGE	**Dynamic factors:** *(in both retraction and wedging phases)*	– Uterine force
		– Cervical resistance
		– Transmission of force onto the cervix
	Mechanics: *(in wedging phase only)*	– Pelvic size and structure
		– Dimensions and attitude of the fetal head
		– Compliance of the fetal head
SECOND STAGE	**Dynamic factors:**	– Force from the abdominal muscles
		– Uterine force
		– Resistance of the pelvic soft tissues

The architecture of the bony pelvis is not the factor, with rare exceptions, that limits vaginal delivery (Chapters 21, 22). The most common cause of secondary protraction and arrest disorders in nulliparous labor is insufficient uterine force (Chapter 21), whereas in multiparas it is mechanical obstruction caused by malposition or relative macrosomia (Chapter 22). The fundamental differences between nulliparous and parous labor will be further elaborated in Chapter 13.

9.5 Summary

- The sigmoid Friedman curve as reference for a normal dilatation pattern is based on arbitrary hypotheses, dubious extrapolations, a miscellaneous population, and erroneous statistics, and is thus incorrect.

- The hypothetical concept of the latent phase of labor has no clinical relevance, is deluding, and should be discarded.
- If graphed against time, normal dilatation proceeds in a straight line.
- Normal labor is short.
- In most cases, it is not so much the mechanical fetopelvic proportions that determine the physiological or pathological course of labor. Rather it is the dynamic interaction between uterine force and the resistance of the cervix and the soft birth canal.
- Although both traction and wedging action contribute to dilatation, there is a clear distinction between the retraction phase (dilatation up to 7–8 cm) and the wedging phase (the final centimeters until the arousal of the reflexive urge to push).
- In the retraction phase adequate uterine force is the sole factor of labor progress, while in the wedging phase it is uterine force in relation to fetopelvic mechanical proportions.
- True fetopelvic disproportion manifests itself only in the wedging phase of first-stage labor through a secondary arrest, never earlier and seldom later.
- The threshold between the first and second stages of labor is redefined: the deciding criterion is not full dilatation but the onset of the irresistible pushing reflex after full dilatation has been achieved.
- The architecture of the bony pelvis is not the factor, with very rare exceptions, that limits vaginal delivery once the natural second stage of labor has been attained.

REFERENCES

1. Friedman EA. The graphic analysis of labor. *Am J Obstet Gynecol* 1954; 68: 1568.
2. Friedman EA. *Labor: Clinical Evaluation and Management*, 2nd ed. New York: Appleton-Century-Crofts; 1978.
3. Cunningham FG, Gant NF, Leveno KJ. Section V. Abnormal labor. In: Williams *Obstetrics*, 21st edn. New York: McGraw-Hill; 2001: 425–67.
4. Hendricks CH, Brenner WE, Kraus G. Normal cervical dilatation pattern in late pregnancy and labor. *Am J Obstet Gynecol* 1970; 106: 1065–82.
5. Chelmow D, Kilpatrick SJ, Laros RK jr. Maternal and neonatal outcomes after prolonged latent phase. *Obstet Gynecol* 1993; 81(4): 486–91.
6. Enkin M, Keirse MJNC, Nellson J, *et al*. Prolonged labor. In: *A Guide to Effective Care in Pregnancy and Childbirth*, 3rd edn. Oxford: Oxford University Press; 2000: 332–40.
7. Cunningham FG, Leveno KJ, Bloom SL. Section IV. Labor and delivery. In: *Williams Obstetrics*, 22nd edn. New York: McGraw-Hill; 2005: 423.
8. Practice Bulletin Number ACOG 49, December 2003. Dystocia and augmentation of labor. *Obstet Gynecol* 2003; 106: 1445–53.
9. O'Driscoll K, Meagher D, Robson M. *Active Management of Labour*, 4th edn. Mosby; 2003.
10. American College of Obstetricians and Gynecologists, Task Force on Cesarean Delivery Rates. Systematic Review and Evidence Based Guidelines: Evaluation of Cesarean Delivery. June 2000.
11. Cunningham FG, Leveno KJ, Bloom SL. Normal labor and delivery. In: *Williams Obstetrics*, 22nd edn. New York: McGraw-Hill; 2005: 422.
12. Sellheim H. *Die Beziehungen des Geburtskanales und des Geburtsobjectes zur Geburtsmechanik*. Leipzig: Thieme; 1906 (in German).
13. De Snoo K. *Beknopt leerboek der verloskunde*. Groningen: Wolters; 1910 (in Dutch).
14. Liao JB, Buhimschi CS, Norwitz ER. Normal labor: Mechanism and duration. In: Chauhan SP, guest ed. Management of First and Second Stages of Labor. *Obstet Gynecol Clin N Am* 2005; 32: 145–64.
15. Norwitz ER, Robinson JN, Repke JT. Labor and delivery. In: Gabbe SG, Neibyl JR, Simpson JL, eds. *Obstetrics: Normal and Problem Pregnancies*, 4th edn. Philadelphia: Churchill Livingston; 2002: 353–94.
16. Fraser WD, Marcoux S, Krauss I, *et al*. Multicenter, randomized, controlled trial of delayed pushing for nulliparous women in the second stage of labor with continuous epidural analgesia: the PEOPLE (Pushing Early or Pushing Late with Epidural) study Group. *Am J Obstet Gynecol* 2000; 182(5): 1165–72.

10

Second-stage labor redefined

From the biological point of view, most aspects of human birth discussed so far can be compared with those seen in other higher mammalian species. The only unique characteristic of human birth, not found in any other species, concerns second-stage labor and is an anatomical one: the internal and external rotation of the fetal head during expulsion as an adaptation to the curved birth tract that resulted from our upright posture.[1] Even apes have a more or less straight birth canal, and rotation of the fetal head does not occur in the birth of these higher primates.[2]

10.1 Passage through the osseous and soft parts of the birth canal

As soon as the fetal head approaches the pelvic floor, the woman's behavior changes dramatically. She experiences an irresistible urge to bear down at each contraction and her hitherto passive role in labor – in terms of working to birth her child – suddenly changes to active work in which she delivers her child. It is not full dilatation but the subsequent irresistible reflex to push that signals the commencement of the second stage of labor. This is the true and natural line of division between abdominal and vaginal delivery.

> *The genuine expulsion stage only begins at the moment the irresistible pushing reflex is activated after full dilatation has been achieved.*

Since anatomical deformities of the pelvic bones are extremely rare these days, an adequate pelvic inlet nearly always coincides with an adequate capacity of the midpelvis and a normal pelvic outlet. The midpelvic ischial spines are the lateral, uppermost attachment sites of the concave levator ani (0-station). It is the impact on this muscle that first activates the expulsion reflex.

10.1.1 Pelvic adequacy

Proximal to the pelvic floor, the shape and size of the birth canal are limited by the pelvic bone structure. This osseous component of the birth canal determines the pelvic capacity. At the pelvic floor, the birth canal curves 90° under the pubic bone and is then directed upward, where it is bounded only by the soft tissues of the vagina, the pelvic floor, the perineum, and the vulva (Fig. 10.1).

Successful completion of the wedging phase of first-stage labor and arrival at the natural and true expulsion stage of labor provide strong evidence of adequate pelvic capacity, because the fetal head has descended at least to 0-station or may even already rest on the pelvic floor. The entire head is now in the pelvis (Fig. 10.2). At this point the largest diameter of the fetal head is well past the pelvic inlet and this means that a safe vaginal birth is a near certainty, since selective pelvic outlet contraction without midpelvic contraction is almost vanishingly rare.[3,4] From this point forward, the woman has only to overpower the resistance of her pelvic soft tissues, which admittedly requires a tremendous amount of force in a first labor.

> *In the true expulsion stage of labor, the entire fetal head is already in the pelvis. Cephalopelvic proportions no longer play a decisive role: at this juncture, a vaginal delivery is a near certainty.*

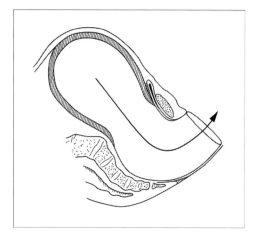

Figure 10.1. Transition of the osseous and soft part of the birth canal at the pelvic floor, where the axis of the birth canal (arrow) curves nearly 90° as it passes under the pubic bone.

The normal position of the occiput at the onset of second-stage labor is in the transverse or oblique diameter of the pelvis until the head passes the level of the ischial spines (0-station), which mark the junction between the midstrait and the outlet of the bony structure. The combined force of the woman's uterus and abdominal muscles propels the flexed fetal head further down and through the opening of the distending levator muscles. At this point, the rectangular curve of the birth canal provokes the internal rotation of the fetal head, followed by extension (deflexion), and the fetal head is born (Fig. 10.2).

10.1.2 Internal rotation and extension

Imagine trying to insert a flexible hose into a stiff pipe with a distant right angle. The hose will get stuck at the rectangular curve unless its end has been cut diagonally. When this is done, the outer cut end will automatically take the inside turn.[5,6] This same principle of plumber's physics applies to the fetal head. The eccentric outer pole, typically the occiput, turns into an anterior position at the level of the pelvic floor or beyond, but not earlier. At this deep level of descent, the axis of the birth canal curves at a near right angle under the pubic bone and at this deep level the head rotates and subsequently extends (Figs. 10.1 and 10.2).

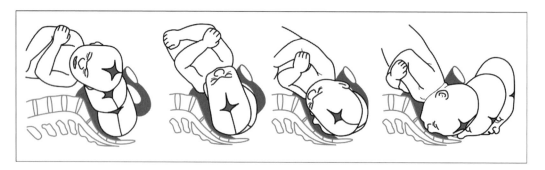

Figure 10.2. Descent and cardinal movements of the fetal head. The occiput turns into the anterior position at the pelvic floor, not earlier. Beyond this point the only resistance lies in the soft tissues. The head is born through extension (deflexion).

It is of fundamental importance that one realizes that internal rotation and subsequent extension of the fetal head are a matter of force. The combination of expulsive force and the direction of the soft birth canal imposes the internal rotation (Fig. 10.2). Since the soft birth canal is oriented upward, extension (deflexion) must occur before the head can pass through it. The expulsive forces push the head against the pelvic floor, forcing the head's extension (deflexion), which brings the base of the occiput into direct contact with the inferior margin of the pubic bone. As the fetal head pushes on the soft division of the birth canal, the perineum begins to visibly bulge and the anus becomes greatly stretched. With increasing distension of the vulva, the head is born by further extension.

> *The fetal head rotates to the anterior position on the pelvic floor at the intersection of the bony and soft tissue portions of the birth canal.*

10.2 Misconceptions

The term "transverse arrest" should be discarded. It is a misnomer attributable to a lack of understanding of the natural process of descent and rotation during the course of normal expulsion. To orthodox obstetricians the term seems to imply a mechanical obstruction, which should be resolved by manual correction, rotational forceps, or vacuum extraction.[7,8] In reality, however, the fetal head is normally in the transverse or oblique diameter of the pelvis when entering the second stage of labor. Internal forward rotation takes place at the pelvic floor (Fig. 10.2). Failure to rotate should be interpreted as an expression of inadequate driving force and should be treated accordingly: by augmentation of uterine force using oxytocin (Chapter 21). Transverse arrest is a problem in the dynamics not the mechanics of birth; "it is not the cause of the delay but rather the result."[9]

> *Internal rotation and subsequent extension of the fetal head are a matter of driving force. Failure of the cardinal movements to occur does not result in but results from protracted expulsion.*

Sonographic studies have shown that two-thirds of all children born with occiput posterior were occiput anterior in first-stage labor.[10] From a physics perspective, however, the expression "faulty internal rotation" is also nonsense. Whenever the fetal head is not flexed (referred to as "sinciput," or "neutral," or "military" attitude) at the moment it reaches the transition of the osseous and soft birth canal, it is the large fontanel that rests in the pelvic axis. In such a position, the expulsive force coerces the fetal head to turn face toward the pubis and the head is born with occiput posterior. This is a physiological phenomenon when the fetal head presents in sinciput attitude.[5,6,11]

> *The term "faulty internal rotation" is a misnomer.*

10.3 Expulsive force versus pelvic soft-tissue resistance

No-one will deny that spontaneous delivery by propulsion is highly preferable to assisted delivery by instrumental traction. Avoidance of traction contributes to a significant reduction in the incidence of birth trauma to both mother and child. The key to a spontaneous expulsion is sufficient driving force in proportion to the resistance of the pelvic soft tissues. The available strength depends greatly on the antecedent events, in particular the duration of first-stage labor. This also applies to the soft-tissue resistance that the woman's expulsive efforts must overcome. Her remaining mental reserves and control determine the extent to which she will be able to relax her pelvic muscles while simultaneously pushing as hard as she can. In conventional practice many women are unable or unwilling to do so after becoming physically and emotionally drained from an overly long and exhausting first stage of labor.

Apart from extremely rare cases involving a selective narrow pelvic outlet, the size and shape of the bony pelvis play no role in the success or failure of expulsion. Women who are carrying an exceptionally large baby or who have an exceptionally small pelvis (contracted pelvis) cease progressing at 7–8 cm when entering the wedging phase and never reach the true expulsion stage (Chapters 9, 21). The true expulsion stage is not part of the "pelvic phase" of labor (Fig. 9.1). Once the fetal head has descended deep enough into the pelvis to activate the irresistible pushing reflex, the only remaining resistance consists of the soft tissues of the pelvic floor and perineum. The key to spontaneous delivery, therefore, is sufficient residual force and relaxed pelvic muscles.

The dynamics of expulsion

$$\frac{Effective}{expulsion} = \frac{Force\ of\ uterus\ and\ voluntary\ muscles}{Resistance\ of\ pelvic\ soft\ tissues}$$

Because the above ratio of force to resistance is more favorable in multiparous births (higher numerator, smaller denominator), women who require the use of vacuum or forceps in their first birth almost invariably deliver their second child spontaneously when given the chance.

10.3.1 Maternal position

In most hospitals, women are encouraged to deliver their babies in the supine position, which is actually quite unnatural. The most common positions for delivery cited in the anthropological literature are squatting, kneeling, and sitting.[2] Squatting during childbirth is common in cultures in which women spend considerable portions of their time in the squatting position while cooking, visiting, caring for infants, and conducting other activities.[12] In western societies, however, very few women have the stamina to remain in this position for the time usually required to deliver a child, and a specialized pillow or birthing stool may be very helpful. The supported squatting position is optimal for allowing a woman's expulsive efforts to work with gravity in delivering her baby, as this position increases intra-abdominal pressure and orients the pelvic outlet more horizontally to facilitate easy extension, crowning, and expulsion.[13,14] These advantages were confirmed by a randomized controlled trial: squatting significantly shortened second stage of labor as compared with the recumbent position, and significantly reduced both instrumental delivery rates and perineal tears, while infant outcomes were similar.[15] This evidence is supported by other, non-randomized studies showing that the semi-upright position of squatting, kneeling, or sitting is the best for expulsion and the most comfortable for the majority of parturient women.[16]

There is no justification for requiring or actively encouraging a supine position during expulsion.

10.4 Summary

- The mechanical possibility of birth depends on the dimensions of the fetal head in proportion to the size and shape of the bony pelvis. Feto-pelvic disproportion becomes manifest only in the wedging phase of first-stage labor, never earlier and seldom later.
- Pelvic deformation is exceedingly rare nowadays in post-industrialized countries.
- The threshold between the first and second stages of labor is redefined. Full dilatation is not the deciding criterion but rather the onset of the irresistible pushing reflex after full dilatation has been achieved. At this stage, the fetal head has at least descended to the midpelvis (0-station), and the largest diameter of the fetal head has passed the pelvic inlet (fetal head fully engaged).

- The mechanical proportion between the bony pelvis and the fetal head no longer plays a role in the second stage of labor, if properly defined. For the expulsion, the parturient has only to overcome the resistance of her pelvic soft tissues, which, admittedly, requires a lot of force.
- Internal rotation and extension of the fetal head during expulsion originate in the driving force. Spontaneous expulsion requires sufficient expulsive force in combination with relaxed pelvic muscles.
- In principle, a child who can be extracted with forceps or a vacuum cup can also be pushed out, provided the woman has sufficient strength remaining.

REFERENCES

1. Naaktgeboren C. The biology of childbirth. In: Chalmers I, Keirse MJNC, Enkin M, eds. *Effective Care in Pregnancy and Childbirth*, vol. 2: *Childbirth*. Oxford: Oxford University Press; 1998.
2. Rosenberg K, Trevathan W. Birth: obstetrics and human evolution. *Br J Obstet Gynaecol* 2002; 109: 1199–206.
3. Norwitz ER, Robinson JN, Repke JT. Labor and delivery. In: Gabbe SG, Neibyl JR, Simpson JL, eds. *Obstetrics: Normal and Problem Pregnancies*, 4th edn. Philadelphia: Churchill Livingston; 2002: 353–94.
4. Cunningham FG, Leveno KJ, Bloom SL. Labor and delivery. In: *Williams Obstetrics*, 22nd edn. New York: McGraw-Hill; 2005: 423.
5. Sellheim H. *Die Beziehungen des Geburtskanales und des Geburtsobjectes zur Geburtsmechanik.* Leipzig: Thieme; 1906 (in German).
6. De Snoo K. *Beknopt leerboek der verloskunde*, Groningen: Wolters; 1910 (in Dutch).
7. Stitely ML, Gherman RB. Labor with abnormal presentation and position. *Obstet Gynecol Clin N Am* 2005; 32: 165–79.
8. Cunningham FG, Leveno KJ, Bloom SL. Dystocia: abnormal labor and delivery. In: *Williams Obstetrics*, 22nd edn. New York: McGraw-Hill; 2005.
9. O'Driscoll K, Meagher D, Robson M. *Active Management of Labour*, 4th edn. Mosby; 2003.
10. Gardberg M, Laakkonen E, Salevaara M. Intrapartum sonography and persistent occiput posterior position; a study of 408 deliveries. *Obstet Gynecol* 1998; 91: 746–9.
11. Pritchard JA, MacDonald PC, eds. *Williams Obstetrics*, 16th edn. New York: Appleton-Century-Crofts, 1980. Chapters 12 and 16.
12. Trevathan W. *Human Birth: An Evolutionary Perspective.* New York: Aldine de Gruyter; 1987.
13. Russell JPG. Moulding of the pelvic outlet. *J Obstet Gynaecol Br Commonw* 1969; 76: 817–20.
14. Ashford JI. Posture for labor and birth. In: Rothman BK, ed. *Encyclopedia of Childbearing*. Phoenix, AZ: Oryx Press; 1993: 313–35.
15. Gardosi J, Hutson M, B-Lynch C. Randomised, controlled trial of squatting in the second stage of labour. *Lancet* 1989; 2(8654): 74–7.
16. Enkin M, Keirse MJNC, Neilson J, *et al. A Guide to Effective Care in Pregnancy and Childbirth*, 3rd edn. Oxford: Oxford University Press; 2000.

11

Definitions and verbal precision

One of the major impediments to improvements in labor care is the lack of clear definitions (Chapter 3). This is true not only of common clinical conditions, of which "normal labor" is a good example, but also of the elementary parameters that describe the basic processes marking the onset and progression of labor. In daily practice, the terms effacement and dilatation are constantly used, but they are seldom accurately defined. In addition, many current expressions such as "the latent phase of labor" usually serve as a cloak for indecision, and ambiguous phrases such as "failure to progress despite good contractions" convey a blatant ignorance of the situation. Most problems encountered in the conduct of labor have their origin in inaccurate diagnosis; unwittingly, these are classified as "dystocia," the most frequently reported indication for operative delivery. Although its common definition – abnormal progress in labor – seems simple, there is an endless variation in the interpretation of what abnormal progress means. This explains the wide variation in the reported incidence and related operative delivery rates in hospitals that appear similar in all other aspects. Dystocia is in fact a complex concept, heterogeneous in its manifestation and causation, and should therefore be examined in detail (Chapters 21, 22). Detailed analysis, in turn, first requires strict definitions of the basic parameters of birth.

> *"Obstetrics is focused on particular elements of abnormal labor and how to surmount problems by operative means, without first defining the basic norms on which such interventions should be based".*[1]

11.1 Elementary parameters of parturition

To avoid semantic debates and confusion about various stages and components of labor, we will formulate unequivocal definitions for such basic phenomena as efficient contractions, cervical effacement, and cervical dilatation. These definitions and their relationship to the definitions of separate clinical events – such as the onset of labor, normal progression, false labor, effective labor, and dystocia – are critical for expert birth care. Evidence-based obstetrics begins with strict definitions.

11.1.1 Labor pains = contractions of labor

Although labor pains are painful contractions, painful uterine contractions are not necessarily labor pains. In Germanic languages (e.g., German and Dutch) different words exist for labor pains (*Wehen*), meaning labor contractions, and uterine contractions in general but not specific for labor (*Kontraktionen*). A similar distinction between "contractions" (of labor) and uterine "contractures" (unrelated to labor) has been suggested in the English literature. In practice, however, these words with explicitly distinctive meanings are being hopelessly mixed up. It is alarming how ambiguously the term "pains" (*Wehen*) is misused, confusing the question whether or not a state of labor exists. Many professionals use extremely unprofessional terminology such as *Vorwehen* (prelabor pains?!), *Übungswehen* (practice pains?!) etc. This confusing use of language can only lead to a lack of clarity and uncertainty at the bedside, because the only thing that counts for the woman in question is that she either does or does not have labor pains because she either is or is not in labor. For her there is no in-between. Absolute clarity regarding the onset of labor is a basic requirement for professional care. Labor pains, i.e., contractions of labor, are by definition uterine contractions that have a progressive effect on the cervix. Pains (*Wehen*) are inherent to labor. There is no labor without labor pains, and a woman does not have labor pains (*Wehen*) without being in labor. Braxton Hicks contractions may indeed be painful, but by definition they are not labor pains (*Wehen*) because they do not have any effect on the cervix. Labor is characterized by pains plus progression.

> Definition
>
> *Contractions of labor (labor pains) are regular uterine contractions with a progressive effect on the cervix, leading to the complete effacement of the cervix followed by dilatation.*

The status of having labor pains can be objectively verified with cervical effacement and dilatation, which are two more everyday terms that are generally used in a careless and often fundamentally incorrect manner. O'Driscoll keenly observed: "In view of the paramount importance of the diagnosis of labor and of the central role of the cervix in this decision-making, surprisingly little attention is generally directed to the understood meaning of the terms used to describe cervical behavior in early labor. Instead, the terms effacement and dilatation tend to be taken for granted and are quickly passed over, as if everyone understood precisely what they meant."[1]

> Cervix in labor
>
> *Effacement and dilatation are consecutive and not simultaneous features of one and the same process: the incorporation of the cervix in the lower segment of the uterus.*

11.1.2 Effacement

Effacement refers to the inclusion of the cervical body into the lower uterine segment. This process begins at the internal os and proceeds gradually downward to the external os, at which juncture the cervical canal disappears and effacement is complete (Fig. 11.1).

> Definition
>
> *Effacement is the shortening of the cervix through its incorporation into the lower uterine segment. With full effacement there is no longer an internal os or a cervical body.*

11.1.3 Cervical accessibility versus dilatation

In nulliparas, the antepartum cervical body is closed, but at term it often becomes weak enough to allow the easy passage of a probing fingertip. It is an endless source of confusion that this finding is considered the equivalent of 1 or 2 cm dilatation in an intact or halfway-effaced cervix. Since dilatation refers only to the external os of the fully effaced cervix, such a conclusion is by definition impossible and counterinformative. One should not call this dilatation but rather cervical accessibility. The term accessibility is intended to convey an inert and temporary static situation, which provides information regarding the extent of prelabor cervical weakening. In contrast, the term dilatation connotes an evolving, dynamic situation resulting from active uterine force. This distinction may seem to be semantic quibbling, but it is actually essential for avoiding the rampant verbal confusion and mistakes that currently occur in the diagnosis of labor (Chapter 14). "Of course, no problem in the diagnosis of labor exists when a well-dilated cervix accompanies regular and painful contractions. As always, the need for verbal precision is greatest in doubtful cases where diagnosis presents a genuine problem."[1]

> *"Accessibility" gives information about cervical ripening, "dilatation" about uterine force.*

11.1.4 Dilatation

The term dilatation relates only to the active opening of the external os by uterine force. The external os can be actively opened only if the cervical body has completely disappeared into the lower uterine segment, i.e., if full effacement has occurred. It is essential to recognize that effacement is, by definition, completed before dilatation begins. To speak about dilatation before effacement is complete involves a direct contradiction in terms.

> Definition
>
> Dilatation *is the diameter of the external os of the fully effaced cervix.*

  This definition holds true for both nulliparas and multiparas. The term dilatation is commonly used incorrectly, especially in relation to multiparas, because most standard textbooks mistakenly teach that the patulous parous cervix simultaneously effaces and dilates. This is a persistent mistake, based on and leading to a careless use of words: cervical accessibility is confused with dilatation. In contrast to the situation with nulliparas, the parous cervical canal is cone-shaped and the external os may freely admit one or two examining fingertips in late pregnancy, while the internal os may still be closed (Fig. 11.1). Thus, by definition, there is still no dilatation, only accessibility. Contractions do not yet stretch the external os, because the body of the cervix must first vanish completely (full effacement) before the external os can be pulled open. Accessibility only then becomes dilatation. In practice, full effacement is the equivalent of 1 cm of dilatation in a nullipara, because the external os is always open to this extent. In multiparas dilatation begins only at 2 or 3 cm (Fig. 11.1) and in grand multiparas the dilatation scale could begin at an even larger value.

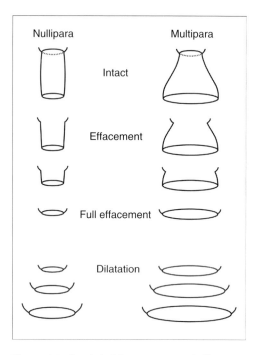

Figure 11.1. Cervix in labor: sequence of effacement and dilatation.

11.1.5 The transition at full effacement

Effacement and dilatation are consecutive and not simultaneous features of one and the same process: the incorporation of the cervix into the lower segment of the uterus. The point at which effacement ends and dilatation begins requires special attention. At this juncture, the presence or absence of painful contractions is decisive and the practical consequence is straightforward: without regular contractions there is no question of labor, whereas a woman with regular, painful contractions and a fully effaced cervix can and must be firmly declared to be in labor (Chapter 14).

> *The significance of complete effacement for the diagnosis of labor is generally overlooked.*

11.1.6 The beginning of labor

One of the most important decisions in labor involves recognizing whether or not labor has started. Many care providers avoid this dilemma by leaving this decision to the woman as a self-diagnosis on the basis of regular, painful contractions, at which point the so-called latent phase of labor begins (Chapter 9).[2] However, this practice avoids a professional distinction between true and false labor. Even leading textbooks, which strongly influence current teaching and practice, still claim that "the confirmation of labor is presumed to be reasonably reliable only once painful contractions have established at least 3 cm dilatation."[3] According to that proposition, the diagnosis of labor is confirmed only after the event, and even worse, primary dysfunctional labor is not recognized at all (Chapters 14, 15, 21). An essential difference between theory and practice is that the doctor – or more likely the midwife – cannot enjoy the luxury of hindsight when an agitated woman presents late at night because she thinks she is in labor.[1] A firm and prospective decision is required in these circumstances, and full effacement plays a decisive role (Chapter 14).

> *The point at which effacement ends and dilatation begins is the practical demarcation line of whether a woman with regular contractions is in labor or not.*

Given the fundamental importance of accurate diagnosis in early labor, separate chapters will address the distinction between true and false labor and the timely recognition of primary ineffective labor (Chapters 14, 15, 21).

11.1.7 Crucial clarity

Poor definitions and resultant conceptual blurring hinder the transfer of knowledge and stand in the way of significant discussion on any aspect of labor. Most studies on labor-related issues in the obstetric and midwifery literature are more or less invalidated by imprecise definitions of elementary parameters of labor such as its onset and thus the duration of normal labor. By inference, systematic reviews on studies of dystocia, amniotomy, augmentation of labor, etc., are often much less evidence-based than they pretend to be.

Even more worrying from the perspective of everyday practice is the use by professionals of ill-defined and equivocal terminology for basic parameters of birth, which hampers adequate transfer of exact patient information. This inevitably leads to inconsistent management by ever-changing staff and hence confusion at the bedside. No one can deny that consistent care requires care providers cooperating within a single practice use the same language and unequivocal terminology.

> *Accurate definitions and verbal precision promote consistency in thoughts and actions and clarity at the bedside.*

Clear and consistent labor management benefits from the proper use of professional language; a woman either is in labor or she is not. Unprofessional phrases, such as practice run, labor not established, rumbling, niggling, nagging, latent labor, slow start, beginning in labor, or moderate labor, serve only as a cloak for indecision or ignorance and are as misleading as saying a little bit pregnant, somewhat sterile, or a little bit dead. Nonetheless, one is regularly faced with a woman who considers herself to have been in labor for more than 24 hours, while her primary birth attendant classifies her first 10–20 hours as niggling, latent, or moderately or gradually beginning, or slowly in labor. Such meaningless jargon only serves as cover for a hesitant and muddling demeanor which, in turn, can only lead to chaos, misery, and despair. Thus, for clarity's sake:

- Strict definitions of the terms effacement and dilatation are the first requirement for the correct diagnosis of the onset of labor (Chapter 14).

- A careful diagnosis of labor onset is a *conditio sine qua non* to define the duration of labor.
- Only a strict definition of labor duration allows for objectively distinguishing between a normal and an abnormal duration, which further supports the criteria for normal progress (Chapter 15).
- A clear definition of normal progress is needed for determining departures from normal and for evaluating treatment (Chapters 21, 27). Clinical science, too, begins with definitions.

> *Most studies on normal labor, prolonged labor, and dystocia are invalidated by imprecise definitions of labor onset, and systematic reviews are consequently less evidence-based than they pretend to be.*

11.1.8 "Good" contractions

The sole purpose of uterine contractions in the first stage of labor is to dilate the cervix and, ultimately, to provoke descent and activate the pushing reflex. The sole objective of contractions in second-stage labor is to prompt the cardinal movements of the fetal head and to expel the fetus. Therefore, the quality of contractions should be evaluated exclusively as it relates to these effects.

Unfortunately, too many care providers lose sight of these effect-criteria. They often use meaningless jargon such as "slow, prolonged, or protracted labor, despite good contractions." This is a contradiction in terms. Careless use of words stems from, and leads to, a failure to recognize dynamic birth disorders in time (Chapter 21). The regrettable result is therapeutic paralysis by dithering and insecure providers in cases of primary ineffective uterine force in early labor, leading to a detrimental waste of time and an unnecessary exhaustion of both the woman and her uterus.

> The effect-criterion
>
> *The quality of contractions must be evaluated exclusively in terms of their effect.*

Impressive uterine action ("super strong contractions"), as judged from the external appearance of the patient, is easily misinterpreted as a manifestation of good contractions. This explains why many orthodox caregivers allow themselves to be misled into a mode of expectation despite minimal progress, which is then discovered too late. Even when the contractions have become a truly painful experience for the woman and feel forceful upon palpation, this does not mean that uterine action is also efficient and effective (Chapter 8). These clinical signs correlate only poorly with labor progress. Uterine action is not the goal, but uterine effectiveness is, and the only "good" contractions are those with a progressive effect on the cervix. Proper evaluation of normality of labor requires accurate assessment of progression in dilatation. In other words, appropriate supervision of labor demands regular vaginal examinations. Four hours of waiting is much too long to discover that labor has hardly progressed (Chapter 15).

11.1.9 Pitfall of intrauterine pressure readings

A similar misconception flourishes in relation to Montevideo units, of which most clinicians mistakenly believe that they evaluate the quality of contractions. By this definition, uterine activity is the product of intrauterine pressure – peak uterine pressure above base-line tone – of a contraction in mmHg multiplied by contraction frequency per 10 minutes. The decision to start or refrain from augmentation of labor is then made depending on an arbitrary amount of Montevideo units, as though uterine pressure were a goal in and of itself. However, it is not the pressure that is relevant, but the net effect of the vector force, i.e., progression in dilatation. Moreover, pressure and force are two entirely different physical entities and uncoordinated dysfunctional contractions can build up pressure without exerting effective, directional force on the cervix (Chapter 8). In fact, insufficient progress of labor is the only criterion on which to base the clinical decision to augment labor, regardless of the amount of Montevideo units, and the same applies to the evaluation of treatment. In reality, Montevideo units are not as useful in the evaluation of uterine performance as they are typically believed to be. The only relevant parameter is labor progression; pressure is not the measure.

> *The only good contractions of labor are those that lead to adequate progression of the birth process, irrespective of painfulness, uterine tone, or Montevideo units. Force is the course; pressure is not the measure.*

11.2 Redefining the stages and phases of labor

Although natural labor is a continuous process, human childbirth traditionally has been divided into the first or dilational stage of labor and the second or expulsion stage of delivery, with full cervical dilatation as the transition point.[3,4] In conventional teaching, first-stage labor is artificially subdivided into the alleged latent phase of labor and the active phase of labor (Chapter 9).[2,3,4] These artificial divisions were originally designed to facilitate study and to assist in clinical management. Ironically, however, most problems in the conduct and care of labor arise exactly from these classic subdivisions. In daily practice, inept management of labor largely results from inaccurate assessment of the transition from one stage of labor to the next: the prelabor transformation phase → the onset of true labor = the first or dilational stage → the onset of the second or expulsion stage.

11.2.1 The latent phase refuted

Imprecision in describing the cervical changes in early labor has led to fundamental and pervasive misapprehensions. There are numerous compelling arguments for radically erasing the concept of the latent phase entirely from our vocabulary and our practice:

- The fact that effacement and dilatation are consecutive and not simultaneous events was generally overlooked in the original studies describing early labor. Similarly, the decisive role of full effacement was entirely neglected.
- In the source studies introducing the concept of latent labor, the term dilatation was ill-defined, so that cervical accessibility was most likely misinterpreted as dilatation. If the fundamental parameters are ill-defined, the subsequent conclusions can be wide of the mark.
- The concept of the latent phase is based on studies flawed with methodological inaccuracies and based on miscellaneous populations not representative of "normal" labor (Chapter 9).
- It is the artificial concept of the latent phase, in particular, that frequently provides an alibi for indecision, ambiguity, and a failure to implement essential policies in early labor.
- Recognition of a latent phase allows birth care providers to circumvent the differentiation between true and false labor and between effective and primary ineffective uterine action in early labor (Chapters 14, 15, 21).
- These omissions are the most common and most pervasive shortcomings in conventional birth care, leading to inept labor management and unnecessarily long labors with all the related complications.

For these reasons, we had better discard the concept of the latent phase of labor completely. Instead, we advocate clear criteria based on accurately defined parameters to confidently assess the clinical onset of labor (Chapter 14) as well as normal progression in early labor (Chapters 15, 21).

> *The latent phase of labor is poorly defined, and it is prudent to discontinue the clinical use of this misguided and misleading concept altogether.*

11.2.2 Normal progress in dilatation

The characteristics of normal first-stage labor are actually far less complex in practice than suggested by Friedman's sigmoid dilatation curve; there is no latent phase and there is no deceleration phase in normal labor. Normal dilatation proceeds in a straight line (Chapter 9) and at a rate of at least 1 cm/h (Chapter 15). Primary slow progression in early labor is a dynamic birth disorder (Chapter 21) and so is secondary slowing down: it occurs only in abnormal labor when the fetal head fails to descend because of inadequate wedging action (Chapter 9). In normal labor, however, the transition from the retraction phase to the wedging phase – a subdivision based purely on physical grounds (Chapter 9) – passes completely unnoticed. There are no distinct recognizable phases in normal first-stage labor, only in abnormal labor.

> *In contrast with the conventional Friedman doctrine, normal labor is characterized by steady progress in dilatation from the outset, without any terminal deceleration phase of dilatation.*

11.2.3 Onset of second-stage labor

In conventional teaching, complete dilatation is the demarcation point between first- and second-stage labor. The unfortunate result of this contention is that mainstream practice dictates that the parturient begin to bear down (push) in concert with each contraction as soon as the cervix attains full dilatation, even if she does not feel the urgency to do so. Here obstetrics strays far from biology; female mammals in nature deliver their offspring without the assessment of full dilatation, and in prehistoric times a cavewoman did not know when she had achieved complete dilatation. The only thing she invariably noticed was the irrepressible pushing reflex as soon as the descending fetal part applied pressure to her pelvic floor and compelled her to bear down.

From a biological and practical standpoint, it is far more logical to distinguish between a passive (dilatation) first stage and an active (expulsion) second stage of labor. The logical dividing line between the two is the reflexive, irrepressible urge to bear down at each contraction near, at, or after attainment of full dilatation. At that point the fetus's head has already descended at least halfway down the pelvis or even rests on the pelvic floor. This terminology is more in accordance with the mother's perception and behavior because she experiences a sudden overwhelming sensation of pressure on her levator and lower rectum. As a natural reflex her hitherto passive role in labor – in terms of working to birth her child – suddenly changes to instinctive, active work in which she delivers her baby. The difference between the newly proposed and the conventional demarcation points is fundamental: absence of the irrepressible pushing reflex at complete dilatation indicates that the active stage of expulsion has not yet begun. Pushing at full dilatation in the absence of the instinctive, irrepressible reflex to do so goes against nature and is relatively ineffective (Chapter 21).

> **Fundamental redefinition**
>
> *The traditional tenet that divides labor into the first (dilatational) and the second (expulsive) stages, with full dilatation as the dividing line, is replaced by the distinction of the first (passive) and the second (active) stages, with the occurrence of the expulsion reflex beyond full dilatation as the transition point.*

This proposition has far-reaching consequences for practice. Firstly, if the fetal head is still high and care providers urge the woman to push in the absence of the reflexive impulse to do so, she is likely to waste her energy and her resolve. The ensuing slow progress and exhaustion or arbitrary time limits will then often result in a failed expulsion resolved by instrumental traction.[5] Secondly, attempts to deliver the fetal head by forceps or vacuum during first-stage labor – even though the cervix is fully dilated – are almost inevitably traumatic for both mother and baby, because the fetal head is still high in the pelvis and the vagina is not yet stretched. If forced extraction is undertaken, the obstetrician has to pull very hard – often too hard – and clinical experience shows that once an effort at rotation and extraction is begun it is very difficult to stop. In contemporary obstetrics, instrumental extraction of a caput from above the inter-spinal line (0-station) should be considered as malpractice (Chapter 22), unless it is done for exceptional circumstances such as acute and severe fetal distress, for example due to (partial) placental abruption.

11.3 The concept of normal labor

Normal labor and delivery is the goal to which all who are concerned with childbirth should consciously aspire. Hence it may come as a surprise to discover that "normal labor" is seldom, if ever, prospectively defined. "Normal" labor and delivery is typically regarded as a conclusion in retrospect: if a healthy baby has been born in good condition without any medical interference. However, a retrospective deduction does not positively inspire care providers toward a sensible rationale for the conduct and care of labor in order to achieve the ultimate prize of spontaneous delivery. The formulation of an agreed and prospective definition of normal labor is therefore an immensely useful and rewarding exercise. "This definition should be posted in a prominent position in every antenatal clinic and every delivery unit, to serve as a clear statement of common purpose."[1] We propose the following:

Prospective definition

Labor is normal if it starts spontaneously, if progress is normal (at least 1cm/h), if the woman gives birth to her baby vaginally, by her own efforts, and without harm to either party.

By inference, labor is classified as abnormal when labor is induced, when labor lasts longer than 12 hours, when labor is concluded by operative delivery, when any harm befalls the baby, or when the mother sustains substantial physical or emo-

tional damage. This is not to say that induction, outlet instrumental delivery, or cesarean delivery should never be practiced, but rather that they should be practiced with utmost discretion as the lesser of two evils.[1]

It should be noted that selective amniotomy and selective use of oxytocin are intentionally not designated as "abnormal," as these are specific measures particularly taken to restore "normalcy" of labor. This view is shared in the consensus statement on normal birth from the UK Maternity Care Working Party consisting of representatives from the Royal College of Midwives, the RCOG, and the UK National Childbirth Trust.[b] A detailed and comprehensive plan specifically designed to offer all women the best chance of a normal delivery is the subject of the next section of this book.

"An agreed, prospective definition for 'normal labor' should be posted in a prominent position in every antenatal clinic and every delivery unit, to serve as a clear statement of common purpose."[1]

11.4 Summary

- Most of the problems encountered in childbirth originate in inaccurate diagnosis, primarily because the elementary parameters describing labor and delivery are poorly defined.
- Most of the literature on labor is invalidated by imprecise definitions of onset of labor, and as a consequence, many systematic reviews about the duration of labor and dystocia are much less evidence-based than they pretend to be.
- New and unequivocal definitions are presented for the basic parameters of parturition, and the conventional teaching of the phases and stages of labor is challenged and fundamentally reassessed.
- Effacement and dilatation are consecutive and not simultaneous features of one and the same process: the incorporation of the cervix into the lower segment of the uterus.

- Dilatation is the diameter of the external os of the fully effaced cervix. Effacement is by definition completed before dilatation begins.
- Critical to rational management of early labor is abolishing the concept of a latent phase, and establishing a clear clinical diagnosis of true labor onset instead.
- The only "good" contractions are effective contractions establishing sufficient labor progress, irrespective of their painfulness, irrespective of uterine tone as determined by fundal palpation, and irrespective of the number of "Montevideo units" assessed with intrauterine pressure monitoring. Pressure is not the measure, only progress counts.
- Adequate uterine force is the deciding factor for a successful birth. The frequently heard clinical conclusion "insufficient progress despite good contractions" conveys a blatant ignorance of the biophysics of labor. Only adequately orchestrated uterine contractions are efficient and only efficient contractions can be effective. Uterine force determines the course.
- The threshold between the first and second stages of labor is fundamentally redefined. Full dilatation is not the deciding criterion, but the onset of the irresistible pushing reflex after full dilatation has been achieved.
- As always, the need for verbal precision is greatest in doubtful cases where diagnosis presents a genuine problem, such as the onset of labor, the distinction between normal and abnormal progression, and the transition point from the first to the second stage of labor.
- Only verbal precision and accurate definitions allow reliable diagnosis and promote consistency in thoughts and action, both prerequisites for expert labor management according to the principles of *proactive support of labor*.

REFERENCES

1. O'Driscoll K, Meagher D, Robson M. *Active Management of Labour*, 4th edn. Mosby; 2003.
2. Friedman EA. *Labor: Clinical Evaluation and Management, 2nd edn*. New York: Appleton-Century-Crofts; 1978.
3. Cunningham FG, Leveno KJ, Bloom SL, *et al*. Normal labor and delivery. In: *Williams Obstetrics*, 22nd edn. New York: McGraw-Hill; 2005: 407–42.
4. Ness A, Goldberg J, Berghella V. Abnormalities of the first and second stages of labor. In: Chauhan SP, guest ed. Management of First and Second Stages of Labor. *Obstet Gynecol Clin N Am* 2005; 32: 201–20.
5. Fraser WD, Marcoux S, Krauss I, *et al*. Multicenter, randomized, controlled trial of delayed pushing for nulliparous women in the second stage of labor with continuous epidural analgesia: the PEOPLE (Pushing Early or Pushing Late with Epidural) Study Group. *Am J Obstet Gynecol* 2000; 182(5): 1165–72.
6. Maternity Care Working Party. *Making Normal Birth a Reality: Image of a Normal Birth*; 2007 (available at: www.appg-maternity.org.uk).

Proactive support of labor

"We are all working to one end, some with knowledge and design, others without knowing what they do."

— Marcus Aurelius

12

Introductory synopsis

Posing the right questions with an open mind often provides answers that are self-evident. A critical analysis of mainstream childbirth practice identified (iatrogenic) long labors and delayed treatment of dysfunctional labor as the main contributors to women's dissatisfaction with their childbirth experience and as the root cause of high operative delivery rates (Section 1). Clearly, prevention of long labor is important. A reappraisal of the fundamental biophysics of parturition highlighted the physiological preconditions required for a smooth, spontaneous, and safe delivery (Section 2). The most significant themes with the most important practical consequences were:

1. The need for care of the laboring mother to be based on a clear understanding of what is going on during labor and to have clear definitions.
2. The rejection of the notion of latent labor.
3. The identification of unnecessary induction as a cause of failed labor and cesarean delivery.

The foregoing analyses touch the very heart of current childbirth practices and implicitly provide the clue to structural improvements: a systematic approach to normal childbirth – *proactive support of labor* – which will be explained in full detail in this section. Before we begin, though, full credit must first be given to the original inventors of this method of care with a brief tour back to its Irish cradle and a comment on some stubborn and widespread misunderstandings.

12.1 The origin

The practical approach to childbirth explained in the following chapters is largely based on the pioneering work of Kieran O'Driscoll and co-workers. In 1969, they published a landmark article in the British Medical Journal entitled "Prevention of prolonged labour."[1] O'Driscoll highlighted his concern that too many women were experiencing traumatic deliveries after prolonged labor, suffering greatly because of exhaustion, confusion, and intoxication with analgesic drugs. Recognizing this physical and emotional stress, he introduced a revolutionary concept of labor management aimed at the normalization and rehumanization of birth by intensively supportive care and proactive prevention of prolonged labor.

12.1.1 Conceptual birth care

As his concept of care evolved through the 1970s and 1980s in the Maternity Hospital in Dublin, O'Driscoll was the first obstetrician to recognize and teach that apt labor management, targeted at spontaneous and rewarding delivery, consists of four strongly interdependent components: pre-labor education of all childbearing women, a clear strategy for the management of labor, sound labor ward organization, and continuous audit of all procedures. Emphasis is placed on continuous, personal, one-on-one supportive care for all laboring women and timely clinical measures to prevent long labor.[2]

With regard to the interventional component, O'Driscoll introduced a strictly pragmatic approach, founded on the empirical evidence that "effective uterine action" is the key to normal labor. He and his co-workers convincingly demonstrated that effective uterine force can be ensured in nearly all cases, with a very high degree of safety, provided a consistent policy is applied with a small number of rules that can be precisely stated. O'Driscoll named his revolutionary concept the *active management of labor*,[3] highly inspiring in nearly all aspects, except for its name.

12.1.2 Misunderstandings and controversy

The name proved to be a source of great confusion, controversy, and cognitive dissonance. In the traditional childbirth world the word "active" is a dirty word and from the midwife's point of view the natural process of birth should not and cannot be "managed" (Chapter 5).[4] Therefore, O'Driscoll's original and challenging treatise was not read at all, or was disputed on the basis of second- or third-hand information, and/or his approach was misapplied and consequently misunderstood and even held up to ridicule as "aggressive management" or "active mismanagement." Negative sentiments were most strongly reflected in midwifery publications. One author, for instance, writes that "the assumption that labor and delivery should progress within a medical framework detracts from the uniqueness of each woman's labor."[5] Although such a statement might arise from a genuine concern regarding women's autonomy, it more likely originates in the false assumption that most women do not desire minor interventions to prevent long labor.[6] A WHO consultant – neither midwife nor obstetrician but a pediatrician with strong connections and influence in the midwifery world – fulminates that "the active management of labor reduces women to a birth machine," and "puts laboring women on the conveyor belt."[7] He even claims that "the active management of labor is a quintessential example of the medicalization of birth, illustrating the inappropriate use of technology."[8] Such lampoons bear

testimony of ignorance, are wide of the mark, and do great injustice to one of the greatest and most inspiring obstetricians ever. In reality, the integral concept of active management – if applied correctly in all its components – effectively restores the current imbalance between natural childbirth and intervention. Readers familiar with the classic treatise by O'Driscoll and Meagher know that the adjective "active" stands for *proactive* and *active involvement*, to enhance the experience of childbirth for the normal healthy mother. This goal should be subscribed to by all right-minded birth care providers worldwide.

12.1.3 Distortion, perversion, confusion

The inventors of the "active management of labor" explicitly warned that no single component of their approach can be safely omitted because, like a jigsaw puzzle, the pieces fit snugly together to form a composite picture. However, the truth of the matter is that most followers to date have only adopted the technical, interventional components – early amniotomy and augmentation of labor – while neglecting all other critical elements. These include adequate prelabor education, continuous supportive care throughout labor, a positive attitude and personal commitment of birth attendants, active involvement of consultant-obstetricians in the supervision of the first stage of labor, and constant peer review of all procedures and relevant outcomes. A stripped and perverted version simply does not work and may even result in contrary effects. In effect, the other supportive elements of care are far more important than the technical procedures, but they cannot be implemented unless early correction of dysfunctional labor is also performed.

Misinterpretation of this method of birth care became a cause of deep concern. The policy was designed specifically for the management of a first labor and it is this essential characteristic that has been widely ignored. The term "active management" has now come to signify different aspects of what may be broadly described as labor management, including parous labor. Confusion and controversy increased further, both in practice and in the literature. Most studies of the active management of labor differed strongly in their individual components compared with the original concept and, consequently, results were inconclusive with regard to the efficacy in reducing cesarean rates. Discussions deviated far from the elementary points O'Driscoll made and finally foundered. His fundamentally important clinical lessons on how to improve women's satisfaction with childbirth fell virtually into oblivion as a result. Evidently, in order to distinguish the basic ideas from the misinterpretations and to regain an understanding of the clear benefits of this form of care, one needs to examine and comprehend the full original concept. Readers are therefore encouraged to consult the classic treatise of O'Driscoll and Meagher and enjoy its vigorous prose.[2] The present book elaborates and complements the original guidelines and provides the solid clinical evidence supporting this concept-based approach to childbirth.

12.1.4 Need for a new name

By now, however, the name "active management" is severely misapplied and widely misused. Aggressive induction protocols, routine amniotomy, excessive use of oxytocin including during parous labor, epidural analgesia, and even operative delivery are actions frequently thought to be synonymous with "active management of labor." Such pervasive misunderstandings led us to the conclusion that by now the apostrophized name has severely worn out, is generally abused, and has proved to be counterproductive, and should therefore be replaced. Orthodox caregivers tend to have closed minds on the subject of labor. Strikingly, as soon as we stopped using the name "active management" in our discussions with the midwives and doctors who work in or refer to our hospital, they started to listen to our arguments in favor of this approach, gradually began to cooperate, and finally grew enthusiastic through experience. This illustrates how deeply the passive attitude toward labor is rooted and how far we have to go to implement fundamental reforms and structural improvements in childbirth.

12.2 Proactive support of labor

The original active management of labor was purely empirical and authority based ("the Dublin experience").[2] Such an apodictic foundation is no longer acceptable in the current era of evidence-based medicine and it is precisely the current confusion and the distortion of the original concept, as well as the scientific requirement of providing independent clinical evidence, that justify the present publication.

12.2.1 Justification and rehabilitation

This book advocates the re-birth of the original concept by showing the need for reforms (Section 1), by demonstrating its natural scientific basis (Section 2), and by providing the clinical evidence (this section). It is an effort to rehabilitate and revitalize the full concept as a means of promoting spontaneous and safe delivery. Every component will be tested following the paradigm of evidence-based medicine. Individual features that could not meet the standards of evidence-based medicine and/or are often conceived as aggressive have been adapted or discarded. Ample, independent evidence of the effectiveness of the overall plan in reducing surgical delivery rates and in improving women's satisfaction with the childbirth experience will be provided. Since the active management of labor was specifically designed for in-hospital births only, we modified this concept of birth care to negotiate healthcare systems that include the possibility of selected home births. Many of O'Driscoll's astute observations and striking statements will be cited, paraphrased, or quoted verbatim. However, not to outdo the pioneering master but to bypass prejudices and to avoid cognitive dissonance that might deter exactly those who would benefit most from reading this manual, we have given this modified and extended version a more cognitively consonant name: *proactive support of labor.*

12.3 The leading principle

The leading proposition is that most pregnant women prefer to give birth by their own efforts and that they want to accomplish this feat in an acceptable manner that is safe both for themselves and for their babies. Despite appearances to the contrary at some critical moments during a difficult labor, only very few women want from the outset to exchange this personal achievement for a surgical delivery by an obstetrician. That is why care – in all its aspects – must be directed toward clear and positive guidance to enhance women's self-reliance and self-confidence. Childbirth is a tremendous challenge and women should therefore begin labor well prepared and as mentally and physically fit as possible. Secondly, they must be positively supported and effectively coached through the arduous dilatation stage in order to reach the expulsion stage with sufficient strength and resolve to deliver their child by their own strength. To this end, prevention of prolonged first-stage labor is critical. This principle has numerous practical implications for prelabor guidance and preparation, for intrapartum moral support, and in fact for all aspects of childbirth including patient education, professionals' working relations, and organization. It leaves no aspect of childbirth untouched. Since the interplay of the various elements of high-quality birth care is seldom or never discussed in standard textbooks, we will emphasize time and again the critical importance of providing the whole package of care. The following paragraphs give a short synopsis.

> Proactive support of labor
>
> *To be able to give birth spontaneously, women must begin labor in a fit condition, and remain fit through the dilatation stage, in order to reach the expulsion stage with enough reserves to deliver their child by their own efforts. Prevention of long first-stage labor is crucial in this respect.*

12.4 Features and benchmarks

While conventional childbirth is culturally shaped and primarily characterized by inconsistencies and a lack of standards for the care of normal labor (Section 1), *proactive support of labor* represents a cohesive conceptual framework of birth care, universally applicable in any professional birth setting.

12.4.1 Purpose and target group

Promotion of normality in childbirth by the enhancement of professional labor and delivery skills is the main objective. The subject is confined strictly to healthy women carrying a single, healthy term fetus in the cephalic presentation. These women represent more than 90% of all pregnancies. The discussion should not be confused by the introduction of severe maternal diseases, hemorrhage, prelabor fetal compromise, or obstetrical abnormalities, especially those that implicate the fetus as a cause of obstruction such as twins or breech and other malpresentations.

> Proactive support of labor *is designed specifically for the conduct and care of healthy women, carrying a single, healthy term fetus in the cephalic presentation.*

12.4.2 An overall plan

Pregnant women are attended these days by several caregivers: obstetricians, residents, interns, midwives, nurses, and so on in random order. Added to this they consult sonographers, birth educators, anesthesiologists, etc. Modern obstetrics is team work. As a result, high-quality birth care has become impossible without a common goal and a central birth-plan that all personnel participating in one practice must agree to and comply with. Such a birth-plan has nothing to do with artificial regimentation of the natural process of birth. To guard pregnant women from inconsistencies in information and care and all their unfortunate consequences is a matter of plain common sense and a mark of respect for women.

12.4.3 Unequivocal information

Consistent information and care require all care providers cooperating within a single practice to use the same definitions and terminology (Chapter 11). Verbal precision is one of the cornerstones of high-quality care. Any science, including clinical science, begins with definitions, and evidence-based care aimed at spontaneous, normal delivery begins with precise criteria for normal and abnormal labor.

12.4.4 Natural scientific basis

The concept of *proactive support* is firmly rooted in natural science. All the following chapters should be read in constant conjunction with Section 2 of this book. Several important issues will be reiterated throughout the present section. This serves to translate the physiological key points into different clinical contexts of daily practice and constant repetition serves educational purposes as well.

12.4.5 Focus on first labors

No plan for birth care can possibly be successful unless it starts from the proposition that the first labor is fundamentally different from all subsequent births. The birth of a first child is one of the most profound experiences, for better or worse, in a woman's life. A smooth, successful, and rewarding first delivery increases the likelihood that there will be few or no problems in a subsequent birth. In contrast, a traumatic first experience is likely to repeat itself, and a first cesarean delivery heightens the chances of a repeat cesarean. Given the critical importance of the first childbirth experience, *proactive support of labor* focuses on the supervision of first labors. The differences between nulliparas and multiparas are even more fundamental than is commonly realized: the frequently occurring

dystocia observed in nulliparas is primarily of dynamic origin (and is not infrequently iatrogenic), whereas the relatively rare problem of dystocia in parous women typically originates in mechanical birth obstruction (Chapter 13).

12.4.6 A clear diagnosis of the onset of labor

The requirement "fit at the start" forces the care provider to make a clear decision regarding the actual onset of labor. In conventional care this is a decision typically left to the pregnant woman, with the inherent hazard of a false start being recognized too late or not at all. When this occurs, the woman becomes exhausted before the actual labor begins. Conversely, when the onset of labor is not properly diagnosed, what constitutes primary dysfunctional labor will also not be recognized as such. This leads to overall indecisive management and creates uncertainties (in both the patient and others), avoidable loss of time, and a counter-productive waste of maternal energy. Thus, one of the most important pillars of *proactive support of labor* is an objective, clinical diagnosis of the onset of labor (Chapter 14). The vague and counterproductive concept of the latent phase of labor is resolutely abandoned (Chapter 11).

12.4.7 Early detection and correction of dysfunctional labor

Equally important is early recognition and correction of dysfunctional labor. This is not an unnecessary interference with natural birth, but a timely correction of abnormally slow labor. Natural or physiological labor is short (Chapter 7). Uterine action is evaluated in terms of labor progression only (Chapter 11). Expert birth care rests on the assertion that efficient uterine contractile force is the key to normal labor and thus effective uterine force must be ensured (Chapter 8). Ineffective uterine powers, reflected by slow dilatation of less than 1 cm/h, must be augmented within one hour by amniotomy and, if necessary, by an oxytocin infusion to avoid unnecessary maternal energy loss and adverse adrenergic responses (Chapter 15). The early correction of abnormally slow labor also guards against exhaustion of the uterus itself (refractory uterus), which is important as uterine responsiveness to oxytocin diminishes strongly when lactate accumulates (Chapter 8). Uterine resistance to oxytocin therapy is a common problem in conventional practices, where dysfunctional labor is mostly treated too late.

12.4.8 A twelve-hour limit

Typically, conventional birth attendants place no time constraints on the first stage of labor, although they do so in the second stage. In contrast, we explicitly limit first-stage labor to 10 hours to allow women to reach the expulsion stage with a sufficient reserve of strength. To this end, we adhere strictly to a minimum dilatation of 1 cm/h as a criterion for normal progression, a criterion that the obligatory partogram reflects in its normality line (Chapter 15). We have already addressed many of the widespread and pervasive misconceptions regarding the meaning of efficient uterine powers (Section 2). In the present section we will unravel the complex syndrome of dystocia in detailed causal diagnoses (Chapters 21, 22) and we will offer an extensive discussion about the facts and myths surrounding early amniotomy and the early augmentation of dysfunctional labor with oxytocin (Chapter 17). Early correction of slow labor does not lead to more interventions. Rather, the exact opposite is the case.

12.4.9 Personal attention and continuous support

Providing supportive care and working to ensure the safety of both mother and child mean that women in labor should never be left alone. To this end, one-on-one companionship in labor is the central component of *proactive support* and the reason why well-trained nurses, possibly supplemented with certified doulas, are invaluable in providing this method of care (Chapter 16). By

limiting the duration of labor, shift changes for all care providers during any given labor can be kept to a minimum. This idea of active involvement and personal continuity also applies to the midwives and obstetricians who are ultimately responsible. These providers should not stay back-stage and run in only when full dilatation has occurred or in the event of an emergency. Furthermore, a woman in labor should not receive care from several different attendants during her labor. Personal continuity and personal commitment of staff are key to a rewarding childbirth experience for mothers and caregivers alike.

12.4.10 Coaching

Ideally, a birth attendant is primarily a coach who helps the pregnant woman to access her innate strength and to navigate the discomforts of late pregnancy and the exertion of labor. This is in contrast to a physician or paramedic who "treats" the patient. Thus, some essential components of being a good coach – and by extension practicing *proactive support of labor* – include:
- Properly preparing each woman for her forthcoming labor and delivery
- Patiently awaiting the natural onset of labor
- Adherence to a clear and consistent birth-plan
- Providing continuous, personal care
- Maintaining a positive attitude and vigilantly warding against demoralizing statements and actions from all persons in attendance
- Preserving safety and acting decisively

In short, one must be as clear and consistent as possible, while conveying the utmost respect for all birthing women and staff who support them.

12.4.11 Prelabor preparation and assurance

With the overall plan, any pregnant woman can now be well prepared for the forthcoming labor and delivery and can be given two firm guarantees: that she will not be in labor longer than 12 hours and that she will never be left without a personal nurse and/ or a doula by her side at all times. These two guarantees completely change the face of women's expectations of labor. Taken together they are at the very heart of the matter and in practice they are entirely dependent on each other.

Prelabor education is best provided on an individual basis through antenatal consultation with nurses or midwives who have ongoing experience in the delivery ward in question (Chapter 19). Prelabor preparation is aimed at reinforcement of women's self-confidence, and firm promises about labor support, short labor, and availability of effective pain relief should be made. Prelabor preparation is relevant and effective only if promises made are kept, which means that all caregivers should agree to and comply with the central strategy in words and deeds. Modern birth care is teamwork and teamwork necessitates strict adherence to agreements.

12.4.12 Coping with labor pain

The pain of labor and delivery puts women's emotional stability to the test. There is no pain and stress from everyday life that is comparable to the physical pains inflicted by the birth of a first child. However, since labor pain is fundamentally different from the pain of wounds or infections, the obstetrical approach to pain must be different from the purely medical approach of using analgesic drugs, sedatives, or epidural block (Chapter 18). The best antidote to labor pain is intensive supportive care on a one-on-one basis, and accelerating a slow labor is generally far more constructive than the provision of medical pain relief alone. In addition, a good bedside manner requires a full appreciation and knowledge of the many methods for coping with the natural pain and discomfort of normal labor, while the potentially negative impact of medical pain relief measures, such as opioid drugs and epidural analgesia, on all other aspects of labor care must be fully appreciated (Chapter 20).

12.4.13 An end to elective inductions

Induction of labor wreaks absolute havoc on the experience and outcome of labor. The duration of labor is artificially prolonged, physical and emotional stress increase, there is a greater demand for analgesia, and operative delivery rates for iatrogenic "dystocia" and "fetal distress" rocket. Induction of labor accomplishes the exact opposite of that for which *proactive support of labor* strives. It is for this reason that we advise obstetricians to practice extreme restraint with this procedure (Chapter 23).

12.4.14 Safety for mother and child

What is good for mothers is mostly good for their babies. Both benefit from care that is specifically and proactively directed toward reducing the possibility of maternal exhaustion, especially when this is typically followed by a potentially traumatic instrumental delivery. Conversely, both mother and child are unnecessarily harmed by an invasive artificial delivery performed on the basis of an incorrect interpretation of a fetal indication. The dictum "when in doubt, get it out" is all too often put into practice, but it represents an oversimplification of a complex set of problems. It is for this reason that we present clear approaches to the identification of the fetus truly at risk and the effective prevention of perinatal hypoxic brain injury (Chapter 24) and associated medicolegal litigation (Chapter 25).

12.4.15 Appropriate working relations

In the final analysis, it is the midwives and labor room nurses who must convert most recommendations into practice. But obstetricians will have to take the lead by creating the proper organization and allowing the conditions needed for nurses and midwives to do their job adequately. With a consistent birth-plan, nurses and midwives no longer remain powerless to influence the course of difficult labor, as the nurse-midwife is authorized to accelerate slow labor according to the strict guidelines (Chapter 17). She is no longer exposed to the possibilities of unfair criticism, because of the agreed guidelines and constant back-up by expert medical staff. Redefinition of professional working relationships and the very existence of a central policy of care greatly enhance team spirit among nurses, midwives, residents, and obstetricians – dynamics that are a prerequisite for good birth care (Chapter 26).

12.4.16 Organization

The welfare of mothers and their babies must not depend on the time of day at which labor happens to occur. All pregnant women have the right to the same optimal birth care, 24 hours a day and 7 days a week. At the same time, care providers have the right to normal working hours and acceptable workloads. Suggestions for an adequate organization wherein both interests are united are discussed in Chapter 26. Poor organization can quickly unravel the best of intentions. In particular, one-on-one nursing support throughout labor is often thought to be utopian because of a lack of financial and/or human resources. However, hospital managers should realize that a substantial reduction in cesarean sections translates into an equal reduction in postoperative care, freeing nurses to work in the delivery rooms. Good birth care and sound economics can surely complement one another. Furthermore, the organization of childbirth should not be subject to territorial disputes between midwives and obstetricians. Provider-centered care must be replaced by patient-centered care (Chapter 26).

12.4.17 Quality control and audit

The creation of optimal birth care is a continuously evolving process that must be maintained by a careful audit of all procedures and outcomes (Chapter 27). This requires a far more exact diagnosis and determination of the problems encountered during labor than the usually imprecise conclusions drawn by current practice such as "dystocia" or "fetal distress" (Chapters 21, 24). The step-by-step approach of *proactive support of*

labor with its clear-cut definitions and specifically causal diagnoses of various birth disorders together form the finest tools for continuous evaluation of all procedures and outcomes.

12.4.18 Evidence-based obstetrics

As events in labor seldom happen in isolation, measures taken in one direction are likely to have consequences in another. Amniotomy is one example of many that will follow in the chapters to come. Information regarding this interconnectedness is generally missing from publications confined to only one narrow aspect of labor. This form of selective reporting and meta-analyses of such studies often conceal a significant distortion of the overall picture. As a result individual "evidence-based" policy proposals – or refraining from measures on the basis of such "evidence" – may very well lead to unforeseen evidence-*biased* mismanagement or evidence-*biased* non-management (Chapter 6).

Clearly, the overall plan must be kept in mind at all times. In effect, the whole package of care proves to achieve far more benefits than the sum of its components. With this in mind, the utility and efficacy of each separate component of *proactive support of labor* will be tested in each chapter, consulting the latest studies and systematic reviews from the international literature. The grading of clinical studies and the hierarchy of evidence used was explained in Chapter 1. Finally, the whole package of care will be incontestably shown to restore the balance between maternal and fetal outcomes (Chapters 28–30). *Proactive support of labor* minimizes the number of traumatic birth experiences and effectively slashes operative deliveries rates without any detrimental effects on the welfare of the babies.

REFERENCES

1. O'Driscoll K, Jackson RJA, Gallagher JT. Prevention of prolonged labour. *BMJ* 1969; 2: 389–477.

2. O'Driscoll K, Meagher D, Robson M. *Active Management of Labour*, 4th edn. Mosby; 2003.

3. O'Driscoll K, Stronge JM, Minogue M. Active management of labour. *BMJ* 1973; 3: 135–7.

4. Kaufman KJ. Effective control or effective care. *Birth* 1993; 20(3): 150–61.

5. Axten S. Is active management always necessary? *Modern Midwife* 1995; 5(5): 18–20.

6. Pates JA, Satin AJ. Active management of labor. *Obstet Gynecol Clin N Am* 2005; 32: 221–30.

7. Wagner M. *Pursuing the birth Machine: the Search for Appropriate Birth Technology*, Sydney & London: ACE Graphics; 1994.

8. Wagner M. Active management of labor. *Birth Gaz* 1996; 93:14–19.

13

Nulliparous versus parous labor

Every discourse on the supervision of labor and delivery should begin with the fundamental distinction between the first and subsequent births. Strangely enough, leading textbooks hardly ever devote a separate chapter to this important issue. In mainstream practice the conduct of labor is troublingly confused because of misplaced extrapolation of nullipara-specific birth disorders to multiparas and vice versa. In reality, the duration of labor, the nature of labor disorders, and the impact of the birth experience differ so radically between the first and subsequent births that they justify the following striking statement made by O'Driscoll:

> *"Nulliparas and multiparas behave like different biological species in nearly all matters relating to labor and delivery."*[1]

13.1 Unique first experience

A woman may have several children but she becomes mother only once. The crucial importance of the course and outcome of a woman's first labor and delivery cannot be overemphasized. The physical and emotional impact of the first childbirth experience determines a woman's expectation and attitude to all later births. A woman with a positive first experience is unlikely to be worried about the next delivery, while the outlook of a woman with a negative birth experience is marred by fears of a repeat performance. The emotional

trauma can have serious consequences outside the narrow range of vision of midwifery and obstetrics as it can haunt a woman for the rest of her life (Chapter 2). A traumatic first birth experience can severely undermine mother–child bonding, affect her marriage, and occasionally have a scarring effect that leads a woman to decide against having a second child despite earlier plans of having a larger family. Typically, the residual effect of a traumatic first birth experience reveals itself during a preconceptional consultation or early during her second pregnancy in an urgent request for prelabor commitment to epidural analgesia or even an elective cesarean section. Ironically, a prompt accession to such requests reinforces her fear about labor, for which there is absolutely no foundation in clinical practice. The sequence of events in first childbirth is generally not predictive of the course of later births.[1]

> In contrast to what most people and even care providers assume, a problematic dilatation stage in first labor does not provide a prognostic sign for troubles in subsequent births. There is no connection.

In fact, long, exhausting labor is a problem specific to first labor. In contrast, parous women do not suffer from dysfunctional labor to a significant extent, provided their parasympathetic condition – which is essential for normal birth – has not been destroyed beforehand by the emotional trauma of an ill-managed previous birth. The message is all too clear: there is only one first birth experience, so invest the utmost in the care and outcome of first labor and few or no problems will be encountered in later births. Conversely, the damage inflicted by a low standard of care and attention the first time round is usually irreversible; birth care for multiparas then becomes a futile and never-ending game of catch-up from the start. All the good intentions in a later birth will founder if the woman was emotionally traumatized during her first labor and/or if her uterus has been scarred by a previous cesarean section.

> *A traumatic first birth experience effectively undermines a woman's future reproductive career.*

13.2 Parity-specific features

The most distinctive feature of first labor compared with all subsequent births is its duration: the first is the worst. More than any other objective measure, the length of a first labor determines the emotional and physical impact of childbirth. Apart from the susceptibility to lasting psycho-emotional trauma, first-time mothers run a significantly greater risk of sustaining physical injury to themselves and their babies than do parous women. This is directly related to the longer duration of the first labor per se and to the consequently higher rate of intrusive interventions including operative deliveries.

13.2.1 Duration of labor

A first birth takes significantly longer than all subsequent births because inefficient uterine power is common during first labor and because the cervix has never been dilated before (Chapter 8). Additionally, there is a direct relationship between the overall length of first labor and the likelihood of emotional trauma, invasive interventions, and operative deliveries.[2–4] In other words, duration

is the key problem of first labors. By inference, effective restriction on the duration should provide the basic solution for most problems encountered in first labors. Short labor is best accomplished by ensuring sufficient progress from the very start of labor. Effective uterine force is the key to normal labor (Chapter 8), and expert labor management rests on this proposition.

> *Duration is the key problem of first labors, leading to operative deliveries and trauma. Proactive prevention of long first labor is the key to the solution of most labor problems.*

13.2.2 Nulliparous dynamics versus multiparous mechanics

The clinical difference between troublesome nulliparous labor and difficult parous labor is analogous to the fundamental distinction in physics between labor dynamics and birth mechanics (Chapter 9). The disorders frequently found in first labors are nearly always primarily rooted in dynamic factors – i.e., inefficient and therefore ineffective uterine force in relation to the resistance of the cervix and the birth tract – and must be treated accordingly. In contrast, occasional dystocia in multiparas typically originates in obstruction caused by fetal malposition or relative macrosomia.[5] These rules of thumb may sound rather dogmatic but are, nonetheless, extremely relevant for daily, intelligent practice.

> *The most common cause of labor protraction and arrest disorders in nulliparous labor is insufficient uterine force, whereas dystocia in multiparous labor usually results from mechanical obstruction.*

13.2.3 Fetal distress

The comparatively long duration of first labors presents significantly more risks for first-borns. Compression of the umbilical cord is the most frequent cause of fetal compromise during labor, and the ability of the fetus to bear these intermittent but recurrent incidents depends strongly on the duration of labor (Chapter 24). The second important hazard for the fetus during labor is uterine hypertonia in the intervals between contractions, leading to fetal hypoxia. This typically occurs when an already exhausted uterus is stimulated with oxytocin (too late), or when labor is being induced (Chapter 8). The third important fetal hazard during labor is intrauterine infection, and the chance of this increases strongly with the duration of labor. Clearly, short labor benefits babies.

13.2.4 Trauma

With common vertex presentations, first-borns suffer perinatal trauma more frequently than subsequent offspring. Birth injuries to the mother or child can be discussed under one heading (Chapter 4): both mainly result from instrumental interventions, in particular forced traction.[6–12] This fundamental truth in clinical obstetrics underscores the importance of *proactive support of labor*, wherein both mother and child benefit from a policy of care that proactively reduces the duration of first labor and avoids forced forceps or vacuum deliveries.

> *The comparatively long duration of first labors presents significantly more fetal risks. First-borns are exposed more and longer to risks of fetal distress, perinatal infection, and birth trauma.*

13.2.5 Rupture of uterus

The ultimate obstetric trauma is rupture of the uterus, which is a rare but dramatic complication that is life-threatening to both mother and child. This potentially catastrophic complication is specific to parous labor.[13,14] The most common cause is a previous cesarean section and the chance of rupture of the uterine scar rises significantly when labor is induced with prostaglandins or (injudiciously) augmented with oxytocin.[15] Clearly, the

best way to prevent this obstetric calamity is to avoid cesarean section the first time round. It should be noted, however, that uterine rupture may occur even in multiparas with an uneventful obstetric history who now experience obstructed labor (due to fetal macrosomia or malposition), and the greater the parity of the woman the greater the vulnerability of her uterus to rupture.[16] In contrast, rupture of a nulliparous uterus is such an exceptional event in western obstetrics that for practical purposes it can be assumed not to occur. Judicious use of oxytocin in first labor does not cause rupture of the uterus even if used to prove or exclude cephalopelvic disproportion (Chapters 21, 22). This immunity from uterine rupture is another fundamental feature of first labor that has important clinical implications.

> *"The nulliparous uterus is rupture-proof; the parous uterus is rupture-prone."*[1]

13.2.6 Specification of the meaning of multiparity

The term multipara or parous labor as it has been used thus far pertains to a woman who has had a previous vaginal birth. As the classification of G2 P1 has historically also been applied to those who have undergone previous cesarean delivery, further specifications are required. In the context of the dynamics and mechanics of labor, it will best serve a woman with a cesarean scar to realize what phase her previous labor had reached. A multipara who had a previous prelabor cesarean section should be considered a nullipara in all aspects of labor (i.e., prone to dysfunctional labor), except for the important fact that she is now vulnerable to uterine rupture as well. This status seriously restricts the possibilities of effective management of a trial of first labor after cesarean (VBAC). This consequence is hardly ever given enough consideration when suggesting a prelabor cesarean in first pregnancy, e.g., for a breech presentation. VBAC success rate is partly dependent on the extent of cervical dilatation reached at the prior cesarean delivery.[17] A parturient women who previously had a cesarean in well-advanced first-stage labor can now be regarded as a cervical and uterine multipara, but a vaginal nullipara: first-stage labor can be expected to progress satisfactorily; the second stage of labor, however, will then be comparable with that of all first deliveries.

> *It best serves the interests of a woman with a cesarean scar to realize how far her previous labor had advanced.*

13.3 Parity-based approaches

The fact that the nulliparous uterus is frequently inefficient in labor but is immune to rupture, added to the information that the parous uterus is generally very efficient but relatively prone to rupture, has significant consequences for diagnosis and treatment of difficult labor:

> **Fundamental distinction**
>
> *Insufficient progress in first labor must be approached as a dynamic birth disorder until proven otherwise, whereas failure to progress in parous labor is strongly indicative of a mechanical birth obstruction until proven otherwise.*

13.3.1 Prolonged labor in nulliparas: a dynamic disorder

The all too common expectant attitude to labor typically results in late augmentation of slow labor and often not before definite arrest and signs of maternal exhaustion are manifest (Section 1). As the functional capacity of the pelvis has not yet been proven by an earlier birth, slow progress of first labor is then considered to point to fetopelvic disproportion. This "mechanistic" (Chapter 3) misconception combined with misplaced anxiety

over potential uterine rupture partly explains the commonly late or half-hearted use of low-dose oxytocin in these circumstances. As time passes, however, the exhausted uterus gradually becomes insensitive to stimulation, thereby rendering the administration of oxytocin ineffective (Chapters 8, 17, 21). As a result, progression remains insufficient despite the use of oxytocin. This observation is then misconstrued as confirmation that a mechanical obstruction exists. This is classic circular reasoning in which the obstetrician figuratively bites his/her own tail, but the consequent pain is for their patient. The correct point of view and fully appropriate management are exactly the opposite of this approach. Failure to progress in first labor must always be regarded as an expression of ineffective uterine force until fetopelvic disproportion has been demonstrated by reaching at least 7 cm dilatation, accompanied by substantial molding, caput succedaneum formation, and extreme hyperflexion of the non-descending head (Chapter 9). The diagnosis of birth obstruction in first labor usually requires timely and proper use of oxytocin. In fact, true mechanical dystocia occurs in less than 1% of all first labors (Chapters 22, 29).

> *Augmentation of first labor – to prove or exclude cephalopelvic disproportion – poses no threat to the welfare of mother or fetus.*

13.3.2 Protracted labor in multiparas: a mechanical problem

The guiding thought in problematic parous labor is exactly the opposite. The experienced uterus is by nature efficient and cervical resistance is low, making ineffective uterine action exceedingly rare in parous labor. However, secondary arrest in the wedging phase (Chapter 9) occasionally occurs and should cause one to be extremely alert, because secondary protraction of parous labor is strongly indicative of unfavorable fetopelvic proportions with potentially dangerous complications. Obstructed parous labor results from malposition of the fetal head or relative macrosomia (Chapter 22).

> *Secondary protraction or arrest in parous labor is highly indicative of mechanical birth obstruction.*

In common practice, however, too many birth attendants assume that mechanical obstruction is unlikely in a parous woman, even if labor is secondarily slow, because the functional capacity of the woman's pelvis has been proven by a previous birth. Nothing could be further from the truth. Protracted multiparous labor should provoke extreme suspicion of obstruction from relative macrosomia or fetal malposition. Because the unscarred parous uterus is by nature effective in labor, and because multiparas are relatively at risk of uterine rupture, the utmost restraint should be exercised when considering oxytocin in a secondary arrest in parous labor (Chapter 21). This is especially true if an epidural, which masks the symptoms of imminent uterine rupture, has been administered.

13.3.3 Correct mindset

One of the fundamental truths in obstetrics is that the etiology of difficult labor differs radically between the first labor and the following labor. This statement might sound rather dogmatic, but it is nevertheless crucial for the correct mindset whenever confronted with a problematic, protracted labor:

> Rule of thumb
>
> *Difficult nulliparous labor → dynamic labor disorder.*
> *Difficult multiparous labor → mechanical labor disorder.*

In the interest of clarity and completeness, we must mention the obvious exceptions to this rule.

Dynamic disorders occasionally do occur in parous labor, but when this happens there are always clearly identifiable causes:

- *Induction.* A woman's fear of recurrence of the protracted course and operative conclusion of her first labor often becomes a self-fulfilling prophecy when the empathetic doctor promises to attend the delivery personally – thereby arranging an elective induction. Such a policy is a common mistake, as the induction procedure in itself usually causes a protracted or failed labor (Chapters 21, 23). Obstetricians would best serve the interests of parous women were they to dispel her fears with a simple but clear explanation of the differences between a first and a second birth, and wait for spontaneous labor to occur.
- *Hypertonic dystocia.* This separate clinical entity, characterized by disorganized, inefficient uterine contractions and fetal distress due to insufficient uterine relaxation, is secondary to a different pathological process altogether involving cytokines production in the myometrium as a result of intrauterine bleeding, passage of meconium, or chorioamnionitis (Chapters 8, 21). Of course, this specific dynamic labor disorder can occur in nulliparous and parous labors alike.
- *Sympathetic arousal.* Primary ineffective parous labor originates in the prior obliteration of the parasympathetic control through anxiety and fear, mostly as a residual effect of the previous adverse birth experience. This results in treating last year's problems, thus rendering the care after the fact and often in vain. Again, the lesson is all too clear:

> Key point
>
> *Invest the utmost in the course and outcome of first labor and few or no problems will be encountered in the following birth. Conversely, irreversible damage may result from a protracted first labor in which the physical and emotional vulnerability of the woman was insufficiently appreciated.*

13.4 Summary

- There are fundamental differences between the first labor and a subsequent labor. The causes of delay and risks of treatment are very different, and proper management rests on this premise.
- Nulliparous labor takes longer because inefficient uterine performance (force) is common and the birth tract has not previously been stretched.
- The main risk-factor for labor disorders is nulliparity. Because of the longer duration of first labors, nulliparas are at greater risk of intrauterine infection, fetal distress, exhaustion, and related cesarean, forceps or vacuum delivery and associated maternal and fetal birth-trauma.
- Problematic parous labor should not be assumed to be an expression of inefficient uterine force. Dynamic dystocia is uncommon in parous labor. The explanation for dysfunctional parous labor should rather be sought elsewhere, beginning with obstruction.
- Nulliparas are proof against uterine rupture, whereas multiparas are vulnerable to uterine rupture, in particular when their uterus has been scarred by a previous cesarean section.
- Oxytocin does not cause rupture of the nulliparous uterus even in the presence of cephalopelvic disproportion, whereas oxytocin may cause rupture of the (unscarred) parous uterus even in normal labor.
- One of the most pervasive errors in obstetrics is the practice of extrapolating from a first to a second labor. This leads to futile treatment of last year's problems. There is virtually no physical connection.
- With optimal care in first labor, subsequent births will pose few or no problems at all. This is the quintessential tenet behind the strategy of *proactive support of labor*.

REFERENCES

1. O'Driscoll K, Meagher D, Robson M. *Active Management of Labour*, 4th edn. Mosby; 2003.

2. Enkin M, Keirse MJNC, Neilson J, *et al.* Prolonged labor. In: *A Guide to Effective Care in Pregnancy and Childbirth*, 3rd edn. Oxford: Oxford University Press; 2000: 332–40.

3. Melmed H, Evans M. Predictive value of cervical dilatation rates, I Primigravids. *Obstet Gynecol* 1976; 47: 1568–75.

4. Chelmow D, Kilpatrick SJ, Laros RK jr. Maternal and neonatal outcomes after prolonged latent phase. *Obstet Gynecol* 1993; 81(4): 486–91.

5. Norwitz ER, Robinson JN, Repke JT. Labor and delivery. In: Gabbe SG, Neibyl JR, Simpson JL, eds. *Obstetrics: Normal and Problem Pregnancies*, 4th edn. Philadelphia: Churchill Livingston; 2002: 353–94.

6. Levine MG, Holroyde J, Woods JR Jr, *et al.* Birth trauma: incidence and predisposing factors. *Obstet Gynecol* 1984; 63: 792–5.

7. Williams MC, Knuppel RA, O'Brien WF, *et al.* Obstetric correlates of neonatal retinal hemorrhage. *Obstet Gynecol* 1993; 81: 688–94.

8. Gebremariam A. Subgaleal haemorrhage: risk factors and neurological and developmental outcome in survivors. *Ann Trop Paediatr* 1999; 19: 45–50.

9. Chadwick LM, Pemberton PJ, Kurinczuk JJ. Neonatal subgaleal haematoma: associated risk factors, complications and outcome. *J Paediatr Child Health* 1996; 32: 228–32.

10. Johnson JH, Figueroa R, Garry D, *et al.* Immediate maternal and neonatal effects of forceps and vacuum-assisted deliveries. *Obstet Gynecol* 2004; 103: 513–18.

11. Uchil D, Arulkumaran S. Neonatal subgaleal hemorrhage and its relationship to delivery by vacuum extraction. *Obstet Gynecol Survey* 2003; 58: 687–93.

12. Johnson RB, Menon BK. Vacuum extraction versus forceps for assisted vaginal delivery. *Cochrane Database Syst Rev* 2000; (2): CD 00024.

13. Kafkas F, Taner CE. Ruptured uterus. *Int J Gynaecol Obstet* 1991; 34(1): 41–4.

14. Vedet A, Hasan B, Ismail A. Rupture of the uterus in labor: a review of 150 cases. *Isr J Med Sci* 1993; 29(10): 639–43.

15. Lydon-Rochelle M, Holt VL, Easterling TR, *et al.* Risk of uterine rupture during labor among women with a prior cesarean delivery. *N Engl J Med* 2001; 345: 3–8.

16. Miller DA, Goodwin TM, Gherman RB, *et al.* Intrapartum rupture of the unscarred uterus. *Obstet Gynecol* 1997; 89: 671–3.

17. Hoskins IA, Gomez JL. Correlation between maximum cervical dilatation at cesarean delivery and subsequent vaginal birth after cesarean delivery. *Obstet Gynecol* 1997; 89(4): 591–3.

14

Diagnosis of labor

Correct diagnosis is the foundation of responsible medical care and this universal truth most certainly applies to childbirth. Yet the expression "diagnosis of labor" sounds rather strange to many ears. A computer search in Medline/PubMed renders no hits. The subject is evaded in the literature, where only cases said to be "in established labor" – thus with a "well dilated cervix" – are included in the scientific reports. Midwives and obstetricians seem to rely on their experience and intuitive skills. In clinical practice, however, many births are attended by younger caregivers who make the decision of admission to the labor ward without clear instructions of how to assess true labor. Textbooks that strongly influence teaching and practice hardly address the subject in detail and seldom formulate strict clinical criteria for early labor. These examples illustrate the general failure to appreciate that the onset of labor may represent a genuine diagnostic problem. The unfortunate consequences can be seen on a daily basis in many hospitals and other birth settings, although these problems are rarely recognized for what they are. If labor is diagnosed in error, inappropriate measurements and interventions are employed. Conversely, if a timely and appropriate diagnosis of labor is not made, primary ineffective labor is not recognized.

Clinical onset of labor

When the diagnosis of labor is incorrect, all subsequent policies are also likely to be incorrect and a troublesome domino effect ensues.

14.1 Professional responsibility

Most pregnant women go into labor without any significant warning, whereas some women may wittingly experience a gradual run-up as they consciously notice the prelabor biological transformation of their uterus due to Braxton Hicks contractions (Chapter 8). A gradual progression to actual labor can last for a number of days but normally allows the woman to go about her everyday tasks and adjust to the intermittent contractility of her uterus. A clear, blood-free cervical mucous plug may break free and there may be periods of mild contractions that come and go. Considering the possibility of such a gradual progression to actual labor, it could be argued that there is no balanced clinical definition – in a strictly academic sense – for the precise moment at which clinical labor begins. This traditional view is all very well but it should not distract from the responsibility to provide clarity if a woman calls upon the professional because she thinks her labor has begun. The ability to pinpoint early a stage when labor can confidently be confirmed is essential for apt supervision of labor and professional conduct and care.

In conventional practice, however, it is commonly assumed that most pregnant women unerringly recognize the onset of their labor by natural instinct. As soon as regular, painful contractions occur, the alleged latent phase of labor, as defined by Friedman, is assumed to have begun.[1] This concept underlies the customary practice that the key decision which forms the basis for subsequent management is left to the mother. She declares herself in labor, with the result that it is she who stipulates birth care and becomes the responsible party for the course of events, including all interventions that might occur thereafter. "This practice, which relinquishes the initiative to patients, is a common but anomalous route without any parallel in regular healthcare."[2] Consider how bizarre it would be to hospitalize a patient for observation who believes she has a hernia and subsequently schedule her for surgery without first performing adequate diagnostics. Clearly, the first step in providing professional care in labor is to confirm or reject the woman's self-diagnosis of labor.

> *The diagnosis of labor is a clinical diagnosis based on objective symptoms, where the full responsibility rests with the professional care provider and not with the pregnant woman.*

14.1.1 A firm clinical decision

Although it could be argued that the diagnosis of labor is fraught with all the difficulties of trying to categorize a continuous variable, patients do not benefit from a semantic academic exercise. The care provider must be resolute when confronted with an agitated woman who declares labor to have begun. It is after all the professional who is (legally) responsible and not the pregnant woman. The declaration of "A" has certain consequences, such as the irrevocable "B" that follows and will direct the course of events. Clarity is essential and this requires a firm clinical decision based on solid diagnostic criteria. For the pregnant woman this is the point of no return. The waiting is over, the physical and emotional challenge begins, and she will not rest until her baby is born.

> *The clinical diagnosis of labor implies an obligatory result: the commitment to delivery.*

From the biophysical perspective, labor begins with the sudden formation of myometrial gap junctions resulting in electrically orchestrated uterine contractions exerting force (Chapter 8). In clinical terms this means that contractions are now rendering a verifiable effect on the cervix.

14.2 Objective symptoms

Painful contractions, at intervals of 10 minutes or less, are essential but not decisive; they must be accompanied by additional symptoms. We adopted the diagnostic criteria pioneered by O'Driscoll and Meagher whereby the only real proof of labor is pains supported by dilatation and thus, by definition, full effacement (Chapter 11). Other criteria that justify a clinical diagnosis of labor include pains supported by a bloody show or pains with spontaneous rupture of membranes. These empirical criteria for factual labor have been evaluated by numerous clinical investigators exploring the active management of labor, and have proved to be correct and very practical: they allow a firm clinical decision in nearly every case.[2–15] Of course, one could ask for references to double-blinded studies, but such information does not exist since it is not feasible to blind a woman on whether she is having labor or not. Given these limitations, we feel confident of the literature and the clinical experience supporting the criteria for labor presented here. As is always the case in clinical decision making, the gratuitous appeal for information from impossible randomized controlled trials does not remove the need to draw conclusions from what we now know.

14.2.1 Pains

Regular painful contractions are a prerequisite for the diagnosis of labor. Without them, labor simply does not exist. Unfortunately, it is a common belief – based on the teaching of Friedman – that persistent painful contractions *alone* provide conclusive evidence of labor. Although this assumption may not seem unreasonable late in pregnancy, the subjective element of pain and discomfort caused by Braxton Hicks contractions might be highly underestimated. Braxton Hicks contractions are a normal start-and-stop phenomenon in late pregnancy and are an early sign of the beginning of uterine transformation (Chapter 8). The pain they cause cannot be differentiated from true labor pains because both are of uterine origin. Consequently, it must be established that the contractions are genuine labor pains, meaning that they have a progressive effect on the cervix.

> *A diagnosis of labor based solely on regular, painful contractions is an elementary mistake.*

14.2.2 Effacement and dilatation

The diagnosis of labor is simple if the woman has regular, painful contractions, a fully effaced cervix, and a few centimeters dilatation. An easy birth can be anticipated with confidence. In practice, about 80% of all nulliparas who make the self-diagnosis of labor on the basis of painful, regular contractions indeed already have a completely effaced cervix and labor can be unequivocally accepted on the basis of this additional symptom alone.[2,16] Considering the decisive importance of effacement and dilatation, it is imperative that the terms be used correctly: dilatation is the diameter of the external os of the fully effaced cervix (Chapter 11).

> Proof of labor
>
> *The transition from full effacement to dilatation is – in the presence of painful contractions – definitive, physical proof that labor has begun.*

Diagnostic problems arise in only 20% of nulliparas who believe themselves to be in labor but in whom the cervix is not yet fully effaced. In these cases imprecise terminology may lead to mistaken conclusions. Cervical accessibility may be wrongly interpreted as dilatation (Chapter 11) and, consequently, labor may be accepted in error. This mistake can easily result in an unnecessarily long ordeal of exhaustion and suffering with a cesarean delivery as the only exit strategy.

14.2.3 Bloody show

If the cervix is not yet fully effaced, a bloody show is of invaluable help because it is an objective sign that contractions are rendering an effect on the cervix and, therefore, represents a symptom very suggestive of labor. A show is a spontaneous vaginal release of blood-stained cervical mucus as a result of uterine contractions. Spontaneous means that it is not the result of a vaginal examination probing the cervical canal. This would be an artifact, just as bloody discharge after amniotomy for induction is an artifact. Blood loss without contractions is not a show, although it is an indication for admission – not to the labor and delivery unit but to the antenatal ward. In contrast, contractions that spontaneously coincide with a bloody show have an objective effect and consequently can be clinically regarded as a convincing sign of labor.

> Definition
>
> *A show is the spontaneous vaginal discharge of blood-stained mucus that results from uterine contractions.*

Approximately 70% of all women who report themselves in labor have a bloody show.[2] This symptom can legitimately – for reasons of consistent and clear practice – serve as a determining sign that labor has begun even in the absence of full effacement of the cervix. Because uterine action might not be optimally effective in this latter condition, progression to full effacement and subsequent dilatation must be monitored closely and if necessary promptly accelerated.

14.2.4 Immediate progress

The diagnosis of labor is even more difficult if painful contractions are supported by neither full effacement nor show. An observation period of no more than one to two hours is advisable during which time legitimate doubts must be communicated. If progression toward complete effacement is established, labor has objectively begun. After two hours without any progress, however, the self-diagnosis of the laboring woman must be firmly rejected. Any blood loss following the first vaginal examination is most likely an artifact.

14.2.5 Ruptured membranes

A clinical dilemma can arise when the membranes are broken. As long as there are no contractions, there is still no question of labor. A vaginal examination is contraindicated because of the risk of introducing infection. That is why we wait – if necessary, as long as 24–48 hours, depending on local protocol – for regular painful contractions to start. However, as soon as regular and painful contractions ("pains") commence, there is every reason to declare the woman in labor. A vaginal examination is then not only justified but indicated. At this point, the only appropriate policy – if necessary with early augmentation – is directed to a delivery within 12 hours regardless of the cervical status at the onset of the contractions. Waiting longer makes no sense, because the woman will not become more fit with the ongoing pains. Waiting is even irresponsible, because uterine contractility might very well be an early sign of intrauterine infection in cases of PROM (prelabor rupture of membranes). It is for this reason that the convenience-motivated practice of sedating women who cannot sleep because of uterine irritability is counterproductive and even dangerous once the membranes are ruptured.

> *By definition, a false start with ruptured membranes is an incorrect diagnosis.*

In about 30% of women who report with painful contractions the membranes have already ruptured spontaneously.[2] This symptom is an even stronger indicator of the onset of labor than is a bloody show. Clinically, the diagnosis of labor is assessed along with all the consequences it implies.

14.3 The objective diagnosis of labor

Clarity is the hallmark of the professional care provider. For this reason a clear, prospective decision must be made in every case and as soon as possible within a maximal time frame of two hours. In the legal world a distinction is made between direct and indirect or circumstantial evidence. The clinical world is no different. Pains with dilatation – and so by definition full effacement   are the only direct proof of labor. A bloody show and rupture of membranes are strong circumstantial evidence.

Clinical evidence of the onset of labor	
Basic prerequisite:	*Painful contractions at intervals of 10 minutes or less.*
Highly suggestive:	*Bloody show or ruptured membranes*
Objective proof:	*Full effacement*

14.3.1 Prelabor education and instructions

Prelabor education in accordance with actual practice is crucial for women to be properly prepared for the challenge of the forthcoming birth (Chapter 19). Therefore, all pregnant women are encouraged to contact their provider and come to the hospital at an early stage when contractions become painful and are accompanied by a show or leakage of fluid or, failing either of these, when the pains – resembling strong menstrual cramping – come at regular intervals of 10 minutes or less for an hour. The need for professional confirmation of their provisional diagnosis of labor should be clearly explained to all pregnant women.

14.3.2 Documentation

The doctor or midwife who is directly responsible for the diagnosis of labor must commit the evidence to permanent record in simple and explicit terms: painful contractions, full efface-ment, a bloody show, or spontaneously ruptured membranes. A simple statement "in labor," without explicitly mentioning the grounds on which this conclusion is based, is not acceptable. Detailed record-keeping ensures that the evi-dence remains available even when the person concerned is no longer on duty.

> *For management and meaningful audit pur-poses, the grounds on which the diagnosis of labor is made must be committed to permanent record in simple and explicit terms.*

The diagnosis of labor constitutes grounds for admission to the labor ward, and in planned home births it is also from that moment that professional responsibility starts and the midwife must remain with her client. The graphic representation of labor progression (partogram) begins at this point, no sooner and no later (Chapter 15). Accurate record-keeping with a partogram forces professional care providers to make an objective diagnosis of labor and subsequently coerces them to undertake timely assessment of progression (Chapter 15). Such exact information is a prerequisite for a rational, responsible policy as well as for mean-ingful audit and scientific evaluation of the super-vision of labor (Chapter 26). Therefore:

- The grounds on which the diagnosis is made are committed to a permanent record including the name of the responsible care provider, thus assuring accountability for the diagnosis of labor and all procedures and interventions that might follow.
- Patients are not admitted to the labor room unless they meet the strict diagnosis of labor.
- No intervention whatsoever is permitted until a firm diagnosis of labor is made.
- There is deliberately no space on the partogram to record the period at home before the professional made the positive diagnosis of labor (Chapter 15).

- The duration of labor is recorded as the interval between the moment the professional confirmed the diagnosis of labor and the birth of the baby (Chapter 15).

> *The labor-record and partogram begin from the moment at which labor is confirmed by the care provider, not before and not after.*

14.4 Indecision

Expert care requires first and foremost insight on the part of the responsible birth attendant. The situation must be crystal clear from the outset in order for that person to convey the necessary information with clarity to the woman and her supporters: either she is or she is not in labor; there is no in-between.

14.4.1 The concept of the latent phase discarded

Unfortunately, conventional caregivers tenaciously hold to the fallacious concept of a latent phase in early labor, although its scientific basis is highly questionable (Chapter 9). The concept is also of little clinical concern and even counterproductive and should therefore be discarded (Chapter 11). The common use of such equivocal terms as "an early start," "latent labor," or "active labor not established" actually evades responsibility. Were a distinction of a latent phase possible in practice, it would still create confusion. Latent labor actually refers to a period of painful contractions that are not yet true labor pains. Such uterine irritability can last from a few to many hours and even, intermittently, for several days. Determining whether or not true labor will actually start is a matter of waiting. Braxton Hicks contractions are normal in late pregnancy and can come and go. Thus, the latent phase of labor is by definition a retrospective diagnosis and therefore has no rele-vance for the uncertain woman who thinks she might be in labor. On the contrary, she needs prospective guidance and a clear answer whether labor has begun or not. A clinical diagnosis must, by nature, be prospective and a diagnosis of labor is a positive decision to commit a woman to delivery. Labor literally means work: from the moment labor commences, the woman will have to work until her baby is born. A birth attendant is a coach, and a good coach is as clear and as resolute as possible. As in the world of sports, where a coach cannot adequately coach a sportswoman without a clear determination of the beginning of the game, the onset of the endeavor of labor must be pinpointed as clearly as possible. Recognition of a latent phase is counterproductive in this respect.

> The "latent phase" is the cover of the insecure and indecisive birth attendant. The fallacious concept of a "latent phase" of labor should be rigidly abandoned.

14.4.2 Avoided diagnosis

Conventional teaching generally overlooks the significance of complete cervical effacement. Consequently, mainstream practice often fails to recognize the early but decisive symptoms of labor and, therefore, remains vague about the clinical onset of labor until it is "well established," meaning dilatation of 3 cm or more. Fear of being deemed an inexpert provider by making a false diagnosis is the unjust excuse made for communicating vague phrases after a first examination that reveals less than 3 cm dilatation. However, in childbirth practice – as in most aspects of life – the biggest problems arise through avoided decisions, not through mistaken ones. "Soft and indecisive doctors make dirty wounds" is a Dutch proverb. An evasive answer or a pseudo-diagnosis of "latent labor" is confusing and counterinformative for all concerned. Vague phrases serve only as excuses whereby the care provider avoids a clear diagnosis of labor. In effect, such behavior places full responsibility on the pregnant woman, where it certainly does not belong.

Even more worrying is that such indecision also delays the second crucial diagnosis – whether uterine action in early labor is effective or not – and thus may lead to an inadvertent, unjustified withholding of treatment. This neglect is the most frequent, most pervasive, and most underrated mistake in the management of first labors (Chapters 15, 21). When clear diagnosis of labor is delayed, several uteri will fail to respond properly to oxytocin in a later stage when dystocia will eventually be undeniable for even the most conservative of labor supervisors (Chapters 8, 21).

> "Most errors in the supervision of labor result from decisions being avoided rather than from decisions wrongly made."[2]

14.5 Errors in diagnosis

No matter how carefully the clinical diagnosis of labor is made, a small chance remains that the course of events will prove it to be incorrect. No clinical diagnostic method is foolproof. Rather, the aim is to reduce the number of errors to a minimum by maximizing objectivity. A mistake can be made either way: a woman's self-diagnosis may be falsely rejected or falsely accepted.

14.5.1 False-negative diagnosis

A woman who is initially determined not to be in labor may report a short time later with an advanced stage of labor. This happens only occasionally given the early state in which labor is recognized by the proposed criteria. Besides, such an initially false-negative diagnosis has no adverse effects for the woman, unless she lives far from the hospital and was sent home. In that case admission to the antenatal ward should have eliminated the possible embarrassment of an unsupported delivery at home or in a car.

14.5.2 False-positive diagnosis

In contrast, a false-positive diagnosis that incorrectly declares the woman to be in labor has far more ominous consequences. She is wrongly admitted to, and retained in, the labor room and exposed to the expectations, pressures, and stresses of that environment. Now there is no way back. Inevitably, after many hours in pain in which no progress is made, the morale – not only of the parturient woman but also that of her partner and the attendant who ought to sit with her – suffers. The woman's motivation weakens rapidly as her physical and mental condition deteriorates. Analgesic drugs and ineffective oxytocin aggravate the problem until the situation reaches a point at which there is but one way out: cesarean section. The indication for the cesarean delivery is likely to be registered as "dystocia,"[17] whereas the truth of the matter is that this woman was not in labor. A critical review of the clinical history is frequently impossible, because the evidence of labor is mostly documented poorly, if at all. In everyday practice the significance of a professional diagnosis of labor is not sufficiently appreciated.

> *All too many women are submitted to cesarean section for the indication dystocia when a state of labor never existed.*

The risk of such a false-positive diagnosis is strongly limited by adherence to the proposed criteria of labor but it can never be totally eliminated. Hence, the small chance that the next hour may prove the initial diagnosis wrong should always be kept in mind. This applies with particular force when the diagnosis of labor is based on contractions accompanied solely by a "bloody show" but unsupported by full effacement or ruptured membranes. Should the contractions subside, then a timely and decisive correction is necessary to re-route the woman from a dead-end track. Professional care requires that a mistake be

not only recognized but also openly acknowledged so that the conduct can be corrected in time – within one hour. The ability to do this is a mark of quality in professional care.

On the other hand, amniotomy is the recommended policy when the frequency or intensity of the contractions subsides after a certain diagnosis of labor is made based on pains supported by full effacement. Likewise, all efforts should be made for a delivery within 12 hours when the diagnosis of labor is supported by spontaneous rupture of membranes. In that case, uterine stimulation must be started immediately – for the reasons explained in section 14.2.5 – if progression fails, regardless of cervical status.

> *The maximum level of objectivity reduces the number of mistakes to a minimum.*

14.6 False start

About 10% of all primigravidas call their care provider or come to the hospital convinced that they are in labor only to find that they do not meet the objective criteria for labor: painful uterine contractions are not accompanied by full effacement and there is neither a "bloody show" nor leakage of amniotic fluid. This is called a false start.

> *A false start is when a woman believes herself to be in labor on the basis of painful contractions that are not supported by other, objective evidence of labor.*

14.6.1 Factors contributing to a false start

Because care providers often offer cryptic answers when asked about how to determine when labor has begun, it is not surprising that inexperienced nulliparas sometimes make a mistake. Indeed, it is remarkable that 90% of first-time mothers-to-be correctly recognize the beginning of their labor. The real problem is for the remaining 10% who have a false start. Ironically, a false start frequently occurs late in the evening when the community-based midwife has just gone to bed and the youngest resident or intern is holding the fort at the hospital. Thus, the agitated woman and her insecure partner may receive vague and evasive answers. She begins to realize that the birth professional from whom she expects to receive clear answers cannot or will not establish whether labor has begun. As a result, she loses trust not only in herself but also in the care provider. Furthermore, this vagueness stymies her partner, nurse, or doula and no-one knows in which direction to guide and coach the woman. A distinctly uneasy atmosphere arises. Uncertainty increases anxiety, lowers the pain threshold, and sets off a vicious circle of anxiety, stress, and pain. The thoughtless care provider will further strengthen any false anticipation by keeping the woman in the labor room and sweeping or stripping the membranes only to worsen the contractility and pain. Now there is a good chance that the presumptive labor will not progress while the important symptom of a show is rendered useless. In the home situation the most disastrous comment late in the evening is "Call me if it gets any worse." That is typically coupled with a failure to check back until morning. A clear decision has been avoided and the woman may reach the point of exhaustion before labor has even begun.

14.6.2 Management of a false start

The first step is to offer a clear explanation that labor has not yet begun. When the reasons for this conclusion are presented with clear arguments, using comprehensible language and with professional and convincing firmness, this information is generally well accepted. A woman must not remain in the labor ward any longer than is necessary to make a diagnosis, in other words, no more than one to two hours. When the woman understands that her labor has not yet begun, and if she is at ease at that moment and does not live

too far from the hospital, she can return home. If she remains anxious and feels insecure, it makes more sense for her to stay the night in the antenatal ward and possibly to be given a sleeping tablet. True sedation – an injection of pethidine combined with a powerful sedative – is necessary only when the agitated woman cannot be convinced that her labor has not yet begun. In our experience fewer than 2% of all nulliparas need this drastic, clinical treatment for a persistent false start.

> *A woman having a false start does not belong in the labor room.*

A woman who chose to give birth at home and is now experiencing a false start should be approached similarly. Her midwife or family doctor should suggest a shower or bath and the bed should be freshened up and rearranged. The woman's partner need not come home from work and the auxiliary maternity nurse need not be mobilized. Tranquility and confidence must be restored. A mild sedative might help. If the woman calls a few hours later, her midwife or family doctor should promptly and personally see her again. Diagnoses via telephone are simply impossible. If the woman is still not in labor, her uneasiness may reach such a state of agitation that admission to the hospital for clinical sedation becomes the most prudent course of action. In the final analysis, patients of community-based midwives or family physicians can be competently treated with clinical sedation on a consultative basis. The woman can then return home the following morning well rested, transferred back to her trusted midwife or family doctor, and deliver her baby under their responsibility (Chapter 26). Prerequisite for this facility, fostering continuity in care, is that the philosophies of home practices and hospital must be on the same wavelength and that policies – from both sides – must be consistently executed. This can occur only if both professions share the same objective criteria for labor.

> *A persistent false start is a serious clinical condition, requiring prompt and rigorous treatment.*

14.6.3 Sedation versus pain relief

The fundamental distinction between sedation and pain relief must be made absolutely clear. Clinical sedation is the ultimate treatment of a tenacious false start. The aim is to break the vicious circle created by false anticipation of birth. Therefore, strong sedatives or narcotics should never be given in the labor room but always on the antenatal ward: the patient must sleep.

Conversely, a woman who is truly in labor must keep her head clear and remain fit. A woman in labor should therefore never be sedated. If effective pain relief in labor is needed, epidural is the method of choice. Clearly an epidural block should never be given before a strict diagnosis of labor and thus a commitment to delivery is made (Chapter 20).

> *There is no place for sedative drugs in the labor room. A woman in labor must keep her head clear.*

14.6.4 Preventing a false start

A critical review of false starts will show that most are directly or indirectly iatrogenic in origin and thus preventable. At the last prenatal visit, false expectations are all too often created by the information that the woman's cervix is already ripe. When the woman is tired of being pregnant and wants to know when it will end, a vaginal examination will generally do more harm than good. If there is no medical indication, one should not do an internal examination!

> *False starts are often iatrogenic in origin and thus preventable.*

Stripping the membranes in late pregnancy is an even worse procedure and in our view is utterly reprehensible. When performed as vigorously as it should be, it is very painful but mostly ineffective all the same. In addition, it raises false expectations, prompts uterine irritability, and invariably leads to artificial blood loss, rendering the symptom of bloody show useless. Doctors have even more means to induce a false start. Along with the influx of modern diagnostic techniques has come an increase in iatrogenic anxiety and uncertainty (Chapter 4). Under the pretext of "better safe than sorry," a decision for priming the cervix for induction with prostaglandins is then easily made. However, the general assumption that "if it doesn't help you, it won't harm you" is absolutely invalid. In reality, cervical priming is the best overture to a disastrous false start and all the related misery, agony, and despair (Chapter 23).

> *Prelabor stripping (sweeping the membranes) is a reprehensible procedure. Cervical priming with prostaglandins is an even more potent means for inducing a disastrous false start.*

Pencilling in or even mentioning a due date is unwise at the outset. The pregnant woman directs her expectations toward this date, and if she goes past it the waiting becomes very difficult. We prefer to speak of the full-term period, which lasts until 42 weeks. If the term woman is nonetheless tired of waiting, then offering explanations is much wiser than a vaginal examination to evaluate cervical ripeness. As soon as she understands the risks of a protracted and failed induction, and that labor and delivery will go much easier – and thus more safely – when her uterus is ready for this process, even the most rigidly scheduled of pregnant women will summon the patience to wait for labor to begin spontaneously. Agreement on a "latest date of delivery," being the date at 42 weeks on which labor will be induced, is a feasible and helpful strategy accepted by most women.[18]

Instead of the routine assessment of "the due date," a pregnant woman is better given the "latest date of delivery."

14.7 Proactive support of labor

Offering true help and support during labor is possible only with absolute clarity of thought and action. Therefore, two early decisions must be made in every case:

1. Whether the woman is or is not in labor; and if she is
2. Whether labor is sufficiently effective (Chapter 15)

If the approach of caregivers to every expectant mother experiencing painful contractions considered these elementary questions and if they took full responsibility for making firm decisions, the majority of protracted, traumatic, and failing labors ending in operative deliveries could be prevented. Any supposedly more subtle approach as defended by orthodox midwives and conventional obstetricians (who, by the way, hardly ever see a patient in the early stages of labor) actually leads to poor (non-)management marred by vagueness and indecision. In contrast, a clear and consistent birthplan involves strict rules that must be put into practice at all times:

Rules governing proper management of early labor

- *No intervention whatsoever is permitted until a firm diagnosis of labor is made.*
- *The responsible midwife or doctor presents the evidence of labor on permanent record in simple and explicit terms: pains, bloody show, ruptured membranes, full effacement.*
- *From that moment on, a partogram is kept in all cases and labor must progress adequately.*

14.8 Summary

- Diagnosis is the single most important issue in the supervision of labor. When the diagnosis of labor is wrong, all subsequent measures and interventions are likely to be wrong as well.
- Clearly, a decision of such consequence should not be left solely to the expectant mother. Therefore, the first step in professional birth care is to confirm or refute the self-diagnosis made by the pregnant woman.
- A reliable diagnosis can be made only on the basis of objective criteria. The occurrence of regular, painful contractions is a prerequisite for diagnosing labor but is not conclusive evidence. Bloody show and ruptured membranes are very suggestive signs. Definitive proof is full effacement of the cervix.
- Considering the decisive importance of effacement and dilatation, it is imperative that the terms be used correctly: dilatation is the diameter of the external os of the fully effaced cervix.
- A woman with painful contractions and a fully effaced cervix is definitively in labor and therefore dilatation must progress.
- The prevalent attitude of expectancy or indecision until dilatation has been well established (by reaching at least 3 cm) overlooks the decisive role of full effacement for the diagnosis of labor and wrongly withholds treatment if early dilatation is too slow.
- A pregnant woman who persistently believes that she is in labor but does not meet the objective criteria is having a false start. This serious condition must be recognized in timely fashion and treated promptly before the only solution is cesarean delivery, which follows much distress and anguish.
- The great majority of disastrous false starts are directly or indirectly iatrogenic and can thus be prevented.

REFERENCES

1. Friedman EA. *Labor: Clinical Evaluation and Management*, 2nd edn. New York: Appleton-Century-Crofts; 1978.
2. O'Driscoll K, Meagher D, Robson M. *Active Management of Labour*, 4th edn. Mosby; 2003.
3. Turner M, Brassil M, Gordon H. Active management of labor associated with a decrease in the cesarean section rate in nulliparas. *Obstet Gynecol* 1988; 71: 150–4.
4. Akoury H, Brodie G, Caddick R, McLaughlin V, Pugh P. Active management of labor and operative delivery in nulliparous women. *Am J Obstet Gynecol* 1988; 158: 255–8.
5. Boylan P, Frankowski R, Roundtree R, Selwyn B, Parrish K. Effect of active management on the incidence of cesarean section for dystocia in nulliparas. *Am J Perinatol* 1991; 8: 373–9.
6. Lopez-Zeno J, Peaceman A, Adashek J. Socol M. A controlled trial of a program for the active management of labor. *N Engl J Med* 1992; 326: 450–4.
7. Frigoletto F, Lieberman E, Lang J, *et al.* A clinical trial of active management of labor. *N Engl J Med* 1995; 333: 745–50.
8. Cammu H, van Eeckhout E. A randomised controlled trial of early versus delayed use of amniotomy and oxytocin infusion in nulliparous labour. *Br J Obstet Gynaecol* 1996; 103: 313–18.
9. Fraser W, Vendittelli F, Krauss I, Bréart G. Effects of early augmentation of labour with amniotomy and oxytocin in nulliparous women: a meta-analysis. *Br J Obstet Gynaecol* 1998; 105: 189–94.
10. Fraser W, Marcoux S, Moutquin J, Christen A. Effect of early amniotomy on the risk of dystocia in nulliparous women. *N Engl J Med* 1993; 328: 1145–9.
11. Boylan P, Parisi V. Effect of active management on latent phase labor. *Am J Perinatol* 1990; 7: 363–5.
12. Masoli P, Picó V, Pellerano 1. Manejo activo del parto. Experiencia en el hospital Gustavo Fricke. *Rev Chil Obstet Ginecol* 1986; 51:223–30.
13. Vengadasalam D. Active management of labour: an approach to reducing the rising caesarean rate. *Singapore J Obstet Gynecol* 1986; 17: 33–6.
14. Hogston P, Noble W. Active management of labor: the Portsmouth experience. *J Obstet Gynaecol* 1993; 13: 340–2.
15. Impey L, Hobson J, O'Herlihy C. Graphic analysis of actively managed labor: prospective computation of labor progress in 500 consecutive nulliparous women in spontaneous labor at term. *Am J Obstet Gynecol* 2000; 183: 438–43.
16. Hendricks CH, Brenner WE, Kraus G. Normal cervical dilatation pattern in late pregnancy and labor. *Am J Obstet Gynecol* 1970; 106: 1065–82.
17. Stewart PJ, Duhlberg C, Arnett AC, Elmslie T, Hall PF. Diagnosis of dystocia and management with cesarean section among primiparous women in Ottowa Carleton. *CMAJ* 1990;142:459–63.
18. Ayers S, Collenette A, Hollis B, Manyonda I. Feasibility study of a Latest Date of Delivery (LDD) system of managing pregnancy. *J Psychosom Obstet Gynecol* 2005; 26(3): 167–71.

15

Prevention of long labor

When a woman asks her antenatal care provider how long her forthcoming labor and delivery might last, she usually receives an evasive answer. Apparently, prospective limits for the duration of normal labor are not clearly set since "normal birth" is still widely considered to be a retrospective characterization made when all has gone well on its own.

> *The lack of prospective norms for the progression and duration of labor is one of the main shortcomings in traditional midwifery and conventional obstetrics.*

This lack of prospective norms has a historical background. After all, women have been giving birth since the beginning of humanity, sometimes after two or three days of agony. In ancient times nothing could be done to resolve the problem of overly long labor without the introduction of extreme hazards. Surgery was almost invariably lethal and was not an option. Hence, the course and outcome of childbirth was a trial by ordeal and was believed to be God's will. The guiding principles of European midwifery evolved over recent centuries. Care throughout a long and slow labor was limited to moral support – an emotionally heavy and sometimes even superhuman task (which might explain why alcohol consumption among midwives was a popular topic, discussed with disdain in the classic world literature of the nineteenth century). Whether the unborn child was still alive was always a question. When the woman finally reached full dilatation, she might be nearly dead from exhaustion. In privileged circles, the "master" would then arrive and save the woman from death with his "iron hands" (forceps). Otherwise, arrested birth meant death for both mother and child. Delivery literally meant mechanical deliverance – a skilled trade. Empiricism helped in the further evolution of this handcraft in the twentieth century. The master became the obstetrician and medical advances in antiseptics, blood typing, and anesthesiology made it much safer to operate in the event of arrested labor. But the perception of the natural birth process remained predominantly mechanistic (Chapter 3) and the expectant, passive attitude in the first stage of labor prevails to this day in many birth settings.

> *Tolerance of long labor goes back in history to when nothing could be done to resolve the problem of protracted labor without the introduction of extraneous hazards for mother and child.*

It would be difficult to exaggerate the beneficial effects of an accurate, prospective working definition of normal duration of labor on everyday practice (Chapter 11), since failure to define what is clearly one of the basic parameters of clinical obstetrics has been a major obstacle to improvements in management for many years. The current cesarean rates for dystocia mainly reflect how long modern women are willing to allow labor to continue. Indeed, the duration of labor determines, more than any other measurable factor, how taxing the birth will be, not only for the parturient but also for her partner, the fetus, and the birth attendants who care for all of them. Preservation of effective progress of labor by ascertaining efficient uterine contractions is one of the major potential benefits of contemporary birth care. Labor need no longer be a slow and nightmarish agony.

15.1 Duration of normal labor

The word "normal" literally means remaining sufficiently within "norms," and such a classification must of course be prospective. To establish limits for the duration of normal labor, and by inference criteria for normal progression, we must first define what is meant by labor duration:

Definition

The duration of labor is recorded as the number of hours between the moment at which the birth professional confirms the diagnosis of labor and the time of delivery.

For hospital births, labor duration is equal to the number of hours a woman spends in the delivery unit, provided that no patient is admitted unless she meets the strict diagnosis of labor as defined in the previous chapter. On practical grounds – in the sense of policy and conduct – the third stage of labor (afterbirth) is not included in this definition.

It is evident that every woman in whom labor is confirmed has been in labor before arriving at the hospital or before the midwife's arrival at the home. However, to estimate duration from such evidence is guesswork. It is pointless to speculate on the presumed "latent phase" or the total time the woman was in labor before she decided to call for professional help. Moreover, it has no relevance for the subsequent supervision of the labor.

Instead, there are strong practical arguments in favor of the above definition:

- The woman decides for herself when she calls for her midwife or will go to the hospital.
- Professional responsibility begins only when a woman elects to place herself in a professional's care.
- The diagnosis of labor is the professional responsibility of the midwife or physician.
- From the moment the diagnosis of labor is confirmed, the birth professional is fully accountable for the maximum duration of that labor.
- Accurate records demand precise information that permits comparisons and allows for meaningful audit of procedures and outcomes (Chapter 27).
- Most women generally tend to recall the duration of their labor in this manner.

15.1.1 Statistics

Using the criteria of the above definition for the duration of labor, half of all nulliparas give birth within six hours (Chapter 9). It is incorrect to calculate the average duration of labor, because the distribution skews heavily to the left. Furthermore, it would make no sense as virtually no births above the 90th percentile of duration are completed without extraneous measures. Given the asymmetrical variance, it would be better to define the boundaries of the duration of normal first labor as twice the number of hours in which half of all nulliparas give birth: $2 \times 6 = 12$ hours. This boundary actually matches or even exceeds the 95th percentile of the database studies reporting on the duration of labor (Chapter 9). In conclusion, 12 hours is the boundary of normality.

Normal labor and delivery last no more than 12 hours.

15.1.2 Impact of prolonged labor

Many orthodox care providers still feel uneasy with or plainly disagree with this proposition. In retrospect, some accept as normal a labor that lasts more than 24 hours, owing to a long "latent phase" or otherwise. Such tolerance of long labor seems to be dictated more by ideology-driven sentiments than by valid arguments (Chapter 5). In reality, long labor is strongly associated with poor outcomes: more fetal distress, more interventions, and more operative deliveries.[1,2] Moreover, to most laboring women the 12-hour norm is close to or even well beyond acceptability.

> *Women have declared their intolerance of long labors by increasingly requesting cesarean delivery when progress is slow.*

The impact of labor duration must be evaluated as much in emotional as in physical terms. Although some women are already unduly perturbed at the point of admission, and others remain apparently unmoved after many hours have passed, most fall somewhere between the two extremes. Nowadays the majority of women typically endure the strain and pain of labor well for between six and eight hours. If a woman is well prepared and well supported and cared for, it is unlikely she will panic. As time passes, however, physical and emotional strength begins to weaken perceptibly. After 12 hours, morale typically deteriorates exponentially. When the end is not yet in sight, "a stage may be reached in which the adult woman is reduced to pleading with anyone standing by for deliverance, unless she is rendered semiconscious by powerful sedatives into a degrading state of indifference or lulled into a would-be sense of security by epidural analgesia."[3] Desperation, dehydration, salt depletion, ketoacidosis, and a humiliating loss of decorum complete her total disablement. The effects of such a trauma are likely to remain with her for the rest of her life (Chapter 2).

> *It is difficult to exaggerate the physical and emotional impact of prolonged labor because it may endure a lifetime.*

15.1.3 Prospective norm for normal progress

The lessons from nature (Chapter 7), undeniable statistics, and the impact of emotional disturbance and physical exhaustion caused by a long labor provide the rationale for a prospective, woman-friendly norm for the duration of labor and delivery. Laboring women normally reach the expulsion stage well within 10 hours and deliver within 12 hours. Taken together with the fact that normal dilatation proceeds at least in a straight line (Chapter 9), this means that the physiological dilatation rate is at least 1 cm/h. In fact, the average dilatation rate of nulliparas who ultimately deliver spontaneously is 1.75 cm/h.[4] These women dilate in a manner that is at the very least linear and mostly accelerative.

> *Normal progress of dilatation is at least linear and proceeds at a minimum rate of 1 cm/h.*

15.2 The partogram

A visual record of progression is exceedingly elucidating and very useful for the supervision of labor (Fig. 15.1). Simplicity is the key. The partogram, as designed by Philpott and modified by Hendricks and O'Driscoll, starts at the well-defined diagnosis of labor (Chapter 14), and progress during the first stage of labor is measured exclusively in terms of dilatation (Chapter 11).

A cervix that is completely effaced is marked at 1 cm (Fig. 15.1) because the external os is always open to this extent. Dilatation in centimeters is plotted against time in hours with an x to y axis ratio of 1:1. The diagonal is the normality line indicating the slowest rate of progress accepted as normal. There is intentionally no space on the graph for the period prior to the point of labor confirmation or for births lasting longer than 12 hours. The partogram covers a period of 10 hours for the first stage and 2 hours for the second stage.

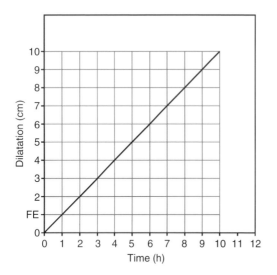

Figure 15.1. The partogram. FE = full effacement. No allowance is made for the time prior to the diagnosis of labor. The diagonal is the line that demarcates the limit of normality.

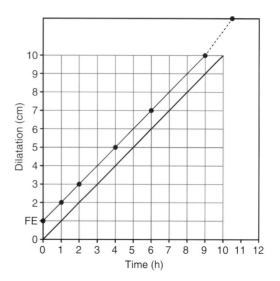

Figure 15.2. Example of a normal labor. FE = full effacement. Spontaneous delivery within 11 hours without any intervention.

15.2.1 A prospective and simple, visual record

The partogram begins at the moment the diagnosis of labor is confirmed by the responsible care provider (Chapter 14). The time prior to diagnosis is not taken into consideration: if the first examination reveals 4 cm dilatation, the partogram begins at 4 cm on the vertical axis, which corresponds with zero hour on the horizontal axis (Fig. 15.3). Such a finding does not mean, as is often suggested, that a woman was in labor long before record keeping commenced; rather it should be viewed as a sign of effective labor.

The partogram is used as a prospective tool in all cases, not as an optional graph to be made in retrospect when arrest of labor is already final. Obligatory sticking to the partogram, on line, keeps the attention of care providers on the task at hand. Labor is considered normal when the graph remains on the left-hand side of the normal line and is at least as steep as this diagonal (Figs. 15.2 and 15.3). Deviations from normal are readily apparent (Chapter 21).

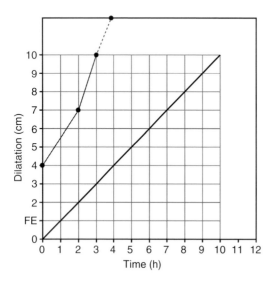

Figure 15.3. Example of the course of a normal labor. FE = full effacement. Spontaneous delivery within four hours without any intervention.

15.2.2 Features of a useful partogram design

The method of partographic labor representation strongly affects obstetric decision making, and the simpler it is the better it is. In the hypothetical situations of Cartmill and Thornton's study the 1:1 x to y axis ratio and the exclusion of a latent phase were associated with the fewest decisions to perform a cesarean section.[5] That is why we strongly advise against the partogram of commercially available electronic dossiers with asymmetrical x to y axis ratios. Cartmill and Thornton's study also supports the decision to discard the concept of the latent phase entirely from obstetric practice (Chapter 11).

We strongly advise against use of the WHO partogram,[6] originally designed to assist labor management in third-world birth centers, or other partogram designs that are similarly crammed with minute details on station and position of the fetal head, contraction frequency, fetal heart beat counts, etc. Such details usually distract from the sole purpose, which is to relate progress to passage of time. Simplicity is the key. Moreover, the WHO partogram is the typical product of a "nonsensus consensus", as it includes a "latent phase of labor," which is allowed to last 12 hours before an action-line is passed and, therefore, disregards a strict diagnosis of labor. Clearly, the result defeats the purpose of keeping a partogram. Indeed, accurate assessment of the onset of labor and control of its total duration within a time frame of 12 hours represent the most important technical measures to avoid prolonged labor and related emotional trauma, instrumental delivery, and cesarean section for dystocia (Chapter 30). To reiterate yet again, recognition of a latent phase of labor is counterproductive in this respect.

> *The partogram designed by the WHO neglects the main purposes of proactive labor management and should therefore not be used.*

15.3 Monitoring progress

Prospective keeping of the partogram in the proposed design forces the care provider to make two early decisions in every case:

- Whether labor has actually begun; and if so,
- Whether uterine action is effective.

The irony is that conventional midwives often avoid these crucial early decisions, whereas many obstetricians, especially in smaller hospitals, conveniently delegate these to a nurse, who must then make these determinations on the basis of the external appearance of the pregnant woman in the absence of a vaginal examination. Obligatory and prospective use of the partogram puts an end to this unprofessional behavior. Proper supervision of labor requires an objective confirmation of labor onset and regular assessments of progress, which is simply impossible without vaginal examinations.

15.3.1 Early assessments

Progress in early labor should be monitored at intervals of one hour, as four hours is much too long to wait to discover that labor has not advanced. Slow progress in the first three hours is a clear indication of ineffective labor, and corrective action must be taken without delay. As soon as dilatation has reached 3 cm, the frequency of vaginal examinations may be reduced to once every two hours. The emphasis placed on cervical assessments in early labor differs fundamentally from conventional practices whereby no worthwhile medical decision is considered necessary until a woman has been in labor for several hours and the threat of complications is imminent. "Such belated decision-making involves primarily the rescue of mothers and babies from potentially dangerous predicaments that develop over a protracted period of time in what were initially normal cases. No serious thought is given to prevention."[3] Keeping a visual record at short intervals from the very onset of labor is the obvious solution. Early diagnosis and correction of slow labor are the key to spontaneous delivery.

> *"Close attention to progress during the early hours of labor is the best insurance against difficulties later."*[3]

15.4 Patient information and guidance

Practice during labor must correspond with the information provided to the woman antenatally (Chapter 19). In contrast to the usual half-hearted instructions, a pregnant woman is best encouraged to come to the hospital at an early stage as soon as she assumes her labor has begun. If she has been taught the importance of the professional confirmation of her provisional diagnosis of labor and of the early assessments of labor progression, then the provider must act accordingly. Prelabor agreements that are not kept in the delivery room strongly undermine a woman's confidence not only in the staff on duty but also in the labor department as a whole.

15.4.1 Prediction of the hour of birth

Care and intrapartum information must be clear and consistent. The use of mystifying medical jargon as a cloak for indecision or the utterance of inanities to the effect that "all is well" or "progress is as good as can be expected" each constitute "an intolerable affront to the intelligence of women."[3] Information must be exact and comprehensible. A clear pattern of dilatation can be established within 2–3 hours and linear extrapolation of the partogram enables the caregiver to predict the hour of delivery in nearly every case. "Since most women are not accustomed to think in terms of dilatation, but are merely anxious to know when their baby will be born, informing them of this expected arrival time – give or take 1 hour – is of paramount importance."[3] The knowledge that there is a predictable end in sight usually boosts morale, not only of the parturient but also of the auxiliary people involved in supporting and comforting her.

> Boosting morale
>
> *Communication must be exact, consistent, comprehensible, and motivating at all times. The expected time of delivery – give or take an hour – can and must be established in the early stages of her labor and should be conveyed to every woman within three hours after admission.*

Despite all these considerations, many orthodox caregivers feel disheartened with the proposed early assessments, claiming that nature must take its course and that vaginal examinations are unnecessarily burdensome for a woman.[7] These caregivers should realize, however, that the proposed early examinations are done only to evaluate dilatation and that these assessments are brief and minimally disruptive. Indeed, the orthodox ritual of checking the fetopelvic relationship by assessing the station and position of the fetal occiput at each vaginal examination is not only burdensome but is superfluous and counterproductive at this stage. During early first-stage labor this routine can only provide irrelevant information of "unfavorable position" such as occiput posterior, to the effect that the supervisor gets off on the wrong foot and imparts a discouraging note to the event (Chapter 22). A pessimistic prognostic assessment tends to self-fulfillment by iatrogenic dynamic birth disorders (Chapters 21). Vaginal examinations in the retraction phase of labor (Chapter 9) should be focused solely on cervical effacement and dilatation and thus should be brief, minimally disruptive, painless, and not unfriendly to the woman. Like a sportswoman's coach, a birth attendant simply cannot supervise and motivate a woman in labor without having a clear determination of its beginning, and certainly not without regular and timely evaluation of its progress.

> *A vaginal examination with the restricted purpose of assessing dilatation is brief and minimally disruptive.*

15.4.2 Crucial bedside clarity

Regular assessments keep the laboring woman posted on her progress. After each vaginal examination the result is conveyed directly to her as it is plotted on the partogram in her presence. At that time it is decided when the next evaluation will be, and that appointment should be strictly kept!

As long as dilatation progresses satisfactorily, labor is normal and progress is monitored exclusively by dilatation rate. Only when the wedging phase becomes manifest by a secondary slowing beyond 7 cm is there good reason to assess the station, position, and attitude of the fetal head, as well as the presence or absence of caput succedaneum and molding (Chapter 9). As long as dilatation progresses normally, however, these data are de facto irrelevant. Incidentally, when one applies the rules of *proactive support of labor*, the total number of vaginal examinations – 3.7 times on average – is actually lower than in conventional practices wherein slow, long labors are tolerated.[8]

> *The result of each vaginal examination is conveyed directly to the parturient as it is being plotted on the partogram.*

15.5 Timely correction

Early dilatation rate strongly determines the course of labor and predicts its outcome. Cardozo *et al.* reported that a normal cervimetric pattern resulted in a vaginal delivery rate of 98.4%, whereas primary dysfunctional labor, which could be improved by oxytocin, had a 93.8% incidence of vaginal delivery.[9] But if there was no improvement in the rate of cervical dilatation when oxytocin was administered, the vaginal delivery rate was only 22.7%. In an Israeli study on the predictive value of dilatation rates, more than 93% of nulliparas who dilated at a rate of ≥ 1 cm/h from the onset of labor succeeded in giving birth spontaneously, whereas more than 70% of more slowly dilating women ultimately

had an operative delivery.[4] Who can maintain that the orthodox, tolerant attitude to slow labor is friendly to women? When asked, no pregnant woman wishes her forthcoming labor to last more than 12 hours. The expectant approach of many autonomous midwives and other conservative providers appears to be based more on territorial interests and/or atavistic ideology, rather than their patients' preferences and needs.

> *A fundamental solution to the inappropriately high cesarean rate will remain impossible as long as midwives and doctors fail to recognize strict criteria for normal progress of early labor.*

15.5.1 Selective but timely use of amniotomy and oxytocin

Proactive support of labor does not medicalize birth but rather ensures a normal course of the process. When dilatation proceeds well, the membranes are left intact. If progress is <1 cm/h, there is justifiable cause for artificial rupture of membranes. This applies to both home and hospital births. If amniotomy does not normalize progress within 1–2 hours, or if at any later stage the rate of progress remains less than 1 cm/h, oxytocin must be started promptly (Chapter 21). At this precise time, a woman who is laboring at home should be transferred to the hospital. The further a woman's course of labor deviates from the norm, the greater the abnormality and the associated chance of exhaustion, emotional trauma, and operative delivery. It follows that in no instance must the partogram be allowed to cross the normality line for more than two hours without corrective intervention. It should be noted that the majority of parturient women supervised according to the principles of *proactive support of labor* do not need oxytocin at all.

If, after institution of timely measures, delivery is not imminent after 12 hours, a cesarean section should be considered. Actually, prevention of emotional trauma is of even greater importance than the avoidance of cesarean delivery. Supportive, proactive direction toward a spontaneous delivery within 12 hours is not aggressive but preemptive and above all friendly to the woman. We have yet to meet a woman who has just given birth by her own strength after 10 hours of labor who complains that the labor was too short.

> *In no instances must the course of labor be allowed to cross the normality line for more than two hours.*

It is important to emphasize that early amniotomy and oxytocin should be employed only when indicated: if labor progression is slow, meaning dilatation rate <1 cm/h. This policy does not lead to more frequent use of oxytocin but rather to more appropriate timing of it. In our Dutch secondary care practice, the use of oxytocin (29% of all labors) matches the 50th percentile of the Dutch National Obstetric Registration for secondary care, and analysis of international figures reveals similar or higher oxytocin treatment rates for all labors (primary plus secondary care). Conservative critics, mostly unaware of the percentage of women receiving oxytocin in mainstream childbirth (but often too late), argue that 30% of women receiving oxytocin is not normal. Such criticism is countered with the question whether the current 50% rate of operative deliveries of nulliparas is normal (Chapter 2).

> *Proactive support of labor does not necessarily mean more frequent use of oxytocin, but rather better timed and better dosed use.*

15.5.2 Advantages to the mothers

The mechanisms by which selective early amniotomy and, if required, subsequent oxytocin treatment effectively accelerate dilatation and shorten labor, will be addressed more comprehensively in Chapter 17. It will additionally be shown that use of early amniotomy and oxytocin, in appropriate

doses, is so effective at accelerating slow labor that the diagnosis of labor must be seriously doubted if these measures fail to produce the desired response. This is commonplace in practices where the woman's self-diagnosis of labor is taken for granted.

Early augmentation is highly effective in reducing the incidence of prolonged labor. An Oxford study analyzed a cohort of 500 actively managed nulliparous labors.[10] The mean cervical dilatation at admission was 1.7 cm and the mean duration of labor was 6.1 hours; all but 2.8% were delivered within 12 hours and the cesarean rate was 5.4%. Two randomized studies on this subject showed highly significant reductions in the incidence of labor lasting >12 hours: from 19% to 5% and from 26% to 9%.[11,12] A meta-analysis of all randomized trials gives a typical odds ratio (OR) of 0.3 (95% CI 0.2–0.4).[13] Reduction in the incidence of prolonged labor is an independent outcome parameter of paramount importance (Chapter 28), since prolonged labor is strongly associated with a traumatizing childbirth. Elimination of such negative birth experiences without resorting to operative delivery is the main objective of *proactive support of labor*.

Early correction of slow labor is a woman-friendly policy indeed. When honestly informed about likely scenarios, parturients with initially slow labor invariably prefer a preemptive IV-line with oxytocin in their arm to a needle in their back, a vacuum-cup or forceps in their vagina, or a knife in their lower abdomen at a later stage.

> *Early correction of slow labor completely changes the face of childbirth.*

15.5.3 Misguidance from poor studies

Since the critical diagnosis of labor has seldom – if ever – been properly addressed in randomized trials comparing early and delayed oxytocin treatment, one might attain a misguided opinion of the effect of early amniotomy and augmentation on cesarean rates (Chapter 17). Most of these studies questioning the benefits of early augmentation only started in the alleged "active stage of labor" after 3 cm dilatation had been reached, so they actually compared late with very late augmentation. However, after a long "latent phase" many a uterus may fail to respond to oxytocin (*refractory uterus*, Chapters 8, 21). The dubious or simply incorrect conclusions of poorly designed or poorly executed studies in this field will be addressed in more detail in Chapters 17 and 30.

For now a warning should suffice: obstetricians and midwives should be cautioned that early corrective action in slow labor may not reduce cesarean rates in the absence of all other fundamental changes to policies and routines. A major benefit of the proactive restriction of labor duration is that more than 80% of all nulliparas deliver within eight hours, the duration of a care provider's duty shifts.[14] This facilitates continuous and personally committed care (Chapter 16). Indeed, *proactive support of labor* means much more than just early augmentation of labor. Prelabor education, consistent practice, and one-on-one supportive care extended to all women in labor are at least as important. Moreover, *proactive support of labor* is a mindset, characterized by a positive, motivating attitude directing all aspects of labor care. The effectiveness of the overall plan in the reduction of operative deliveries will be discussed in detail in the final chapters.

> *Early augmentation of slow labor is highly effective in the prevention of prolonged labor and associated traumatizing birth experiences (Evidence level A).*

15.5.4 Advantages to the caregivers

O'Driscoll and Meagher keenly observed that long duration of labor strongly affects the attitude of professional staff: "[in conventional obstetrics] . . . a shared sense of impotence in the face of widespread physical suffering, and even moral degradation, frequently colors the attitude of nurses, midwives, and doctors from their early student days. As a result, many birth care providers either tend to avoid the delivery room as much as possible, or tend to resort to excessive use of analgesia to alleviate otherwise intolerable personal stress."[3] Indeed, *proactive support of labor* completely changes the face of childbirth for all concerned.

> *Control of labor duration is almost as important for staff as it is for their patients.*

15.6 Summary

- An accurate working definition for the duration of labor has significant advantages in everyday practice. Duration of labor determines the impact of childbirth on patients and attendants.
- The duration of labor is best defined as the interval between the professional, objective diagnosis of labor and the eventual delivery of the baby.
- Childbirth should never be allowed to last more than 12 hours. Control of labor duration without resort to cesarean section represents the major advantage of *proactive support of labor* for all concerned.
- Progress in dilatation is the only criterion of normality in the first stage of labor. Normal dilatation proceeds at a minimum rate of 1 cm/h and the care provider must ensure that progression is and remains normal.
- Emphasis is placed on early labor. Regular assessments at one-hour intervals should be mandatory. As soon as dilatation has reached 3 cm the frequency of vaginal examinations can be reduced to once every two hours. Four hours is much too long to discover that labor has not advanced.
- Keeping a visual record of progress is eminently feasible for detecting deviations from normal and prompting corrective measures without delay.
- Normal dilatation proceeds in a straight line, the direction of which forecasts time of delivery. To

boost morale, expected time of delivery should be conveyed to every woman in the early stages of her labor.

- Early augmentation of slow labor is highly effective in reducing the incidence of traumatizing, prolonged labor but may not achieve the goal of reducing cesarean rates when all other propositions of fundamental changes to policies, conduct, and care in childbirth are neglected.

REFERENCES

1. Chelmow D, Kilpatrick SJ, Laros RK Jr. Maternal and neonatal outcomes after prolonged latent phase. *Obstet Gynecol* 1993; 81(4): 486–91.

2. Enkin M, Keirse MJNC, Nellson J, *et al.* Prolonged labor. In: *A Guide to Effective Care in Pregnancy and Childbirth*, 3rd edn. Oxford: Oxford University Press; 2000: 332–40.

3. O'Driscoll K, Meagher D. *Active Management of Labour*, 4th edn. Mosby; 2003.

4. Melmed H, Evans M. Predictive value of cervical dilatation rates, I Primigravids. *Obstet Gynecol* 1976; 47: 1568–75.

5. Cartmill R, Thornton J. Effect of presentation of partogram information on obstetric decision-making. *Lancet* 1992; 339: 1520–2.

6. World Health Organization partograph in management of labour. World Health Organization Maternal Health and Safe Motherhood Programme. *Lancet* 1994; 343(8910): 1399–404.

7. O'Regan M. Active management of labour; the Irish way of birth. *AIMS J* 1998; 10(2) (http//www.aims.org.uk/Journal).

8. Impey L, Boylan P. Active management of labour revisited. *Br J Obstet Gynaecol* 1999; 106: 183–7.

9. Cardozo LD, Gibb DM, Studd JW, Vasant RV, Cooper DJ. Predictive value of cervimetric labour patterns in primigravidae. *Br J Obstet Gynaecol* 1982; 89(1): 33–8.

10. Impey L, Hobson J, O'Herlihy C. Graphic analysis of actively managed labor: prospective computation of labor progress in 500 consecutive nulliparous women in spontaneous labor at term. *Am J Obstet Gynecol* 2000; 183: 438–43.

11. Lopez-Zeno J, Peaceman A, Adashek J, Socol M. A controlled trial of a program for the active management of labor. *N Engl J Med* 1992; 326: 450–4.

12. Frigoletto F, Lieberman E, Lang J, *et al.* A clinical trial of active management of labor. *N Engl J Med* 1995; 333: 745–50.

13. Fraser W, Vendittelli F, Krauss I, Bréart G. Effects of early augmentation of labour with amniotomy and oxytocin in nulliparous women: a meta-analysis. *Br J Obstet Gynaecol* 1998; 105: 189–94.

14. Hogston P, Noble W. Active management of labor: the Portsmouth experience. *J Obstet Gynaecol* 1993; 17; 340–2.

16

Personal continuity and continuous support

Giving birth is a parasympathetic process, a physiological condition that requires a feeling of ease, rest, comfort, confidence, and security. When these environmental conditions are not met, anxiety and fear inevitably trigger a stress response that inhibits uterine contractions and increases the likelihood of prolonged, dysfunctional labor (Chapter 7). Parasympathetic dominance in labor is best promoted by a one-on-one female companion and the personal attention of a trustworthy professional who watches over the parturient's safety and ensures that labor progresses. This is a double-edged sword: the demanding requirements of non-stop presence, personal commitment, and continuous labor support are strongly correlated with a fixed limit on the maximum duration of labor, because neither is possible without the other. Work schedules exceeding 12 hours are unrealistic.

16.1 Lack of supportive care

Until 50–60 years ago, childbirth was primarily a woman's world, one in which women of all cultures were attended and supported by other women during labor and delivery. Over the past 5–6 decades, however, hospitals have replaced the familiar environment of home. Physicians have replaced midwives for low-risk births and nursing staff have replaced female family members as supporters during birth. Childbirth in modern maternity centers currently subjects women to institutional routines, a lack of privacy, unfamiliar personnel,

work shift changes, and other conditions as highlighted in Chapter 4 that inevitably undermine the parasympathetic process of birth. These conditions usually have an adverse effect on the physiological course of the labor process, increase the chances of obstetric excess, and set a vicious circle into being.

16.1.1 Discontinuous care

The ability of nurses and midwives to provide unstinting labor support is usually limited by their simultaneous responsibility for more than one laboring woman. Added to this, they may very well begin or end work shifts in the middle of a woman's labor, usually work in short-staffed institutions, and spend a large proportion of their time managing technology and keeping records (Chapter 4).

> Continuous and personal supportive care during labor has become the exception rather than the rule.

16.1.2 Post-modern trends

Legitimate concerns about the "dehumanization" of a woman's birthing experience in the modern maternity unit have led to calls for a return to home deliveries attended by independent midwives.[1–5] This post-modern trend presumes the superiority of autonomous midwifery care during normal labor, but the documented results of formal midwifery-centered childbirth practices argue against this proposition (Chapter 5). Unlike the midwives of earlier times – who worked around the clock and stayed with their laboring clients from beginning to end – contemporary midwives have their own family life, disallowing duty shifts longer than eight hours. Additional tasks for other "clients" further prevent them from providing continuous labor support at home or in alternative birth centers. As a result, periodic visits at intervals of three hours or more during the first stage of labor are now common practice in autonomous midwifery care. Clearly this situation is far from ideal and is, in fact, irresponsible, as shown by the Dutch example (Chapter 5). Clearly, advocates of home births should be cautioned not to replace obstetric excess by non-attendance.

> *Many midwives no longer sit with their laboring clients throughout the entire process of labor, thus nullifying the alleged superiority and safety of their care.*

16.1.3 Birth environments

The key issue is not the location of birth – be it the hospital, a primary birth center, or the home – but rather what supports the best chance of a safe and rewarding delivery. Improvement of basic care can only be brought about through radical changes in both secondary and primary care and in the close cooperation between them (Chapter 26). In countries with a fully medicalized childbirth system, the evidence supports midwifery-led care for low-risk women, and obstetricians providing unduly interventionist care should accept this evidence.[6–13] On the other hand, the often encountered antipathy of fundamentalist midwives against prudent obstetricians is foolish as well.

Apart from territorial disputes between midwives and obstetricians (Chapter 5), the prime necessity for rehumanizing childbirth is adequate and continuous support for women by women during all labors regardless of the place of birth. In addition, every effort should be made to ensure that a woman's birthing environment is non-stressful, empowering, communicative of respect, private, and not dictated by routines that may be experienced as harsh and add risk without discernible benefit.[14] At the same time, fetal well-being must be monitored and adequate progress must be ensured. These obligatory assessments and measures might be experienced as disruptive, but the consequent potential stress is best counteracted by adequate prelabor preparation (Chapter 19), personal commitment and continuity of care from the provider, and continuous support from a well-informed, female one-on-one companion in labor. The organizational implications of this system will be addressed in Chapter 26.

> *Not the location of birth, but personal attention, commitment, and continuous support are the key factors in rehumanizing childbirth and providing effective, safe, and rewarding birth care.*

16.2 Personal attention and personal continuity

Paradoxically, the tolerance of long labors by conventional midwives wreaks absolute havoc with this basic requirement of continual presence throughout the entire labor and delivery. The midwife attending a home birth should never leave her laboring client. If continuous attendance cannot be guaranteed, then home birth becomes irresponsible (Chapter 5). On the other hand, hospitals must take positive steps to prevent several members of staff from simultaneously attending the same parturient. Personal attention and continuity of care require that every woman in labor has face-to-face attendance by one midwife or one resident who is known to her by name. The provider must appreciate that in every individual case giving birth is a unique life event for each woman, and a casual or impersonal approach is experienced as insensitive and is counterproductive. While a midwife or a resident may attend more than one laboring woman, the attention of a nurse is preferably confined to a single patient. Nurses should be selected on the basis of supportive skills and should be trained to be sufficiently aware of the constant need for such skills. A woman's experience of labor depends largely on the quality of the relationship established with the nurse assigned to her personally.[14] Clearly, "personal attention does *not* mean a group of nurses caring for an equivalent number of patients on a collective basis."[15]

> *In the labor and delivery unit, the nurse's attention should be confined to one patient only.*

16.2.1 Mutual dependency

In the final analysis it is the labor room nurses and the midwives who must convert most recommendations into practice (Chapter 26). Although few consultants will dispute the importance of personal attention and continuous support, many continue only to pay lip service to the ideal while taking no interest in the implementation of a labor protocol that truly enables the frontline birth attendants to provide such intensive care. By intentionally limiting the duration of labor to a maximum of 12 hours, the shift changes of the care providers during labor are kept to a minimum. When the rules of *proactive support of labor* are applied, 80% of all nulliparas give birth within the timeframe of one duty-shift[16] and the disadvantage of the inevitable personal discontinuity in the other 20% is buffered by the knowledge that only one shift change will occur and that the succeeding care provider will follow exactly the same, consistent policy for the conduct and care of labor.

> *Continuous personal presence and limitation of labor duration are mutually dependent; neither one is feasible without the other.*

Reliance on the endeavors of the personal nurse is no excuse for the midwife or physician to stay "back-stage" and to enter the room only on full dilatation or in the event of an emergency. The midwife and physician must also be actively involved and commit themselves to regular assessments of labor progress, the woman's physical and emotional status, and the well-being of the fetus. A redefinition of the responsibilities and proper working relations between nurses, midwives, and physicians is absolutely mandatory and will be addressed in Chapter 26.

16.3 Continuous support during labor

Women report that one of the most disturbing prospects of labor is the fear of being left alone, and unfortunately such fears of isolation are only too well founded in common childbirth practices.[17] Effective provisions must be made to resolve this situation. One-on-one companionship in labor forms the cornerstone of *proactive support of labor*.

> *A central feature of proactive support in childbirth is the promise that the woman will not be left alone during her labor at any time.*

Mere physical presence is not enough. Supportive care involves eye contact, friendly touch, reassurance, encouragement, consistent information and advice, emotional support, words of praise, comfort measures, and advocacy, which means helping the woman articulate her wishes to the medical staff.[14] The one-on-one female companion in labor – the personal nurse and/or certified doula – carries out this important task.

16.3.1 The evidence for continuous support

Continuous support by women for women effectively reduces anxiety and fear and associated adverse effects during labor. The latest systematic Cochrane review of the scientific evidence on continuous support for women during childbirth clearly proves that women who experience one-on-one supportive care are:[18]

- Less likely to have a cesarean section: (15 trials, $n = 12\,791$; RR = 0.90, 95% CI 0.82–0.99)
- Less likely to have a forceps or vacuum delivery: (14 trials, $n = 12\,757$; RR = 0.89, 95% CI 0.83–0.96)
- Less likely to report dissatisfaction with their childbirth experiences: (6 trials, $n = 9824$; RR = 0.73, 95% CI 0.65–0.83)
- More likely to give birth without use of analgesia or anesthesia: (11 trials, $n = 11\,051$; RR = 0.87, 95% CI 0.79–0.96)
- More likely to have a spontaneous vaginal birth: (14 trials, $n = 12\,757$; RR = 1.08, 95% CI 1.04–1.13)

The outstanding meta-analysis did not detect any adverse effects and none are plausible. The effects of continuous support were consistently positive in all trials, but the degree of benefit varied among institutions owing to differences in standard practices. Institutions varied in policies as to whether or not routine electronic fetal monitoring was used, whether or not epidural analgesia was available 24/7, whether or not they allowed additional support people of the woman's own choosing to be present, and whether or not early labor augmentation was standard policy. Indeed, a clear labor management protocol is critical and in fact the whole package of *proactive support of labor* achieves far more than the sum of its individual components (Chapters 29, 30).

> *One-on-one supportive care during labor has been shown to confer important benefits without attendant risks (Evidence level A).*

The Cochrane review included both multiparas and nulliparas and, therefore, the beneficial effects of continuous labor support on first labor outcomes – the main group of interest – were probably diluted. Another systematic meta-analysis by Zhang *et al.*[19] specifically focused on first labors (4 trials, $n = 1349$) and all advantageous effects of continuous labor support were demonstrated to be far more pronounced, including a significant shortening of first labor:

> **Beneficial effects of continuous labor support on first labors (Evidence level A)**
>
> 1. *Shortening of first labors by 2.8 hours on the average (95% CI 2.2–3.4 hours)*
> 2. *Reduction of the need for labor augmentation; RR 0.44 (95% CI 0.4–0.7)*
> 3. *Doubling of the spontaneous delivery rate; RR 2.01 (95% CI 1.5–2.7)*
> 4. *Reduction of cesarean deliveries by half; RR 0.54 (95% CI 0.4–0.6)*
> 5. *Reduction of instrumental vaginal deliveries by half; RR 0.46 (95% CI 0.3–0.7)*

16.3.2 Early support

The Cochrane meta-analysis also provides evidence of a "dose–response" phenomenon.[18] A strong and prolonged dose of continuous support is the most effective and the benefits are strongest when one-on-one support begins in early labor. This is an important finding because it confirms and emphasizes the necessity of an early, clear-cut diagnosis of labor and early assessment of uterine effectiveness as discussed in the previous two chapters.

16.3.3 One-on-one companion in labor

All trials included in the systematic reviews involved one-on-one support provided by experienced women who had given birth themselves or/ and had received education and practiced as nurses, midwives, doulas, or childbirth educators. An additional finding of the Cochrane meta-analysis was that the effects of continuous support appear to vary by type of provider.[18] The effects of continuous support are stronger when the provider is not a member of the staff and thus has no obligation to anyone other than the parturient woman. The reduction in operative births may be less when women receive support from nurses or midwives whose training, role, and/or identity involve responsibilities that extend beyond labor support.

Divided loyalties and duties in addition to labor support as well as the constraints of institutional policies and routines may all play a role. This emphasizes the need for reevaluation of all well-intended nursing rituals (Chapter 4), which will undoubtedly show that many of these can be safely discarded, freeing nurses to focus on their primary task: supportive care.

> *Continuous labor support is most effective when it begins in early labor and when it is provided by a caregiver who has an exclusive focus on this task (Evidence level A).*

The hospital delivery unit should be designated an intensive care area, not with regard to high-tech equipment but rather with regard to intensive one-on-one nursing. But hospital managers advocating "managed care" – and mostly unencumbered by insight into the essential requirements for high-quality childbirth – often preclude such a provision because of lack of funds. These hospital administrators should realize, however, that a substantial reduction in cesarean deliveries translates into an equally substantial reduction in postoperative care, thus freeing nurses to work in the delivery rooms. Good birth care and sound economics can surely complement one another (Chapter 26).

> *The hospital delivery unit should be designated an intensive care area, not with regard to high-tech equipment but rather with regard to intensive one-on-one nursing.*

In the authors' [P.R., A.F.] hospital, one-on-one nursing is practiced and all employees are trained in the principles of *proactive support of labor* aimed at a spontaneous delivery within 12 hours. With this overall policy, the highest spontaneous vaginal delivery rate for years in a row has been achieved in the national league tables, without any adverse effects on perinatal outcomes (Chapter 29).

Admittedly, it is increasingly difficult to optimize nursing staff quotas as is the case in most maternity centers where economists increasingly dictate the rules. This is another reason why specific attention should be given to the possibility of labor support by well-trained but non-institutional staff.

16.3.4 Doula services

Over the past decade several initiatives to employ the services of women with special training in labor support have begun in some countries. This new member of the caregiver team is commonly known as a doula (δουλη is the Greek word for "female slave" or "handmaiden"). She may, however, also be called a labor companion, birth partner, labor support specialist, labor assistant, or birth buddy. In the model pioneered chiefly in middle-class circles in the USA and Canada, the mother selects her doula during pregnancy; they establish a personal relationship that is likely also to involve the woman's partner, and they discuss the mother's preferences and concerns before labor. The pregnant woman may have other priorities besides medical help, because she does not leave her work, community, life-experiences, and family responsibilities behind when she enters the hospital to give birth. Her doula has detailed knowledge of the particular circumstances and is, therefore, likely to be in a better position to provide personal care and comfort than unfamiliar hospital staff.

The doula brings her experience and training, often to the level of certification, to the labor support role during childbirth. She rallies the mother's own powers and improves morale. There are several training workshops and guidebooks to teach nurses and doulas how to help a woman cope with the natural pain and discomfort of normal labor and delivery and to improve her labor environment (Chapter 18).[20] The evidence clearly dictates that there should be serious medical and political efforts not only to promote continuous support of all laboring women by a doula or nursing equivalent but also to provide resources for its universal implementation. In most places a lot of improvements still need to be made.

> *Continuous, personal support during labor should be the norm rather than the exception.*

16.3.5 Presence of partners and other people

No controlled trials have evaluated the effects of women's partners, family members, or friends as providers of labor support. Insights into the nature and value of such support have been gleaned from observational studies, but self-selection presents a major problem in the interpretation and the potential for making generalizations on the basis of the results of such studies.[21]

In practice, hospitals vary greatly in the extent to which they permit people of the woman's own choosing in labor wards, but it would be imprudent to assume that the presence of several people will provide additional support. Family and friends such as husbands and partners may be there to share the experience rather than to provide support. When there are major tensions in the couple's relationship, practical and emotional support in labor by the partner may be difficult to provide or to accept. Paradoxically, loving partners may feel powerless and suffer as much as the laboring woman who is experiencing pain and exertion and thus may unwittingly undermine the woman's ability to cope with labor and delivery. It should be noted that allowing fathers into the labor rooms coincides historically with the staggering increase in the use of epidural analgesia, other interventions, and operative delivery rates. These facts are difficult to reconcile.[15] The assumption that rigid policies about the birth environment lead to an increase in interventions may not necessarily be true.[15–21] Husbands/partners are often bad doulas indeed.

> *It would be unwise to rely on the supportive skills of expectant fathers, women's relatives, or friends.*

Nevertheless, the presence of fathers in the labor room is now the norm in most hospitals, and many departments even permit other lay people to be present as well. Indeed, where women have strong preferences for who should be with them at this time, these should be respected. However, given the difficulties of generalizing, the proper policy must be one of sensitivity by the professional staff to the possible negative effects of the presence of fathers and relatives or friends. In some cases, a café around the corner might be a better place for the husband/partner to wait, not only for the sake of the woman giving birth but for the sake of everyone involved. In the labor room women generally have far more to gain from the presence of a female companion who is not only sympathetic but also well-informed and therefore in a much better position to provide the type of firm support and guidance that are needed. Effective support by nurses or doulas, however, is always strongly dependent on a clear and consistent conduct of labor by the midwife or physician. In effect, continuous labor support cannot be implemented unless early correction of dysfunctional labor is performed as well. Contemporary childbirth is teamwork, and teamwork requires an overall, consistent birth-plan: *proactive support of labor.*

16.4 Summary

- Positive steps are necessary to prevent several members of staff from simultaneously attending the same woman in labor.
- Personal commitment means that each woman in labor is attended face-to-face by one midwife or one resident, who is known to her by name.
- Continuous nursing support on a one-on-one basis during labor should be the norm rather than the exception.
- One-on-one companionship in labor forms the cornerstone of *proactive support of labor.*
- The evidence shows that continuous labor support by a personal nurse or doula significantly shortens first labors, reduces the need

for labor augmentation, reduces a woman's likelihood of asking for pain medication, and increases both her chances for spontaneous birth and her satisfaction with the labor experience.

- The benefits of continuous support are strongest when it begins in early labor. This emphasizes the importance of a strict and early diagnosis of labor.

- The requirements of personal continuity and non-stop labor support demand a limit on the duration of labor to a maximum of 12 hours. Neither precondition for a rewarding childbirth experience is feasible without the other. Duty shifts exceeding 12 hours are not realistic.

- The whole package of *proactive support of labor* achieves more beneficial effects than the simple sum of its components.

REFERENCES

1. Osbourne A. A culture of fear: the midwifery perspective. Association of Radical Midwives; *Midwifery Matters Issue* no 100, Spring 2004.

2. Wagner M. Fish can't see water: the need to humanize birth. *Int J Gynaecol Obstet* 2001; 75: S25–37.

3. Block J. *Pushed: The Painful Truth about Childbirth and Modern Maternity Care.* Cambridge, MA: Da Capo Press; 2007.

4. Wagner M. *Born in the USA: How a Broken Maternity System Must Be Fixed to Put Women and Children First.* Berkeley, CA: University of California Press; 2007.

5. Lake R, Epstein E. *The Business of Being Born.* A documentary film (2007) www.thebusinessofbeingborn.com/about.htm.

6. Rooks J, Weatherby NL, Ernst EK, *et al.* Outcomes of care in birth centers. The National Birth Center Study. *N Engl J Med* 1989; 321: 1804–11.

7. Murphy P, Fullerton J. Outcomes of intended home births in nurse-midwifery practice: a prospective descriptive study. *Obstet Gynecol* 1998; 92(3): 461–70.

8. Hundley V, Cruickshanh R, Lanf G, *et al.* Midwifery managed delivery-unit: a randomised controlled comparison with consultant led care. *BMJ* 1994; 309: 1401–4.

9. Turnbull D, Holmes A, Shields N, *et al.* Randomised controlled trial of efficacy of midwife managed care. *Lancet* 1996; 348: 213–18.

10. Brown S, Grimes D. A meta-analysis of nurse practitioners and nurse midwives in primary care. *Nurs Res* 1995; 44: 332–9.

11. Wagner M. Midwifery in the industrialized world. *J Soc Obstet Gynaecol Canada* 1998; 13: 1225–34.

12. Hinds M, Bergeisen GH, Allen DT. Neonatal outcome in planned vs unplanned out-of-hospital births in Kentucky. *JAMA* 1985; 253: 1578–82.

13. MacDorman M, Singh G. Midwifery care, social and medical risk factors, and birth outcomes in the USA. *J Epidemiol Community Health* 1998; 52: 310–17.

14. Hodnett ED. Pain and women's satisfaction with the experience of childbirth: a systematic review. *Am J Obstet Gynecol* 2002; 186: S160–72.

15. O'Driscoll K, Meagher D, Robson M. *Active Management of Labour,* 4th edn. Mosby; 2003.

16. Hogston P, Noble W. Active management of labour: the Portsmouth experience. *J Obstet Gynaecol* 1993; 13: 340–2.

17. Enkin M, Keirse MJNC, Neilson J, *et al.* Social and professional support in childbirth. In: *A Guide to Effective Care in Pregnancy and Childbirth,* 3rd edn. Oxford: Oxford University Press; 2000.

18. Hodnett ED, Gates S, Hofmeyr GJ, Salaka C. Continuous support for women during childbirth. *Cochrane Database Syst Rev* 2003; (3): CD003766.

19. Zhang J, Bernasko JW, Leybovich E, Fahs M, Hatch MC. Continuous labor support from labor attendant for primiparous women: a meta-analysis. *Obstet Gynecol* 1996; 88(4): 739–44.

20. Klaus M, Kennel JH, Klaus PH. *Doula Book; How a Trained Labor Companion Can Help You Have a Shorter, Easier, and Healthier Birth.* Cambridge, MA: Da Capo; 2002.

21. Enkin M, Keirse MJNC, Neilson J, *et al.* Hospital practices. In: *A Guide to Effective Care in Pregnancy and Childbirth,* 3rd edn. Oxford: Oxford University Press; 2000.

Amniotomy and oxytocin

Clinical practice with regard to augmentation of labor is often difficult to comprehend. In many maternity units there is no protocol for the diagnosis and treatment of slow labor and each physician seems to have fixed preferences for which there is no factual basis. In effect, some obstetricians criticize midwives or residents for rupturing the membranes (especially late in the evening), whereas others criticize those who dare to consult them for slow labor when the membranes are still intact. Timing and dosage of oxytocin treatment also vary widely. While some obstetricians forbid any measures in the alleged "latent phase of labor," others order the administration of oxytocin without prior amniotomy. One consultant may feel that an IV drip with 2.5 U of oxytocin best accelerates labor, whereas another may prefer to use 5 U and yet another 10 U. To complicate matters even further, some doctors use all three doses consecutively on the same woman. No wonder residents and nurses become utterly confused. In such capricious circumstances, mistakes are bound to happen. Clearly, high-quality care demands an overall plan and explicit rules for the timing and execution of augmentation of labor, and criticism should be directed toward those who do not comply.

17.1 The truth about amniotomy

Although amniotomy is among the most commonly performed procedures in obstetrics, there is a lack of reliable data on this issue. The literature is confusing because amniotomy cannot be studied in isolation. Action taken in one direction is likely to have repercussions in another, and such information is generally missing from publications on this subject, thus diminishing their relevance.

17.1.1 Selective versus routine amniotomy

By the time a diagnosis of labor is made, spontaneous rupture of the membranes has already occurred in 30% of women (Chapter 14). Management of the 70% who begin labor with intact membranes remains controversial in general practice. Routine amniotomy is advocated by interventionist doctors, while others attempt to preserve the membranes as long as possible. The latter approach is also typical for midwives. As in most disputes, wisdom lies somewhere in between.

Several randomized trials have compared routine amniotomy at the onset of labor with selective amniotomy performed "only if indicated," but not specified. The first Cochrane meta-analysis (now withdrawn) demonstrated a reduction in labor duration of between 60 and 120 minutes by routine amniotomy, a decrease in the use of oxytocin (OR = 0.79; 95% CI 0.67–0.92) and fewer low Apgar scores (OR = 0.54; 95% CI 0.30–0.96).[1] These findings were not confirmed in the second Cochrane meta-analysis (2007).[2] The second review also failed to detect a tempering effect on cesarean section rates and even discerned a trend (though not statistically significant) toward an increase in the risk of cesarean delivery after routine amniotomy (OR = 1.26; 95% CI 0.98–1.62). The reviewers speculated that this trend might result from amniotomy-related abnormalities, as detected by CTG, or early recognition of meconium, thus lowering the threshold for operative delivery. Another explanation might be clinical suspicion of infection when long labor is still tolerated after routine early amniotomy. Indeed, the major concern after artificial rupture of membranes is intrauterine infection, but the risk of this is directly related to the amniotomy–delivery interval. Thus, amniotomy should be part of an overall plan that includes appropriate timing and concomitant policies. However, this essential information is missing in the trials reviewed by the Cochrane groups. In fact, the problem of infection is as good as nonexistent when labor and delivery are concluded within 8–12 hours. Intrauterine infection is a problem specifically of prelabor rupture of the membranes (PROM), of long inductions, and of conservatively (non-)managed long labors. As always, the results of a meta-analysis can be no stronger than the studies that contribute to it; indeed, there was no consistency between the studies reviewed regarding the timing of amniotomy during labor in terms of cervical dilatation and the amniotomy–delivery intervals were not reported. Despite or because of the lack of information on the total package of care in the studies reviewed, the Cochrane reviewers concluded that amniotomy should not be used routinely as part of standard labor management and care.

> *The policy of routine amniotomy in all cases of labor should be abandoned (Evidence level A).*

This viewpoint is in accordance with the principle of *proactive support* that any intervention should be performed only when indicated but that, when it is, action must be definite. Amniotomy should therefore be reserved for women with abnormally slow progress of labor. Such abnormal progress must of course be defined. This diagnosis should be made during the course of labor whenever

dilatation is less than 1 cm/h, and even so in the early stage of spontaneous labor (Chapters 15, 21).

17.1.2 Indication for selective amniotomy

Naturally, there are women in whom labor, when given the chance, will accelerate spontaneously after an initially slow onset. However, birth attendants do not possess a crystal ball; with that same chance, expectancy might very well result in an overly long labor and related agony. In this context, we remind readers that the mean duration of the "latent phase" as defined by Friedman was 8.6 hours (+2 SD 20.6 hours) for first labor and that the range was 1 to 44 hours, with a maximum of 20 hours still accepted as statistically "normal" (sic).[3] Clearly, it is better to dismiss the concept of the latent phase altogether (Chapter 11). There is no doubt that timely amniotomy can convert slow labor to normal progression. If the uterus fails to respond, it prevents further delay in oxytocin treatment, as oxytocin is preferably not given within one hour after artificial rupture of membranes. Its effect should first be evaluated, as oxytocin started instantly after amniotomy may lead to prompt overstimulation.

To assure a delivery within 12 hours, prospective criteria for normal progress are needed and early diagnosis and prompt treatment of slow labor are mandatory. For this reason, we rupture the membranes whenever progress is less than 1 cm/h at any stage of labor, even at 1 cm dilatation (full effacement). Like the diagnosis of labor itself, amniotomy embodies a firm commitment to delivery. There is no way back and policies must be clear and must be followed.

> *The membranes should be ruptured whenever progress of labor is less than 1 cm/h, even if dilatation is only 1 cm (= fully effaced cervix).*

17.1.3 Safety of amniotomy

A floating fetal head is the only pertinent contraindication for amniotomy. When the fetal head is in the pelvic inlet but is unstable, care should be taken to avoid dislodging it. An assistant who applies fundal and suprapubic pressure will eliminate the risk of umbilical cord prolapse. These precautions are particularly relevant when inducing multiparous labor but seldom or never in first labors that began spontaneously. A variety of other potential hazards have been postulated but never substantiated. It has been suggested that increased pressure differences around the fetal skull, combined with a reduction in amniotic fluid after amniotomy, predisposes to fetal skull deformity, an increased incidence of decelerations in fetal heart rate, and fetal distress. However, studies intended to show these harmful effects are subject to considerable selection bias and do not permit reliable conclusions.[4] Only one prospective, randomized study identified increased mild and moderate umbilical cord compression patterns on the CTG as a result of amniotomy, but no severe fetal heart rate decelerations were found and the rate of cesarean delivery for fetal distress was unaffected.[5] Fetal surveillance during (augmented) labor will be addressed in Chapter 24.

17.1.4 Evidence-based conclusions

After evaluating the evidence, we can confidently conclude that amniotomy for acceleration of slow labor is a safe and effective procedure, provided that it is employed as a component of an overall plan aimed at spontaneous delivery within 12 hours. Additional measures to restrict duration of labor effectively prevent the development of intrauterine infection.

> *Amniotomy for correction of slow labor is an effective and safe procedure (Evidence level A).*

There is no rational justification for postponing amniotomy when labor is slow. Neither the fetus nor the mother benefits from long labor, and restriction of duration of labor enables personal and continuous support during the entire labor,

both of which are interdependent features of high-quality birth care (Chapter 16). Moreover, amniotomy provides valuable information on the possible causative involvement of passage of meconium whenever uterine force is inefficient (hypertonic dystocia, Chapters 8, 21). All of these considerations apply equally to home births. There is no valid reason to forbid midwives to rupture the membranes at home if early labor is too slow. On the contrary, criticism should be reserved for those who do not. An unengaged head is the only contraindication for amniotomy at home, but this situation at labor onset is in itself reason enough for immediate transfer to the hospital.

17.2 Judicious use of oxytocin

Pervasive misconceptions about the risks and benefits of oxytocin stubbornly persist in the minds of many providers as a result of adverse experiences with oxytocin used for labor induction. Added to that, oxytocin therapy in spontaneous but slow labor is often started too late and at too low a dosage. The literature is similarly blurred and marred by misinterpretations and inaccuracies. Many recommendations, even in official guidelines, are rooted in shallow soil.

17.2.1 Misunderstandings

- Firstly, many studies confuse induction with augmentation, and even the most influential American textbook casually states that "there is only a semantic difference between labor induction and augmentation",[6] whereas nothing could be further from the truth (Chapter 8). The fundamental difference between induction and augmentation needs constant reiteration.
- Secondly, most if not all studies and guidelines assume a recognizable "latent phase" and consequently focus on labor subsequent to entering the so-called active phase of labor after 3 cm dilatation. In truth, the greatest benefits of augmentation are often achieved at an earlier

stage in slow labor. To reiterate: the concept of the latent phase should be abandoned.

- Thirdly, in most publications the problem of the exhausted, refractory uterus (Chapter 8) is insufficiently appreciated, neglected, or plainly unknown to the authors.
- Finally and most importantly, most if not all studies and guidelines on protraction and arrest disorders fail to recognize the fundamentally different causes in nulliparous and parous labor. In fact, oxytocin is safe and effective in the former, but may be hazardous in the latter.

> *The literature on augmentation of labor is blurred and marred by inaccuracies. As a result, many recommendations, even in formal guidelines, are in part founded on quicksand.*

17.2.2 Basic considerations

- Oxytocin is a powerful uterine stimulant, provided the myometrium has been transformed, in other words, that there are sufficient CAPs (contraction associated proteins, see Chapter 8) present. This explains why oxytocin is highly effective in accelerating spontaneously begun labor and why it acts unpredictably in labor induction.
- Slow progress in early labor points to an incomplete operating system that still can be established rapidly by oxytocin therapy. The biophysical explanation for the effectiveness of amniotomy and oxytocin in speeding up early labor is an accelerated completion of the myometrial gap junction system, improving the electrical orchestration of the contractions and recruiting the maximum number of myometrial cells for contractile action (Chapter 8).
- A prerequisite for the effective use of oxytocin in spontaneous labor is either spontaneous or artificial rupture of the membranes. Amniotomy reduces the need for oxytocin, and so-called "dry" stimulation is ineffective and not rooted in any logical framework. Once the diagnosis of labor is established, a point of no return has been

reached; if progress is slow, the first step is amniotomy.

- Oxytocin increases PGE_2 and the total intracellular calcium concentration in the myometrium, thereby provoking an increase in uterine force (Chapter 8). This explains its ability to correct protraction and arrest disorders in both the first and second stages of labor (Chapter 21).
- Oxytocin improves both the efficiency and frequency of uterine contractions resulting in increased force per contraction and increased cumulative force per unit time (Chapter 8).
- Appropriate timing is crucial. Prolonged labor results in accumulation of lactic acid in the uterus, as well as myometrial desensitization through a loss of oxytocin-binding sites. The effect of oxytocin in these circumstances may be decreased uterine responsiveness or, paradoxically, uterine tetanic spasms may occur, each of which is a feature of stimulating an exhausted, refractory uterus, loaded with lactic acid (Chapter 8).
- It cannot be overemphasized that the proposed protocol for the use of oxytocin must be restricted to nulliparas at term with singleton vertex presentation and a reassuring fetal status.
- Misapplication of the method to other, wholly unsuitable categories of patients has given rise to reports of obstetric disasters, such as fetal acidemia, trauma, complicated breech delivery, or uterine rupture in parous women, including those laboring after previous cesarean delivery.

> *Judicious use of oxytocin is highly effective in reducing the incidence of traumatizing, prolonged labor (Evidence level A).*

17.3 Evidence-based augmentation

The purpose of labor augmentation is the restoration of normal progression and prevention of prolonged labor. The two largest randomized studies on this subject showed highly significant reductions in the incidence of labor lasting >12 hours. Lopez-Zeno and colleagues reported a reduction from 19% to 5%,[7] and Frigoletto and co-workers reported a reduction from 26% to 9%.[8] A meta-analysis of all randomized trials by Fraser and colleagues demonstrated a typical OR of 0.3 (95% CI 0.2–0.4).[9] A striking detail is that in each of the controlled trials a high proportion of the women who served as controls ultimately received oxytocin for persistent failure to progress. These studies thus indicate that most women who are not initially treated with oxytocin for inadequate progress will still require an oxytocin infusion to deliver in a later stage. The fact that after an initial delay higher than usual doses are often required provides further proof of the need for timely use. Even more importantly, one large randomized controlled trial (RCT) compared augmentation begun at two, three, and four hours to the right of the WHO partogram alert line and explored the women's views on the experience.[10] Mothers whose augmentation began after two hours were significantly more satisfied with their labor than those in whom augmentation began later (*p* < 0.001). Evidently, pregnant women themselves prefer proactive measures to effect short labor.

As stated earlier, oxytocin will not achieve its goal of reducing cesarean rates when all other propositions for *proactive support of labor* are neglected. Augmentation of slow labor is but one component of the overall birth-plan. In fact, most women treated according to the principles of *proactive support of labor* do not receive oxytocin at all.

> Proactive support of labor *does not mean more frequent use of oxytocin, but rather its better timed and better dosed use. In fact, if all components of the overall birth-plan are implemented, most parturients do not need oxytocin at all.*

17.3.1 Safety

The octapeptide oxytocin is one of the most specific therapeutic agents there is and has no side effects, aside from its intrinsic antidiuretic effect.

Table 17.1. Rules governing the safe use of oxytocin

1. Use only in nulliparous women with a single fetus in the vertex position
2. Start of labor is spontaneous
3. Membranes are ruptured and the amniotic fluid is clear
4. The fetus is in good condition
5. Oxytocin is started on time
6. A standard concentration is used at all times
7. The only variable is the infusion rate
8. Direct and non-stop nursing supervision of each woman is mandatory
9. By their own authority, nurses/midwives may increase oxytocin to a pre-fixed maximum of 40 mU/min

To the best of our knowledge, anaphylactic reactions have never been described. Danger of water intoxication arises only after administration of extremely high doses along with intravenous salt-free fluid loads of more than 3 liters.[6] Water intoxication cannot occur when the rules of *proactive support of labor* are followed.

The effect of oxytocin causes the cervix to dilate and, eventually, the head to descend. If oxytocin is used judiciously, this sequential action is almost invariably achieved. However, a good therapeutic agent is safe only in good hands. Danger hides not in the agent but in the ineptitude of users who do not follow a protocol that provides a highly effective series of safeguards. When the execution of labor augmentation is left to junior residents, midwives, or nurses, the rules must be explicit and rigidly enforced (Table 17.1).

Oxytocin is always administered intravenously. To avoid bolus administration, the infusion should be inserted into the main intravenous line close to the venipuncture site. A fixed, standard concentration of oxytocin must be used at all times and preferably administered by an electronically safeguarded IV pump. The only variable is the infusion rate. However, lack of sophisticated infusion equipment is not an excuse for inept labor management, because a simple infusion gravity feed may perform equally well, provided it is carefully monitored by a personal nurse. This is an issue of great practical importance in third-world hospitals where infusion pumps may not be sufficiently available.

17.3.2 Studies on dosage schemes

Oxytocin is administered incrementally to titrate dose to effect because it is not possible to predict a woman's response to a particular dosage.[11] Most large North American and European obstetric units use low-dose oxytocin, whereas the evidence strongly supports the higher-dose regimens.[12] Numerous protocols for the initial dose, incremental increases, and time intervals between doses have been studied. In a blinded RCT comparing a high-dose protocol (4.5 mU/min, with 4.5 mU/min incremental increases every 30 minutes) with a low-dose (1.5 mU/min every 30 minutes) protocol for augmentation, the high-dose regimen was associated with a significant shortening of labor without any adverse perinatal effects.[13] In another large RCT, use of high-dose oxytocin for augmentation benefited women by decreasing the mean time to correct progression of labor by nearly two hours and by decreasing the need for cesarean delivery (10.4% of patients compared with 25.7%).[14] In a prospective trial involving 1676 women that compared a high-dose protocol (6 mU/min every 20 minutes) with a low-dose regimen (1–2 mU/min every 20 minutes) for augmentation of labor, the women who received the higher dose had a three-hour reduction in mean time to delivery, significantly fewer forceps deliveries, fewer cesarean sections for dystocia, and fewer occurrences of intrapartum chorioamnionitis and of neonatal sepsis.[15] The high-dose regimen was associated with an increase in hyperstimulation but no adverse fetal effects were observed. Hyperstimulation was managed by discontinuance of the oxytocin, followed when indicated by resumption of the infusion using only half of the dosage that was used on discontinuance. In a RCT involving 258 nulliparas, a starting dose of 4 mU/min was compared with 10 mU/min.[16] It was demonstrated that the high starting dose is as safe as the low dose but is significantly more effective. In another randomized trial, a high-dose regimen was associated with a shorter second-stage labor and no measurable differences in neonatal outcomes.[17] These studies highlight the importance of *how* oxytocin is used, not simply *whether* oxytocin is used. In many a practice, however, oxytocin is still used in a dose so low that 20 hours would be needed to reach the average target dose intended to ensure delivery within 12 hours. There is now sufficient evidence to suggest that the customary low-dose regimens may actually contribute to the high cesarean delivery rate.[18,19]

> *The evidence supports a high-dose oxytocin regimen (Evidence level A).*

17.3.3 Safe and effective dosage scheme

The purpose of labor augmentation within the overall framework of *proactive support of labor* is to restore progression within one to two hours. The evidence-based benefits favor a high-dose regimen, with incremental increases at short intervals. It is for this reason that we recommend the protocol shown in Table 17.2 for the augmentation of slow labor.

Table 17.2. Safe and effective dosage schedule for oxytocin

- A standard concentration of 5 IU oxytocin in 50 ml balanced salt solution is used at all times
- IV pump starts with 3 ml/h = 300 mU/h = 5 mU/min
- The dose is titrated to its effect at intervals of 15 minutes with dose increments of 3 ml/h = 5 mU/min
- Tachysystole – a frequency of seven or more contractions per 15 minutes – is reason to decrease the dose by half
- The maximum dose is 24 ml/h = 40 mU/min
- Evidence of fetal distress is the only absolute bar to oxytocin treatment

This regimen is safe and can be delegated without reservation to an adequately trained nurse or midwife who stays at the bedside and monitors the frequency of contractions.[20] Following this step-by-step protocol, progress of labor is almost invariably restored within one hour and the maximum dose allowed is attained at the shortest possible time: 75 minutes. This regimen is safe and effective only when the rules are rigidly enforced. Birth attendants should not reduce the rate of infusion simply because the mother complains of pain, which is to be expected. Questioning the established infusion rate is a common manifestation of a low level of confidence in the system and usually derives from lack of knowledge and imprecise instructions. Suggestions that women regard oxytocin with suspicion and frequently decline acceleration because of the pain are the result of serious misunderstandings originating in centers where, paradoxically, induction rates are high.

> *The protocol-directed administration of oxytocin can be left to the responsibility of an adequately trained nurse or midwife.*

17.3.4 Oxytocin and pain

Every birth attendant who has worked in a hospital is familiar with the so-called oxytocin contractions characterized by a rapid increase in intrauterine pressure followed by a sharp peak and a rapid decrease on the monitor. It is common to hear statements that these contractions are more painful than others. This is probably true. However, people forget that such sharply peaked oxytocin contractions are, without exception, specific to induction. In contrast to induction, labor augmentation normalizes contractions, including the normal, intrinsic pain and there is no reason to assume that these contractions should be any more painful. It is important to note that because augmentation shortens labor, there is in fact a decreased need for pain relief measures (Chapters 18, 20).

17.3.5 Duration of oxytocin administration

There are only sparse data to recommend a maximum duration for the augmentation of dysfunctional first-stage labor. The "two-hour rule" of ACOG in diagnosis of dystocia[12] has been successfully challenged in two trials, one using a four-hour limit[21] and the other a six-hour limit[22] to define failed augmentation. Extending the period of oxytocin augmentation beyond two hours was found to be safe and effective in reducing cesarean rates for dystocia in both trials. In fact, the most important issue is early timing to forestall an exhausted uterus that is unresponsive to oxytocin.

For these reasons, we do not use fixed time restraints for augmentation, but we also never allow augmented labor to transgress the partographic normality line for more than four hours. If progress remains inadequate despite high-dose oxytocin, the woman is subjected to cesarean delivery. If dystocia has been treated in time and with the proper dose, continuing to augment labor makes no sense; such a prolonged but ineffective augmentation is unduly harsh and even needlessly traumatizing for the parturient woman. An inescapable cesarean delivery is best performed on time, before emotional trauma arises. Moreover, complication rates relate directly to the pre-cesarean length of labor. Therefore, cesarean delivery is suggested to every woman for whom an easy vaginal delivery is not near at hand after 12 hours of labor. A delivery within 12 hours constitutes the guiding principle of *proactive support of labor*. Despite these seemingly drastic measures, overall cesarean rates for dystocia are effectively kept low (Chapter 29).

> *By design, cesarean delivery is offered whenever an easy vaginal delivery is not near at hand after 12 hours of adequately supported labor.*

17.3.6 Poor response

Provided oxytocin is used in appropriate doses and only in nulliparas who are spontaneously in labor

Table 17.3. Causes of poor response to oxytocin

- Error in diagnosis of labor (or induction)
- Intact membranes
- Delay in oxytocin
- Inadequate dose
- Appropriate dose but hesitant use

and whose amniotic fluid is clear, the frequency and force of contractions will invariably increase. Poor response to oxytocin results from inexpert or hesitant labor management (Table 17.3).

17.4 Maternal and fetal surveillance during augmentation

The goal of augmentation is to correct ineffective labor rapidly while avoiding uterine hyperstimulation that may endanger the fetus. Thus, progression in labor is the only parameter by which to evaluate the efficacy of oxytocin therapy (Section 2), and a doubtful fetal status is the only indication to decrease or discontinue the oxytocin infusion. Therefore, the personal nurse must evaluate both uterine action and fetal heart rate on a regular basis. Oxytocin must be halved or discontinued if contractions persist as more than seven in a 15-minute period, if they last longer than 60 seconds, or if the fetal status is disconcerting. Again, no special equipment is needed for these assessments. During labor augmentation, fetal condition can be monitored as in any normal labor (Chapter 24) and the bedside nurse can easily assess the frequency and duration of contractions by uterine palpation. Intrauterine pressure catheters are not needed and are preferably not used.

> Safeguards
>
> *Oxytocin must be halved or discontinued if contractions occur more frequently than seven times in a 15-minute period, if they last longer than 60 seconds, or if fetal status becomes doubtful.*

17.4.1 No pressure catheters

Intrauterine gauges may be helpful in extremely obese patients, but there is no evidence to demonstrate any improvement in perinatal outcome attributable to the routine use of intrauterine pressure measurements.[23,24] On the contrary, intrauterine pressure monitoring is usually counterproductive, because it easily becomes a technical substitute for personal nursing attention and care. Moreover, intrauterine pressure catheters are an unnecessary annoyance, are not without complications, are a source of infection, and are expensive. Above all, evaluation of uterine performance by pressure measurements may lead obstetricians along the wrong track (Chapter 11); a certain number of Montevideo units is then misconstrued as the criterion for adequate uterine action, which typically leads to a therapeutic deadlock despite insufficient progress. Progress of labor is the only criterion upon which to diagnose dystocia and on which to decide to augment labor and to evaluate its effect (Chapter 11). Pressure is not the measure; only progression counts (Chapter 8).

17.5 Hyperstimulation

Oxytocin improves the efficiency of uterine contractions, resulting in increased force per contraction. Additionally, oxytocin increases the frequency of contractions, thereby increasing uterine force as well.[25] The term tachysystole is used to distinguish hyperstimulation without corresponding fetal heart rate abnormalities from uterine hypertonia associated with fetal heart rate decelerations. The former certainly occurs on occasion, but the latter is hardly ever seen when the above-mentioned inclusion criteria for augmentation of labor are met and the protocol is strictly followed.

> *Intrauterine pressure catheters are not needed and are preferably not used.*

17.5.1 Uterine tachysystole

Tachysystole (seven or more contractions per 15 minutes) is easily managed. Immediate discontinuance of oxytocin almost instantly decreases the frequency of contractions, as the mean half-life of intravenous oxytocin is only 3–5 minutes. Oxytocin might be resumed at half the latest dose if needed. In our experience, hyperstimulation is never an unmanageable problem, nor was it found to be a real problem in any of the previously discussed studies.[12]

> *When the protocol is followed, tachysystole is easily managed.*

17.5.2 No additional fetal risks

Inability to give oxytocin for augmentation of slow labor because of fetal intolerance is a straightforward indication for cesarean delivery. For the sake of proper insight and completeness, the following aside is important: dose–effect titration is problematic only in labor inductions and in unduly delayed augmentations where the uterus may have become refractory to stimulation (Chapter 8). Typically there is no effect initially, despite high doses of oxytocin, while a subsequent dose-increment results in hypertonia with fetal distress. It goes without saying that the responsibility for induction and delayed augmentation should rest with the obstetrician, and in such clinical circumstances intrauterine pressure monitoring might indeed be helpful; a resting pressure of more than 20 mmHg and/or the appearance of prolonged, biphasic contractions (bigemini, or "camel humps") on the monitor are the first signs of imminent fetal danger. Fetal intolerance is a compelling reason to refrain from oxytocin.

> *Hyperstimulation resulting in fetal distress is specific to induction of labor or to unduly delayed augmentation. It is not related to judicious use of oxytocin in spontaneous labor.*

Hypertonic dystocia is a completely different clinical entity (Chapters 8, 21). In this case the cells of the myometrium are randomly excited by chorioamnionitis, meconium, or intrauterine blood to the extent that the coordination and hence the efficiency and effectiveness of contractions are lost. This can lead to a hazardous and vicious circle involving dysfunctional labor and fetal distress. Intrauterine monitoring might be useful in such situations, and an experienced obstetrician must directly supervise such risky labor. If the fetus does not tolerate the uterine powers required for normal progress, a prompt cesarean is the only rational option. As always, policies must be clear and action must be resolute.

> *Hypertonic dystocia is a separate clinical entity altogether and unrelated to oxytocin.*

A healthy fetus with a normal placental reserve capacity is well-equipped to tolerate the stress of normal labor and normalized labor with appropriate augmentation, unless accidents such as umbilical cord compression occur (Chapter 24). This happens as frequently in augmented contractions as it does in spontaneous labor and the impact of such accidents on fetal well-being is the same in both cases. Since the purpose of oxytocin is to normalize labor, it inevitably contributes to the normal chance of fetal distress in labor. Augmentation does not, however, increase the risk of fetal hypoxia. Several randomized studies and a structured meta-analysis incontestably demonstrate that Apgar scores, neonatal blood gases, number of infants transferred to the neonatal intensive care unit, and neurological morbidity are not adversely influenced by judicious augmentation of labor.[9]

It has been taught for many years that oxytocin increases the risk of fetal trauma, especially where there may be an element of fetopelvic disproportion, but there is no factual basis for this proposition, at least in nulliparas (Chapter 22). In first labor the opposite is true, because restoration of effective labor reduces the need for instrumental delivery, which is the main cause of fetal trauma.

> *When used correctly, acceleration of slow labor poses no greater risk of fetal distress or trauma than any other normal labor (Evidence level A).*

17.6 Patients outside the protocol's inclusion criteria

It must be stressed that the rules outlined above apply only to healthy, term nulliparous women with a single fetus in good condition and in the vertex position. Oxytocin should be administered to other patients only under the direct supervision of an obstetrician and heeding the following considerations.

17.6.1 Nulliparas

- In an augmentation that is begun too late, higher doses of oxytocin are generally needed and hypertonia between the contractions is not uncommon (*refractory uterus*, Chapters 8, 21).
- In case of passage of meconium, one should be aware of the risk of hypertonic dystocia.
- When fetal condition is in question, stringent surveillance and additional diagnostic procedures are required (Chapter 24). If the fetus cannot tolerate the contractions needed for adequate progression, a prompt cesarean delivery is the only rational option.
- Although the basic principles of labor management are universally valid, the augmentation guideline cannot be automatically applied to breech or twin births.
- In a multiple pregnancy the uterus is under greater strain than in a singleton pregnancy and therefore might react less predictably.
- During the wedging phase of a breech birth, oxytocin is not without risk, because secondary protraction may be the first sign of unfavorable fetopelvic proportions with dire consequences for the after-coming head. In case of a secondary protraction disorder in a breech delivery, the strict rule applies: resort to a cesarean.

> *Oxytocin treatment of patients who do not meet the strict inclusion criteria of the protocol presented must always be explicitly and personally approved and supervised by the consultant on duty.*

17.6.2 Multiparas

Although multiparous women are prone to uterine rupture – *a fortiori* in the presence of a uterine scar – amniotomy does not pose an increased risk. Whenever indicated, the membranes must be ruptured, after which the contractions will, almost without exception, be sufficiently effective, making oxytocin rarely if ever necessary. After critical analysis, primary ineffective parous labor appears to occur only in multiparas who are induced, who are incorrectly declared in labor, who are negatively conditioned by a traumatizing previous birth, or whose labor is compromised by intrauterine meconium, blood, or pus (Chapter 13).

A secondary protraction and arrest disorder in parous labor is highly suggestive of fetal obstruction (Chapter 9). Use of oxytocin in such circumstances increases the risk of both maternal and fetal trauma and catastrophic uterine rupture. We therefore allow late augmentation of parous labor only in the relatively rare cases when cephalopelvic disproportion and malposition of the fetal head are explicitly ruled out (Chapter 22), and uterine contractions are too infrequent and/or appear to be too weak. Reassurance about such conditions must be definitively demonstrated by absence of molding, absence of caput succedaneum, and absence of extreme hyperflexion. Augmentation of parous labor must always be explicitly and personally approved and supervised by the consultant on duty.

> *There is a grave obligation on the part of the physician to ensure that fetal obstruction has been excluded before augmentation of slow* parous *labor is authorized.*

17.7 Avoiding territorial disputes

In countries with healthcare systems that include the possibility of selected home births led by independent midwives, the issue of augmentation of labor needs special agreements. Midwives attending home births are not allowed to administer oxytocin. That is why patients whose labor at home progresses unsatisfactorily need to be transferred to the hospital without delay. However, labor can be accelerated, without any rational objection, on a consultative outpatient basis. By having labor progression normalized, the parturient woman can remain in the hospital under the care of her chosen and trusted midwife. The stipulation for this possibility is mutual trust and respect between community-based midwives and obstetricians, as well as a legal contract defining the responsibility and legal accountability of each (Chapter 26). Furthermore, home-working midwives and hospital-bound obstetricians must be in absolute agreement regarding the criteria for normal (early) progression and adhere to the same time-specific indications for augmentation. A midwife who transfers a woman to the hospital far too late must not be surprised if the obstetrician – in an effort to catch up after the fact and confronted with a by now exhausted, refractory uterus – takes over the subsequent care of the woman. On the other hand, the midwife must be able to trust that on transferring the parturient to the hospital in due time the woman will remain under her continuing care and responsibility (Chapter 26). The obstetrician who first waits a couple of hours before drawing any conclusions, or worse yet, orders sedatives and does not see the woman until the following morning, undermines the necessary continuity of care and does nothing to generate trust in and respect for hospital care.

> *Clinical augmentation of slow labor can be provided, without any rational objection, on a consultative basis for midwife-led labors.*

17.8 Summary

- The fundamental difference between induction and augmentation requires constant iteration: induction creates slow labor whereas augmentation corrects slow labor.
- As long as labor is normal the membranes should be left intact.
- Amniotomy is the first step to normalizing spontaneous but ineffective labor.
- Augmentation of a nulliparous labor is safe and effective in correcting dysfunctional labor, provided oxytocin stimulation is started in time, i.e., whenever progress of labor is less than 1 cm/h at any stage of labor, even at 1 cm dilatation (= complete effacement).
- In the event of delayed augmentation, oxytocin is both less effective and less safe.
- There are strict inclusion criteria and dosage rules that govern the safe and effective use of oxytocin in labor.
- A properly trained midwife or nurse can independently perform and oversee standard augmentation of labor in a nullipara with a single fetus in the vertex position and in good condition, provided that the rules are rigidly followed.
- The evidence supports high-dose oxytocin regimens. In fact, the widespread use of low-dose oxytocin for labor augmentation contributes to the current high cesarean rates for dystocia.
- When used judiciously, oxytocin does not lead to an increased incidence of fetal distress.
- Signs of fetal hypoxia are the only pertinent contraindication for oxytocin therapy.
- Augmentation of parous labor should only be undertaken on a strictly individual basis, under the careful observation and direct supervision of an obstetrician.

- Augmentation of slow labor is only one component of the overall policy of *proactive support*. In fact, most women cared for following the principles elucidated in this manual do not receive oxytocin at all.

REFERENCES

1. Faser WD, Turcot L, Krauss I, Brison-Carrol G. Amniotomy for shortening spontaneous labor. *Cochrane Database Syst Rev* 2000; (2): CD000015.
2. Smyth RM, Alldred SK, Markham C. Amniotomy for shortening spontaneous labour. *Cochrane Database Syst Rev* 2007; (4): CD006167.
3. Friedman EA. Primigravid labor; a graphicostatistical analysis. *Obstet Gynecol* 1955; 6: 567–89.
4. Enkin M, Keirse MJNC, Chalmers I. Prolonged labour. In: *A Guide to Effective Care in Pregnancy and Childbirth*. Oxford: Oxford Medical Publications; 1990.
5. Garite TJ, Porto M, Carlson NJ, Rumney PJ, Reimbold PA. The influence of elective amniotomy on fetal heart rate patterns and the course of labor in term patients: a randomized study. *Am J Obstet Gynecol* 1993; 168: 1827–32.
6. Cunningham FG, Gilstrap LC III, Gant NF. Induction and augmentation of labor. In: *Williams Obstetrics*, 21st edn. New York: McGraw-Hill; 2001; 469–81.
7. Lopez-Zeno J, Paeceman A, Adashek J, Socol A. A controlled trial of a program of active management of labour. *N Engl J Med* 1992; 326: 450–4.
8. Frigoletto F, Lieberman E, Lang J, *et al*. A clinical trial of active management of labor. *N Engl J Med* 1995; 333: 745–50.
9. Fraser W, Vendittelli F, Krauss I, Bréart G. Effects of early augmentation of labour with amniotomy and oxytocin in nulliparous women: a meta-analysis. *Br J Obstet Gynaecol* 1998; 105: 189–94.
10. Lavender T, Wallymahmed AH, Walkinshaw SA. Managing labor using partograms with different action lines: a prospective study of women's views. *Birth* 1999; 26(2): 89–96.
11. Satin AJ, Leveno KJ, Sherman ML, McIntire DD. Factors affecting the dose response to oxytocin for labor stimulation. *Am J Obstet Gynecol* 1992; 166: 1260–1.
12. Dystocia and augmentation of labor. ACOG practice bulletin no 49. *Obstet Gynecol* 2003; 102: 1445–54 and *Int J Gynecol Obstet* 2004; 49: 315–24.
13. Merill DC, Zlatnik FJ. Randomized double-masked comparison of oxytocin dosage in induction and augmentation of labor. *Obstet Gynecol* 1999; 94: 455–63.
14. Xenakis EM, Langer O, Piper JM, Conway D, Berkus MD. Low-dose versus high-dose oxytocin augmentation of labor: a randomized trial. *Am J Obstet Gynecol* 1995; 173: 1874–8.
15. Satin AJ, Leveno KJ, Sherman ML, Brewster DS, Cunningham FG. High- versus low-dose oxytocin for labor stimulation. *Obstet Gynecol* 1992; 80: 111–16.
16. Majoko F. Effectiveness and safety of high dose oxytocin for augmentation of labour in nulliparous women. *Cent Afr J Med* 2001; 47: 247–50.
17. Bidgood KA, Steer PJ. A randomized control study of oxytocin augmentation of labor. I. Obstetric outcome. *Br J Obstet Gynaecol* 1987; 94: 512–17.
18. Dudley DJ. Oxytocin: use and abuse, science and art. *Clin Obstet Gynecol* 1997; 40(3):516–24.
19. Kotaska AJ, Klein MC, Liston RM. Epidural analgesia associated with low-dose oxytocin augmentation increases cesarean births: a critical look at the external validity of randomized trials. *Am J Obstet Gynecol* 2006; 194; 809–14.
20. Clayworth S. The nurse's role during oxytocin administration. *MCN Am J Matern Child Nurs* 2000; 25(2): 80–4.
21. Arulkumaran S, Koh CH, Ingemarsson I, Ratnam SS. Augmentation of labour: mode of delivery related to cervimetric progress. *Aust N Z J Obstet Gynaecol* 1987; 27: 304–8.
22. Rouse DJ, Owen J, Hauth JC. Active-phase labor arrest: oxytocin augmentation for at least 4 hours. *Obstet Gynecol* 1999; 93: 323–8.
23. Chua S, Kurup A, Alkumaran S, Ratnam SS. Augmentation of labor: does internal tocography result in better obstetric outcome than external tocography? *Obstet Gynecol* 1990; 76: 164–7.
24. Lucidi RS, Chez RA, Creasy RK. The clinical use of intrauterine pressure catheters. *J Matern Fetal Med* 2001; 10(6): 420–2.
25. Allman AC, Genevier ES, Johnson MR, Steer PJ. Head-to-cervix force: an important physiological variable in labour.1. The temporal relation between head-to-cervix force and uterine pressure during labour. *Br J Obstet Gynaecol* 1996; 103: 763–8.

18

Labor pain in broader perspective

A significant feature of customary birth care is the emphasis placed on the physical element of labor pain and its relief. "Many maternity units seem to operate from the belief that the most important contribution caregivers can make to the comfort of women in labor is to ensure that their pain is relieved by epidural analgesia or opioid drugs."[1] In effect, only a minority of women in western countries currently give birth without pain medication; in the USA fewer than 17%.[2] The overall results, however, are far from impressive, even in the short-term sense of immediate consumer satisfaction.

18.1 The nature of labor pain

Giving birth is the only physiological process in nature that causes pain, and the reasons for this have been "explained" with philosophical and religious arguments. Even so, the biological functions of pain in childbirth are clear: pain provides the warning sign to search for a safe birth environment, and endorphins promote effective and mutual mother–child bonding (Chapter 7).

Most women instinctively feel that pain in childbirth is part of life and are justifiably proud of their achievement. Being a link in procreation since *Genesis*, women know that they are responsible for the continued existence of the human species. Moreover, birth increases their pain threshold for the rest of their lives to an unequalled level; if men had to bear birth pain humankind would have become extinct long ago. Clearly, the natural pain of labor is fundamentally different from pain associated with surgical wounds or other forms of injury. Accordingly, birth attendants' attitude to labor pain should be fundamentally different from that of a strictly medical approach. Use of epidural analgesia or opioid drugs is the easiest solution for doctors, but is largely unsatisfactory in its effects. Effectively easing the strain and pain of childbirth requires an overall plan of care characterized by clarity, limiting of the duration of labor, and above all respectful, personal, and continuously supportive care.

> *Pain in childbirth requires a fundamentally different approach from that of standard medicine, which is using drugs.*

18.1.1 Insecurity, anxiety, and pain

It is not the pain of labor that traumatizes women, but rather the lack of personal care in modern maternity centers, the feeling of not being heard, or the fear of being abandoned in so vulnerable a state (Chapter 4). Fear and anxiety are strongly associated with increased pain during labor and modify labor pain through psychological and physiological mechanisms.[3–8] When a woman in labor is insufficiently prepared and supported she may experience a mounting sense of frustration because she feels herself to be a helpless victim of powerful natural forces that she cannot actively influence.

Swept along on a tide of events that she may not fully comprehend, she may lose self control, *a fortiori* when progress is slow and no one can or will tell her when her ordeal is likely to come to an end. Meanwhile, various birth attendants come and go, while for her the problem of protraction seems to begin all over again. Inconsistent and discontinuous care only works to exacerbate the insecurity and anxiety, and fear of the unknown aggravates the pain. The inevitable sympathetic stress response further undermines uterine efficiency and thus progress, and a vicious cycle ensues. A state of panic may develop that very well may trigger a lifelong post-traumatic stress syndrome (Chapter 2). Clearly, large amounts of opioid drugs or an epidural block are not the first measure of prevention.

> *Nothing is more demoralizing and traumatizing than enduring intense pain with no end in sight.*

18.1.2 The physical element of pain in labor

That there is a physical element in the discomfort and pain of labor is beyond question and should never be denied. Delivery is not a bodily pleasure, rather a challenge. Most women are willing to accept pain in childbirth but they do not want the pain to overwhelm them. The character of labor pains is a cramp resembling intense dysmenorrhea, with which most women are at least somewhat familiar. Contractions last about a minute – within which the pain is intense for around 30 seconds – followed by a rest period in which the pain ceases completely. The pains recur every three minutes, somewhat less frequently at the beginning and more frequently toward the end. This amounts to 10 minutes of intense pain per hour and translates into less than one hour of intense pain during the course of a first labor of average duration (6 hours, Chapters 9, 15) and a maximum of one hour and a half for a dilatational period of 10 hours, the limit of normal first-stage labor duration. If prepared properly and as long as clarity and adequate labor

support are maintained, the majority of women will manage without pain medication. The ability to restrict labor duration is crucial in this regard, since the time exposed to the stress, discomfort, and pain is the dominant element in the problem of labor pain.

> *Labor duration is one of the key problems with regard to labor pain.*

Pain in labor is essentially a problem of the first stage, with pain (nociceptive) stimuli arising from mechanical distension of the cervix and lower uterine segment.[9] Although the nociceptive stimuli are even more prevalent during the second stage of labor – because the pelvic floor, vagina, and vulva are now being stretched – a woman is generally better able to cope because she now regains control of her situation. She senses that the conclusion of birth is near and that it can be accelerated by her own efforts. In this "active stage" of birth the tremendous physical exertions required in pushing generally distract her attention from the sensation of pain.

18.1.3 The spectrum of behavioral responses

Owing to the subjective element of discomfort and pain, women's individual reactions to labor vary enormously. Hence, the full spectrum of emotional behavior can be observed in every busy delivery unit every single day. Nonetheless, a standard sequence of reactions progressing with variable velocity can be outlined. A woman initially reacts with startled surprise (it has finally begun), followed by conscious efforts to cope with the contractions. This increasingly requires concentration, which becomes more difficult the stronger and the more frequent the contractions become. In time, she tends to withdraw completely from contact with her surroundings during contractions, keeping her eyes tightly closed in extreme concentration. Up to this point there are no insurmountable problems. As time passes, however, the intensity of the reaction grows with successive pains. The woman may become agitated and restive. She may react unreasonably to the well-meaning efforts at comfort and advice from her partner and her birth attendants. Finally, after what for her is an excessively long period of pain, she can no longer concentrate during the contractions and, what is worse, she can no longer relax during the contraction intervals, let alone recover. Now, the intensity of the pains, and above all the duration of labor, threaten to unhinge her into violent and unmanageable behavior. She can become truly panicked and reach the point of life-long traumatization. "This scenario, where a woman continues to react long after a contraction is over, should never be allowed to develop, because once contact is lost it is hard to reestablish."[1] Permanent loss of women's faculty for real communication is most often the product of insufficient preparation, lack of personal support, and inept labor management, in which no one is paying attention to the simple fact that the duration of labor exceeds the woman's stamina for endurance.

> *The scenario of a woman continuing to react to pain between contractions so that she cannot recover must be avoided in all circumstances.*

Again, simple reliance on drugs for pain relief is not the appropriate policy. Personal supportive care and timely correction of slow labor are usually far more constructive. A dramatic easing of the throes of labor occurs as the impasse of ineffective labor is overcome and normal progress is established, despite the fact that accelerated contractions are much stronger. An additional benefit of early augmentation is the ability to predict the approximate hour of delivery and this is of paramount importance to the morale of all participants in the birth process. At the same time, this approach shows more respect for the woman because it allows her to retain her dignity, mobility, and full control over her body and promotes her giving birth by her own efforts.

18.1.4 Medical pain relief

The ideal technique for pain relief in labor does not exist (Chapter 20). Opioids seem to be the best systemic drugs available, but the amount of analgesia that can be achieved is directly proportional to unpleasant side effects such as orthostatic hypotension, dizziness, nausea, and – worst of all – loss of mental acuity.[10] In addition, opioids cross the placenta and may cause neonatal respiratory depression.[11] Epidural analgesia is generally far more effective and allows the woman to be awake and aware while the baby is alert at birth. Besides these obvious advantages, however, epidural block is more dangerous and involves several co-interventions and unintended effects on the course of labor.[12–14] No good cause is served by pretending otherwise. The benefits and drawbacks of opioids and epidural analgesia will be addressed extensively in Chapter 20.

18.1.5 Psychosocial and environmental influences

"Labor pain occurs in the context of an individual woman's physiology and psychology and of the sociology of the culture surrounding her. That culture includes not only the beliefs, morals, and standards of her family and community but also those of the healthcare system and its providers."[15] In a recent review, no studies were found in which the affective dimensions of labor pain were compared across cultural groups, but the author noted that pain behaviors vary greatly among cultural and subgroups as a result of learned patterns of expected behavior.[15]

The complexity and individuality of the labor experience suggest that a woman and her caregivers may have a limited ability to anticipate her labor pain experience before labor, and that standardized and limited approaches to labor pain management do not meet the needs of many women. Modifiable factors include above all labor duration and adherence to a well-defined birthplan, as well as environmental conditions, coping strategies, fear, anxiety, expectations about the labor experience, and a woman's sense of self-efficacy or confidence in her ability to cope. Care and resources available to women as they look toward their birthing experiences and during the time of labor and birth strongly influence whether the sensory intensity of pain is experienced in a fundamentally negative or positive manner.[15]

> *"Education and policy initiatives can influence a host of factors, such as fear, anxiety, self-efficacy, coping strategies, and care practices, that are important to the pain experience of childbirth."*[15]

Given the customary practice of abundant use of pharmacological pain relief, there seems to be a popular belief that labor pain is bad and that the parturient should be relieved of her pain as soon as possible. Some even suggest cesarean delivery is an option to avoid the pain and stress of labor and the burden of birth.[16] Nancy Lowe, renowned expert in the field of labor pain research, keenly noted the paradoxical element of these beliefs in a society that celebrates individuals who endure great pain and distress in pursuit of mountain peaks or completion of a marathon race.[15] She further comments: "Childbirth has deep significance for everyone; it is a profound physiological, psychosocial, and spiritual event. It is this context of the experience of childbirth that drives some women to experience all of labor, even its pain, and challenges many providers to create and protect a birthing environment in which a broad spectrum of non-pharmacological and pharmacological approaches to pain relief are incorporated, and in which pain is viewed as only one component of the totality of the woman's labor and birth experience."[15]

18.2 Non-pharmacological pain relief measures

Many alternatives are tried to help women who prefer to cope with labor without using drugs:

maternal movement and position changes, mind–body techniques, biofeedback, counterpressure or superficial heat and cold applied to the low back, sterile water injections in the skin overlying the sacrum, transcutaneous electrical nerve stimulation (TENS), bathing, touch and massage, attention focusing and distraction, music, white noise, aromatherapy, herbal medicines or homeopathy, hypnosis, and so on. Several of these measures might be beneficial, but the scientific evidence is generally poor.[10,17,18] TENS has been subjected to more controlled trials than any of the other modalities of non-pharmacological pain relief, but the results remain inconclusive.[10] The Cochrane review found frugal evidence that acupuncture and hypnosis might help in easing labor pain but concluded that more research is needed on these and the other complementary therapies.[18] Another thorough systematic review by Simkin and O'Hara[17] focused on five simple methods of pain relief: continuous labor support, baths, touch and massage, maternal movement and positioning, and intradermal water blocks. The reviewers concluded: "Despite the need for further research we now know enough of these simple and effective methods to recognize that laboring women should have both the opportunity and the encouragement from staff to use them. These methods are safe, effective, and satisfying for many women, but are generally unavailable or underutilized because of almost total reliance on a limited variety of pharmacological methods of pain relief."

18.2.1 Evidence-based recommendations

To effectively incorporate these alternative methods into maternity care, hospitals and caregivers will need, in their usual care, to make the allowances and alterations suggested by Simkin and O'Hara:[17]

1. Make appropriate equipment available, such as bathtubs, areas where women can walk, side rails along the walls to lean on, rocking and straight chairs, birth balls, stools, and other positioning aids, telemetry units, and rolling IV poles.

2. Develop policies that allow women to be out of bed; utilize intermittent instead of continuous fetal monitoring; welcome trained doulas to provide continuous labor support; and ensure safe and appropriate use of the bath.

3. Train maternity staff to ensure that they are skilled, knowledgeable, and open-minded to the safe and appropriate use of these techniques by the women. They should be given training in the use of the birth bed to support a variety of positions, massage skills, appropriate use of the bath, ways to reassure and encourage a distressed woman, ways to communicate empathy and kindness; and for doctors and midwives, ways to assist with births in a variety of positions.

> *Access to and use of drug-free pain relief measures appear to be quite limited and far from commensurate with their universal relevance.*

A major advantage of these methods is that they do not interfere with apt labor management according to the rules of *proactive support of labor*, and they may be used together, with the possibility of producing a greater overall beneficial effect than is provided by any single method. Evidently, it is in particular the personal attention associated with these methods of pain relief and the continuous labor support by a well-motivated, sympathetic, female companion, that are critical in truly helping women to cope with the pain of childbirth (Chapter 16).

18.2.2 Individualization

Clearly, a standardized and limited approach to labor pain management with opioid drugs or epidural block does not meet the needs of many women; so choice among a variety of methods of pain relief and individualization of pain-related care are highly desirable. This consideration is especially important in light of evidence suggesting that vivid and largely accurate memories of the childbirth experience endure through women's lives.[19,20]

> *Individualization of pain-related care is a prerequisite for high-quality maternity care.*

18.3 Pain and women's labor experience

Pain relief and satisfaction with the birth experience are not the same thing, although many doctors tend to equate them. The perspective of women themselves about the role of pain and pain relief in their satisfaction with childbirth was recently analyzed by Hodnett in a landmark systematic review.[21] The meta-analysis involved more than 45 000 women and – although satisfaction is a complex, multidimensional construction, and researchers used a variety of methods to measure it – results were remarkably consistent in all studies reviewed. The reviewer concludes that pain and pain relief do not generally play major roles in women's satisfaction with their childbirth experience unless expectations regarding either are not met. When women themselves evaluate their childbirth experiences, four factors prove to be of predominant importance:

> **Evidence-based contributors to women's childbirth satisfaction**
>
> 1. *The amount of support a woman receives from caregivers*
> 2. *The quality of her relationship with her caregivers*
> 3. *Her involvement with decision-making*
> 4. *Her personal expectations*
>
> *(Evidence level A–B)*

These conditions are so important for the childbirth experience that they override the physical component of pain. This finding is independent of maternal age, socioeconomic status, nationality, ethnicity, and even the influences of the physical birth environment, immobility, and medical interventions.[21]

> *Pain is not the primary determinant of women's sense of satisfaction with their birth experience.*

Focusing on the relationship of medical intervention (not specified) and women's birth satisfaction, Hodnett's systematic review showed either no effect or an effect that favors medical intervention over expectant care.[21] The only large randomized controlled trial that specifically investigated the relation between duration of labor and women's contentment by comparing augmentation begun at two, three, and four hours to the right of the WHO partogram alert line, indisputably showed that mothers whose augmentation began after two hours were significantly more satisfied than those in whom augmentation began later ($p < 0.001$).[22] Evidently, women themselves prefer proactive management ensuring short labor (Evidence level Ib).[23] Women with longer, more difficult, more complicated labors are more likely to request pharmacological analgesia. Conservative critics should accept this evidence supporting the care strategy advocated in this manual, including the intensive one-on-one supportive care and timely correction of dysfunctional labor.

> *Women themselves prefer proactive management ensuring short labor (Evidence level A).*

18.3.1 Support and patient–caregiver relationship

Continuous labor support and the patient–caregiver relationship were addressed extensively in Chapter 16. These essential components of quality birth care are closely correlated with the prevention of long labor because unstinted personal attention cannot be provided for everyone unless the duration of the birth process is limited. Duty-shifts exceeding 12 hours are unrealistic.

> *Personal one-on-one attention is the best antagonist for the pain and strain of labor.*

18.3.2 Personal expectations

The important issue of a woman's involvement with decision-making is strongly related to her personal expectations. Both of these evidence-based contributors to a positive birth experience emphasize the critical importance of adequate prelabor information that must correspond with actual practice. Pregnant women deserve to be treated as adults and have the right to know what to expect during their labor and delivery. The subject of pain should, therefore, never be dismissed but should be openly discussed during pregnancy and, most importantly, always in the wider context of labor support and a consistent policy of care. Prelabor information suffers serious loss of credibility when birth educators are unable to state the overall plan, the available support facilities, and the maximum duration of labor without the customary evasions. Fear of the unknown aggravates stress and pain, while a woman who knows what lies ahead and who has confidence in herself and her birth attendants usually requires less pain medication, and her labor is more likely to progress smoothly. The crucial importance of adequate and honest prelabor preparation cannot be exaggerated. That is the subject of the next chapter.

18.4 Summary

- Women's contentment with their childbirth experience is not contingent upon the absence of pain.
- A motivating, one-on-one personal attendant is the best antidote against the pain of labor.
- The influence of pain, pain relief, and intrapartum interventions on women's satisfaction is neither as obvious, as direct, nor as powerful as

the influence of the attitudes and behaviors of the caregivers and the adherence to a consented birth-plan.

- Individualization of care, continuous support, and a choice among several pain-relief methods are the hallmarks of high-quality birth care.
- Positive steps are needed to allow such individualized care and to make appropriate equipment available to all women in labor.
- Restriction of labor duration is decisive for the birth experience, because the pain-exposure time is the dominant problem of labor. This holds for both the woman giving birth and her caregivers.
- Pain should never be discussed in isolation from available labor support and a well-defined labor plan.
- Prelabor education that corresponds with actual practice is crucial to the enhancement of women's childbirth experience and the alleviation of pain in labor.

REFERENCES

1. O'Driscoll K, Meagher D, Robson M. *Active Management of Labour*, 4th edn. Mosby; 2003.
2. Marmor TR, Krol DM. Labor pain management in the United States: Understanding patterns and the issue of choice. *Am J Obstet Gynecol* 2002; 186: S173–80.
3. Lowe NK. Differences in first and second stage labor pain between nulliparous and multiparous women. *J Psychosom Obstet Gynaecol* 1992; 13: 243–53.
4. Astbury J. Labour pain: the role of childbirth education, information and expectation. In: Peck C, Wallace M, eds. *Problems in Pain*. London: Pergamon; 1980: 245–52.
5. Connolly AM, Pancheri P, Lucchetti, *et al.* Labor as a psychosomatic condition: a study on the influence of personality on self-reported anxiety and pain. In: Pancheri P, Zighella L, eds. *Clinical Psychoneuroendocrinology in Reproduction*. London: Academic Press; 1978: 369–79.
6. Lowe NK. Individual variation in childbirth pain. *J Psychosom Obstet Gynaecol* 1987; 7: 183–92.
7. Reading AE, Cox DN. Psychosocial predictors of labor pain. *Pain* 1985; 22: 309–15.
8. Waldenstrom U, Bergmann V, Vasell G. The complexity of labor pain: experiences of 278 women. *J Psychosom Obstet Gynaecol* 1996; 17: 215–28.
9. Rowlands S, Permezel M. Physiology of pain in labour. *Baillieres Clin Obstet Gynaecol* 1998; 12: 347–62.
10. Enkin M, Keirse MJNC, Neilson J, *et al.* Control of pain in labor. In: *A Guide to Effective Care in Pregnancy and Childbirth*, 3rd edn. Oxford: Oxford University Press; 2000.
11. Bricker L, Lavender T. Parenteral opioids for labor pain relief: A systematic review. *Am J Obstet Gynecol* 2002; 186: S94–109.
12. Mayberry LJ, Clemmens D, De A. Epidural analgesia side effects, co-interventions, and care of women during childbirth: a systematic review. *Am J Obstet Gynecol* 2002; 186: S81–93.
13. Liebermann E, O'Donoghue C. Unintended effects of epidural analgesia on labor: a systematic review. *Am J Obstet Gynecol* 2002; 186: S31–68.
14. Leighton B, Halpern SH. The effects of epidural analgesia on labor, maternal, and neonatal outcomes. *Am J Obstet Gynecol* 2002; 186: S69–77.
15. Lowe NK. The nature of labor pain. *Am J Obstet Gynecol* 2002; 186: S16–24.
16. Waters DC. *Just take it out.* Mt Vernon, IL: Topiary Publishing; 1998.
17. Simkin P, O'Hara M. Nonpharmacological relief of pain during labor: systematic reviews of five methods. *Am J Obstet Gynecol* 2002; 186: S131–59.
18. Smith CA, Collins CT, Cyna AM, Crowther CA. Complementary and alternative therapies for pain management in labour. *Cochrane Database Syst Rev* 2003; (2): CD003521. DOI: 10.1002/14651858.
19. Simkin P. Just another day in a woman's life? Women's long-term perceptions of their first birth experience. Part I. *Birth* 1991; 18: 203–10.
20. Simkin P. Just another day in a woman's life? Women's long-term perceptions of their first birth experience. Part II. *Birth* 1991; 19: 64–81.
21. Hodnett ED. Pain and women's satisfaction with the experience of childbirth: a systematic review. *Am J Obstet Gynecol* 2002; 186: S160–72.
22. Lavender T, Alfirevic Z, Walkinshaw S. Partogram action line study: a randomised trial. *Br J Obstet Gynaecol* 1998; 105(9): 976–80.
23. Lavender T, Wallymahmed AH, Walkinshaw SA. Managing labor using partograms with different action lines: a prospective study of women's views. *Birth* 1999; 26(2): 89–96.

19

Prelabor preparation

In spite of convincing evidence that women's expectations and involvement in decision-making are critical to their satisfaction with the childbirth experience,[1] many obstetricians still neglect prelabor preparation as a topic of real interest. Practitioners rather appear to rely on the assumption that everything will turn out okay and, should this prove not to be the case, that there seem to be few problems that cannot be handled with pain medication or cesarean section. Women's preparation for birth is generally left to antenatal classes conducted by self-employed birth educators or institutional physiotherapists. These teachers, however, are mostly far removed from actual childbirth practice. Left to themselves, professional status and job satisfaction suffer greatly. As a result, some birth educators even appear to be in open conflict with practitioners because they have developed little or no common ground. It is difficult to imagine how lessons in such circumstances could be reassuring to childbearing women.

19.1 Antenatal classes

The widespread popularity of antenatal classes attests to the desire of expectant parents for childbirth education and training programs for labor coping strategies. Despite the best of intentions, these classes may be counterproductive because certain expectations about labor support facilities may be roused that are unmet at labor and delivery. Classes vary widely in content, ranging from psychoprophylaxis to yoga, from the use of birth balls to specific breathing and pushing techniques, from reflexology to aromatherapy, and so forth.[2,3] At birth, however, labor room staff frequently turn a blind eye and a deaf ear to what women were taught previously by "outsiders," and then the discrepancy between expectations and practice inevitably spoils women's labor experiences.

> *A mismatch between lessons and practice undermines women's satisfaction with childbirth.*

Independent antenatal classes organized by official health agencies or coordinated by large consumer groups suffer from a loss of credibility when birth educators are unable to state the labor management policy at the hospital and the available support facilities. Information provided in institutional classes will be more in line with actual practice, but antenatal classes in poorly organized centers may be worse than none at all because women are often left even more apprehensive than before. Institutional staff who cannot agree on a common policy of labor management represent the main impediment to improved standards of care, and in such circumstances class information may raise more questions than will be answered. Clearly, prelabor preparation is of paramount importance, but this can be effective only when educators and practitioners concur with an overall birth-plan: *proactive support of labor.*

> *It is only if all care providers concur with and comply with a consistent birth-plan that clear and honest information and instructions can be given and firm promises can be made.*

Parous women prejudiced by adverse previous experiences tend to have closed minds on the subject of labor. They often set the wrong tone in classes with mixed parity. Group attention is then readily distracted by horror stories about individual bad experiences (elsewhere), and will inevitably be directed toward medical complications and artificial deliveries. For obvious reasons we prefer individual birth education, preferably through nursing consultation where ample time is taken for information on normal labor. Visits to these childbirth educators are easily incorporated in antenatal clinics.

19.2 Purpose and practice

The main objective of prelabor preparation is to define the woman's own role in childbirth and to offer her tools to fulfill it.[4] In order to enhance her sense of self-efficacy and confidence in her ability to cope, each childbearing woman must be able to rely on the promise that all efforts and help will be directed to a normal labor and delivery within a reasonable time.

19.2.1 Prelabor education and training

A distinction should be made between the provision of information and training facilities: information on the labor management strategy – and how women themselves play a crucial role in achieving the prize of spontaneous delivery – is preferably given at the individual level. General training programs to teach women how to cope with the exertion and pain of first-stage labor, and how to reinforce the natural expulsive forces at the second stage, are suitable for group training.

19.2.2 Mutual responsibilities

It could easily be overlooked that getting pregnant is primarily a woman's own responsibility, and so is giving birth. Thus, a serious obligation rests on all expectant mothers to be well-prepared for the forthcoming birth. Nulliparas especially should take full advantage of the prelabor educational service on offer, which must be readily available and relevant in content. It is much too late to begin education in the labor and delivery room.

> *Pregnant women should be made aware that childbirth is primarily their responsibility.*

On the other hand, if more than lip service is to be paid to the proposition that education is an essential component of a maternity center with pretensions of high-quality care, then practitioners must cease to regard such facilities as optional extras. All doctors and midwives should subscribe to the importance of women's preparation for labor and delivery, and should be aware of its content. They should actively encourage their patients, as well as the partners, to use the educational services.

> *All care providers should acknowledge the importance of prelabor education, which should be readily available and relevant in content.*

19.3 Personal education

Above all, what is taught must be seen to correspond with actual practice. Therefore, explicit information on the forthcoming birth is best provided by a labor room nurse or midwife who has ongoing practical experience in the maternity center where the woman will give birth. No teacher should be engaged exclusively in this area because this, inevitably, leads to a condition of isolation, which is one of the main reasons why birth educators are virtually ignored by those in positions of greatest influence, the practitioners.

> *Childbirth education is best provided on an individual basis by labor room nurses or midwives who have ongoing experience in the delivery unit in question.*

19.3.1 Individual educational service

Institutional labor room nurses and/or midwives are in the best position to explain the process of birth and the actual care the woman can count on. Being directly involved in birth attendance in the unit in question, they know exactly what they are talking about. No two pregnant women are the same and personal consultation enables birth educators to tailor their information to the individual in understandable language, trying to help each woman to overcome her personal fears and answering her specific questions. They explain the available provisions for labor support and pain relief methods as mentioned in the previous chapter. The woman's preferences and her wishes are put on record in their chart, knowing that labor room staff will honor these, but unrealistic expectations are adjusted to match real practice. The keynote is mutual confidence and the unstinted message is: "We take you seriously."

> *Prelabor education must correspond with actual practice.*

In our hospital, most nulliparas visit the birth educator several times during pregnancy, starting at 12 weeks. Much more time is allotted for these consultations than the usually short visits to the doctor. The first consultation focuses on general health advice. The emotional shifts of pregnancy may be explored, and issues of sexuality and relationship with the spouse or partner may be discussed as well. Education in late pregnancy is focused primarily on labor and delivery but may be expanded with information on breast feeding and smooth postpartum adjustment to new

motherhood. These consultations allow unique opportunities to provide a favorable image of the entire obstetric service to the consumers, and, most importantly, to obtain a meaningful and legally valid informed consent for the integrated labor management strategy, including epidural analgesia if required. Informed consent sought during the throes of labor is meaningless.

> *Personal one-on-one counseling allows meaningful informed consent with the labor management protocol, including additional measures that might be needed such as epidural analgesia.*

19.4 Content

The guiding principle for adequate prelabor preparation is to convince each woman that she has nothing to fear and that she is perfectly capable of giving birth normally. A motivating spirit is consciously nurtured, not only by the birth educators but by all personnel, including doctors, midwives, residents, and sonographers. Black cloud psychology (Chapter 4) must be rigidly avoided.

19.4.1 Prelabor information

Our birth educators aim to provide accurate and reliable information about labor and delivery and the experiences that women will undergo or encounter. The elementary mechanisms of the natural birth process are clearly explained. A sharp distinction is made between induction of labor and treatment of abnormally slow progress after labor has begun spontaneously. The due date is established as a subsidiary item to avoid the pregnant woman directing her expectations toward this date because, if she goes past it, waiting often becomes increasingly difficult. Instead, we emphasize the full-term period, which lasts until 42 weeks. Information includes the relationship of late pregnancy symptoms such as Braxton Hicks contractions to underlying prelabor processes

(Chapter 8), and suggestions for ways of alleviating these symptoms are given. Clear instructions as to when the pregnant woman should contact the maternity unit are essential. The subjective symptoms of the onset of labor are explicitly explained as well as the need for professional confirmation of her provisional diagnosis of labor (Chapter 14). Each woman is taught the principles of the labor management strategy, including the importance of early assessments and early measures to ensure normal progress (Chapter 15). The use of the partogram is explained and how it is utilized to predict time of delivery.

19.4.2 Promises and reassurances

Pain is discussed openly, but a positive sense of self-reliance is consciously nurtured. This is possible only if prelabor information is accompanied by three firm promises:

1. That she will be continuously supported by a well-informed, sympathetic, female, one-on-one companion in labor.
2. That her labor will not be allowed to last more than 12 hours.
3. That epidural analgesia will always be available as soon as she finds it truly necessary.

The first two guarantees alone completely change the face of women's expectations. Taken together they are at the very heart of the matter and in practice they are entirely dependent on each other. In some cases epidural analgesia has an invaluable contribution to make to the management of first labor, but the indication should always be individually assessed (Chapter 18).

> *The subject of pain in childbirth should never be discussed as a separate problem in isolation from all other relevant aspects of labor support and management.*

We strongly advise against a prelabor commitment to epidural analgesia, because such a promise prior to the event implies a tacit confirmation of the premise that the natural pain of labor will be unbearable. Dark cloud psychology is counterproductive and must be avoided at all times. Prelabor preparation should be aimed at reinforcement of women's coping ability and self-confidence. The very guarantees of *proactive support of labor* – which both the woman and the prelabor educator know will be honored at the critical moment – positively increase the woman's threshold for pain and reduce the need for pharmacological pain alleviation measures. If well-informed, most expectant mothers want to deliver their babies by their own efforts in full mental awareness, and do not wish to be deprived of that sense of achievement by intoxication with opioid drugs or adverse effects of epidural block on the course and outcome of their labor and delivery (Chapter 20).

In the authors' hospitals fewer than 10% of all women in labor need and receive epidural analgesia, even though this service is readily available around the clock. Women in our practice who wish to avoid opioid drugs or epidural analgesia are neither misinformed nor martyrs. On the contrary, they are well-prepared and know exactly what to expect during their labor and delivery, and, consequently, they put trust in themselves and in the staff who care for them.

> Proactive support of labor
>
> *The clear policy and prior assurances are in themselves half the work required to avoid pain medication and to achieve a spontaneous and non-traumatic birth.*

Frank and honest prelabor information, including firm assurances, drastically change the outlook of all pregnant women in our practice. Our childbirth educators have yet to meet the first pregnant woman who fundamentally disagrees with the offered plan and who refuses to sign the informed prelabor consent.

19.4.3 Parous rehabilitation

All nulliparas are encouraged to visit the birth educator several times during their pregnancy.

The importance of this service for parous women depends on their obstetric history. If a woman previously gave birth vaginally to a child in good condition, she is likely to be confident with regard to the course and outcome of the forthcoming birth. Even if she underwent an instrument-assisted delivery, a smooth labor and spontaneous delivery are now a near certainty.

If, in contrast, her first labor was a traumatic experience (elsewhere), prelabor education will be primarily an exercise in rehabilitation. The fundamental difference between the first and the next birth should be clearly explained. The main purpose is to convince her of the certainty that her second labor will not be comparable in any way with her first. While her first labor might have needed acceleration, perhaps an epidural, or even an instrument-assisted delivery, the second birth can confidently be expected to proceed smoothly and to be concluded by herself. "Uncritical prelabor commitment to epidural analgesia – to solve a problem that will not occur – undermines the woman's self-confidence even further, no matter how grateful she may appear to be."[4] Incidentally, women who are scheduled for elective surgery because of a uterine scar, a breech presentation, or any reason, are also invited to visit the antenatal educator, who will painstakingly inform them about the procedure and related routines, including postoperative care.

19.5 Prelabor training groups

All educators in our hospital are acquainted with the prelabor training courses on offer in the proximate neighborhood. They restrict their recommendations to those courses that are geared to the institutional provisions and that do not interfere with the principles and practice of *proactive support of labor*. The recommended group training programs – often including partners – attempt to impart skills for coping with the natural pain of labor and may include yoga, psychoprophylaxis, specific breathing patterns, and other labor coping techniques (Chapter 18). Mutual feedback between the independent but affiliated trainers and the institutional educators and practitioners is taken care of on a regular basis so as to prevent mismatches between training programs and actual practice.

19.6 Standard debriefing

Ideally, all women revisit the educators six weeks after delivery to evaluate their childbirth experience. Without exception, women appreciate this opportunity to show their baby and to share their satisfaction or discontent with the care received throughout labor. This debriefing procedure provides invaluable information for personal feedback to individual caregivers (Chapter 27).

> *Continual evaluation of patients' satisfaction is the foundation of* proactive support of labor.

19.7 Summary

- The evidence shows that women generally consider pain and its relief as subsidiary to intensive labor support unless their expectations regarding either are unmet.
- This emphasizes the crucial importance of frank prelabor information, guidance, and training that must correspond with actual practice.
- Prelabor education is best provided on an individual basis through antenatal consultation by nurses or midwives with ongoing experience in the delivery rooms in question.
- Prelabor preparation should be aimed at reinforcement of a woman's sense of self-efficacy and confidence in her ability to cope, and promoting or generating trust in the caregivers.
- Firm promises about labor support, short labor, and if necessary effective pain relief should be made.
- Prelabor preparation is effective only if all providers agree to and comply with a consistent labor management strategy. Modern birth care is

teamwork and effective teamwork necessitates strict adherence to agreements.

REFERENCES

1. Hodnett ED. Pain and women's satisfaction with the experience of childbirth: a systematic review. *Am J Obstet Gynecol* 2002; 186: S160–72.

2. Simkin P, Enkin M. Antenatal classes. In: Chalmers I, Keirse MJNC, Enkin M, eds. *Effective care in pregnancy and childbirth*. Oxford: Oxford University Press; 1998.

3. Smith CA, Collins CT, Cyna AM, Crowther CA. Complementary and alternative therapies for pain management in labour. *Cochrane Database Syst Rev* 2003; (2), CD003521. DOI: 10.1002/14651858.

4. O'Driscoll K, Meagher D, Robson M. *Active Management of Labour*, 4th edn. Mosby; 2003.

20

Medical pain relief revisited

Many investigators have attempted to evaluate the pain of labor, and two findings have consIstently been reported: first, that there is a wide variation in the pain experienced by women; and, second, that the average level of pain experienced by women in labor is high.[1] Nowadays, women, resigned to the routines of customary birth care, increasingly request pain medication. However, the ideal technique for pain relief in labor does not exist despite claims to the contrary made by certain obstetricians and anesthesiologists. In fact, "the strongest arguments in favor of medical pain relief in childbirth with systemic opioid drugs or epidural analgesia are generally advanced by doctors who do not spend much time in the labor rooms themselves."[2] In reality, opiates can make labor and delivery far more unpleasant than it otherwise would have been, while various aspects of the use of epidural analgesia deserve far more serious attention than they usually get.

> The ideal technique for pain relief in labor does not exist.

20.1 Systemic opioid drugs

The opium derivate pethidine (INN) or meperidine (USAN) was first used in labor in the early 1940s and has become the most commonly used analgesic drug in labor worldwide. A recent survey of obstetric anesthetic practice in US hospitals showed that the use of parenteral opioids in labor was 39% to 56%, depending on the number of births per year: 39% if >1500 births, 56% if 500–1500 births, and 50% if <500 births.[3] In the UK the practice is similar, with 38% of women receiving opiates in labor.[4] Pethidine is commonly used either as first-line labor pain medication that may preclude or precede epidural, or as an inferior alternative for epidural analgesia in settings where epidural service is not available around the clock.

20.1.1 Poor effectiveness

Pethidine has the alleged advantages of familiarity, ease of administration (intravenously or intramuscularly) and low cost, but its widespread use in labor is not supported by strong evidence about its effectiveness for pain relief. A systematic review as comprehensive as it is thorough by Bricker and Lavender[5] casts serious doubts: 48 randomized controlled trials were included for meta-analysis; 35 trials compared opioid with opioid, including different opioid agents, dosages, routes, or techniques of administration, and opioid with co-drug added; 11 trials compared intravenous opioid with epidural analgesia, one compared intravenous opioid with paracervical block, and overall only one trial was placebo-controlled.[6] In this double-blind trial comparing pethidine with placebo (n = 224), more women were dissatisfied with pain relief in the placebo group (71% vs. 83%), but the pethidine results were far from impressive. No convincing research evidence indicates a significantly better effectiveness of other, more recently developed opioids, including the μ-opioid agonist remifentanil.[5,7] In all trials comparing opioids with epidural analgesia, the latter is consistently found to be far more effective.

> *Existing evidence provides very limited support for widespread use of opiates for labor pain relief (Evidence level A).*

20.1.2 Adverse maternal side effects

Opiates may cause more discomfort than they relieve. Administration of any opioid drug is invariably associated with troubling side effects, in most publications briefly and euphemistically described as nausea, vomiting, and sedation. The true clinical meaning of these effects in labor was vigorously articulated by O'Driscoll and Meagher:

Some women suffer from intractable nausea and vomiting, sufficient to turn childbirth into a miserable experience. Some become profoundly depressed, introspective, and so overwhelmed with self pity that they lapse eventually into a state of stupor, from which they are roused only by contractions, to make aimless protests and demand more and more drugs, until . . . a vicious circle is established. Some become [downright stoned,] disorientated and so confused that they are unable to cooperate with their attendants, especially during the second stage of labor, when cooperation is essential if spontaneous delivery is to be achieved. . . . In practice, many women in labor are deeply intoxicated . . . and likely to suffer from a hangover [and sometimes even partial retrograde amnesia], a most undesirable sequel to such a joyous occasion as the birth of a first child. All these adverse effects may follow even a small dose of pethidine given to a person who has had no previous exposure to hard drugs.[2]

> *"Giving birth represents a unique and joyous experience of which mothers should not be deprived by intoxication with opioid drugs."[2]*

Opiates may also pose dangerous medical risks to mothers. All opiates aggravate the already increased gastric acid secretion and decreased gastrointestinal motility during labor.[8] This results in an increased risk of regurgitation and pulmonary aspiration in the unforeseen event of general anesthesia for emergency cesarean section, afterbirth problems, surgical repair of fourth-degree lacerations, and so on.[3] Indeed, "there is a gray area between anesthetics and obstetrics into which not a few disasters of childbirth fall."[2]

20.1.3 Confusing fetal assessment

All opiates readily cross the placenta and reduce fetal heart rate beat-to-beat variability (Chapter 24), simulating an unreassuring fetal status. This may inadvertently lower the threshold for cesarean delivery.

20.1.4 Neonatal hazards of opiates

Opiates build up in the fetus because the neonatal half-life of opioids is considerably longer than the maternal half-life – for instance, the half-life of pethidine is 15–23 hours in the child versus 3–6 hours in the mother.[9,10] This may lead to neonatal respiratory depression, causing serious hypoventilation in the critical minutes to hours after birth.[11–14] Other undesirable effects are decreased neonatal alertness, lower neurobehavioral scores, inhibition of suckling, and a delay in effective feeding.[15–21]

Neonatal respiratory depression from pethidine can be reversed by naloxone (a specific opiate antagonist) administered shortly after birth,[22] but there is no agreement whether naloxone should be given routinely or only in the presence of clinically evident neonatal respiratory depression.[23,24] Some neonatologists caution against routine and indiscriminate use of naloxone immediately after birth because this may distract from the priorities of airway management and adequate oxygenation. More importantly, the adverse effect of opioids on neonatal respiration and neurobehavior lasts significantly longer than the naloxone reversal, which has been shown to be transient,[14] and there is serious potential to miss hazardous neonatal hypoventilation a few hours after birth when the naloxone has worn off.[4]

> *The most hazardous effects of opioids in labor are on the child.*

The critical question remains whether opioids, however small the dose, are totally safe for the child.[3] This concern holds true for any opium derivative used in labor. We wonder how many parturients, if honestly informed, would consent to opioid drugs. In our hospital, none.

20.1.5 Long-term effects

An extremely worrying aspect of the use of opiates during labor is the concept of genetic imprinting at birth for self-destructive behavior such as suicide and hard-drug addiction in later life.[25,26] A Swedish study of known opiate addicts and control siblings showed that a significant proportion of mothers of subjects who subsequently became hard-drug addicts had received opiates in labor.[27] The risk of becoming an addict was confirmed after controlling for confounding variables. When the subjects were matched with their own siblings, the estimated relative risk was 4.7 (95% CI 1.8–12.4, p = 0.002) for three administrations of opioid in labor compared with no drugs. This alarming observation was confirmed in a cohort study of drug abusers in North America.[28] For obvious reasons, a prospective trial to confirm these findings is unlikely to be undertaken.

> *Intrauterine exposure to opioids might lead to a 5-fold increase in self-destructive behavior and hard-drug addiction in later life (Evidence level B).*

20.1.6 Opioids and co-drugs

A number of co-drugs, such as sedatives, tranquilizers, and antiemetics are widely used, in the idle hope that they might enhance the pain-relieving effect of pethidine or antagonize its undesirable effects. None has proved successful and data on neonatal effects are lacking.[5] Although promethazine might reduce some side effects of opioids, it is associated with profound sedation, which is helpful in the treatment of a tenacious false start (Chapter 14) but totally unacceptable in labor; women in labor should keep their heads clear.

20.1.7 PCA with remifentanil

Intravenous patient-controlled analgesia (PCA) with short-acting remifentanil is a new approach in systemic opioid analgesia during labor.[29–32] Parturients self-dose the drug by controlling the IV infusion pump, which allows top-ups with lockout times to prevent overdose. The apparent benefits that accrue from PCA seem to derive at least as much from women's sense of self-control as from the direct analgesic effect of the drug itself. On the basis of limited and small studies, remifentanil has been claimed to be far more effective than pethidine for pain relief in labor, but like all opiates it may cause severe nausea, heavy sedation, and above all maternal respiratory depression.[27,30–32] The clear advantage of remifentanil over pethidine is its short half-life, so that the short-term adverse effects wear off within 10 minutes. It must be stressed, however, that the safety profile of remifentanil in labor has not been established and the overt short-term side effects, such as loss of mental acuity, are at least as worrying as those of pethidine.[29–33] The respiratory depressant effect on the mothers is most troublesome and mandates continuous respiratory supervision or pulse oximetry and stand-by oxygen supplementation and mask ventilation facilities. Remifentanil also crosses the placenta, which may lead to neonatal respiratory depression, whereas other neonatal and long-term potential hazards due to imprinting at birth are still unevaluated.[34,35] In conclusion, there are insufficient data so far to support the widespread use of this form of analgesia in labor. Use should be restricted to selected cases only, where epidural analgesia turns out to be ineffective or where an epidural is counterproductive or contraindicated, such as in women approaching full dilatation or in patients with blood clotting diseases.

> *PCA with remifentanil is no real competitor for epidural analgesia and its short- and long-term hazards have been insufficiently explored and are likely to equal or surpass those of pethidine.*

20.1.8 Balancing the trade-offs

The truth of the matter is that it is practically impossible to administer enough opioids systemically to effectively relieve the woman's labor pain without introducing serious negative effects on both mother and child. The pain-relieving effect of pethidine is so dubious and the list of adverse effects and hidden dangers of systemic opioids is so formidable that the best advice is to ban pethidine from the labor and delivery room completely and to restrict use of remifentanil to strictly selected cases only. Alternative methods of relief – prelabor preparation, personal support, comfort measures, control of labor duration and, if necessary, use of epidural block – offer much brighter and safer prospects of success. The better are the conduct and care of labor, the less is the need for systemic opioid drugs.

> *The disadvantages and potential dangers of systemic opioids in labor outweigh the seeming advantages to such a degree that the use of opiates should best be discontinued during labor.*

20.2 Epidural pain management

Although the overall policy of *proactive support of labor* effectively reduces requests for pain relief, some women, for a variety of reasons, will desire or need, and subsequently experience, great benefits from epidural analgesia. This technique affords complete relief of labor pain in all but a few cases and has the additional advantage that it is not associated with any of the side effects of pethidine; the mother retains her mental acuity and the baby is alert at birth.

20.2.1 Popularity

Because epidural analgesia dramatically changes the degree of medical intervention and maternal–fetal surveillance required, this technique has garnered both advocates and opponents of its use. As a consequence, rates vary widely, and are as high as 98% in some hospitals,[36] or as low 8% in the authors' hospital (P.R., A.F.), despite 24-hour availability of epidural service (Chapter 29). In the USA, overall epidural rates have been estimated to be as high as 50%,[37] but rates may vary substantially between hospitals even within the same region, indicating that other factors are at work than patient requests. In some institutes, anesthesiologists have managed to gain access to prenatal classes where they preach the wonders of epidural block and usually say little or nothing about the risks of this invasive procedure or its possible adverse effects on labor outcome. Moreover, the question remains whether high rates of epidural analgesia are really based on patients' preferences or rather on the advantages of convenience for the caregivers, as epidural may easily serve as a substitute for intensive personal labor support.

> *Twenty-four-hour access to epidural service is imperative for any hospital with pretensions of providing high-quality care, but high rates of its use may actually reflect low standards of labor support.*

20.2.2 Effectiveness of epidural block

Although none of the numerous epidural studies has assessed its impact on childbirth satisfaction or any other psychological outcome, the potential benefits are self-evident in selected cases: few sights are more impressive than the instant resolution of maternal distress that follows a successful epidural block. Unfortunately, this does not always occur. There are connective-tissue bands that form septae within the lumbar epidural space, whose presence helps explain cases of disappointing windows or unanesthetized unilateral areas despite proper epidural placement.[38,39] This occurs not infrequently and women should be told that this might happen. Overall, 85–95% of women rate their pain relief as good to excellent.[40,41] Conversely, in 5–15% of women epidural analgesia proves inadequate. A mismatch between a woman's expectations of pain-free labor and the disappointing effect may further hamper feasible labor coaching and precipitate requests for cesarean delivery as a result.

> *Epidural analgesia is generally effective in the alleviation of labor pain, but there are several underestimated drawbacks as well.*

20.2.3 Potential hazards of epidural analgesia

Placing an epidural block is a highly invasive procedure, entering the space around the dura mater surrounding the spinal cord. Owing to the pregnant woman's altered anatomical state, her restlessness during contractions, and the pregnancy-related swelling of the epidural venous plexus, the procedure can be technically challenging, especially in obese women. The most common complication involves accidental entry of the cerebrospinal space, which is estimated to occur in 2% of all epidural punctures.[42] The resultant leakage of cerebrospinal fluid results in severe, often incapacitating headache which may last for several days. This usually requires a second puncture after delivery to apply a blood patch to stop the leakage. However, if the initial spinal tap is not recognized, spinal injection of the anesthetic agent in the amount meant for

epidural analgesia results in acute and profound depression of vital functions: circulatory collapse and respiratory arrest. Even though this life-threatening complication is rare and can be effectively prevented by the standard use of small test doses, the very possibility of such a calamity necessitates the stand-by presence of resuscitation and ventilation facilities. Inevitably, because of these precautions, the setting and atmosphere of epidural placement are highly medical, which some women may experience as a disruption of the intimate birthing surrounding.

> *Epidural makes labor much more technology-intensive than it otherwise need be.*

20.2.4 Direct adverse effects

An effect inherent in the epidural technique is vasodilatation from sympathetic blockade and decreased cardiac output, resulting in maternal hypotension and reduced uteroplacental blood flow, which may compromise fetal well-being (Chapter 24). In the supine position, hypotension is compounded by obstructed venous return from uterine compression of the abdominal great veins. Even in the absence of maternal hypotension measured in the woman's arm, uteroplacental blood flow may still be significantly reduced.[39] Despite precautions with IV fluid preloads, hypotension is the most common complication of epidural analgesia, severe enough to require treatment with vasopressors in one-third of women.[43] Women receiving epidural analgesia have a 20-fold increased risk of hypotension compared with those who receive systemic pain medication (RR = 20.09; 95% CI 4.83–83.64).[44]

> *Maternal hypotension and related placental blood flow impairment occur in 30% of patients.*

Other inadvertent effects such as voiding difficulties, nausea, pruritus, and shivering during labor are common, but they are usually mild and only infrequently necessitate treatment.[45] Far more worrying is the 4-fold increased risk of intrapartum maternal fever of at least 38°C related to epidural analgesia (RR = 3.67; CI 2.77–4.86).[44] This occurs in 10–15% of all women with epidural.[46] The mechanism remains unclear. As the epidural origin cannot be distinguished from beginning intrauterine infection, newborns are usually admitted to the neonatal ward for observation and treatment with antibiotics as a precaution, but mostly unnecessarily in retrospect. Apart from undue parental worries and fears, baby and mother are separated for the first days after birth, which are vital for a smooth mother–child bonding. In the great majority of cases, sepsis evaluation turns out to be negative because the intrapartum fever was simply attributable to epidural analgesia and was thus iatrogenic in origin.

> *Epidural increases the incidence of maternal fever and the likelihood of neonatal sepsis evaluation and antibiotic treatment.*

In spite of the advent of newer low-dose epidurals, the extent of impaired motor ability remains a cause for concern. An estimated 20% of women decline to stand up and complain of dizziness or sensation of motor weakness, despite normal blood pressure and motor ability tests.[47] For this reason, the appropriateness of the term "light" epidural is called into question.[45] The term "walking" epidural is also misleading and should be discarded, because evidence shows that a large proportion of women (34–85%) who receive what has been called a "light" or "walking" epidural do not spend much time out of bed at all.[45] Possible reasons for this general finding include that the motor block interferes with ability and stability, and that opiates given by the epidural route may contribute to drowsiness and fatigue. Furthermore, women are confined to bed by tubes and cords connecting them to various devices, and nurses have other responsibilities and are not available to assist with ambulation. Finally, caregivers may

simply discourage ambulation, as anesthesia protocols in many labor and delivery units prohibit women from getting out of bed because of safety issues and liability concerns. Women should be informed of this.

> *The terms "light" and "walking" epidural are misleading and should be discontinued.*

20.2.5 Indirect adverse effects

Several outstanding systematic reviews on epidural analgesia have been published recently, using varying study inclusion criteria for meta-analysis and addressing various co-interventions and unintended outcome variables.[44,46,48] The evidence is consistent about the following adverse outcomes:

- Epidural analgesia prolongs the first stage of labor.
- Epidural analgesia increases the need for oxytocin.
- Epidural analgesia turns natural labor into a fully medicalized event.
- Epidural analgesia prolongs the second stage of labor.
- Epidural analgesia increases instrumental delivery rates.
- Epidural analgesia increases third- and fourth-degree perineal lacerations.

> *Epidural analgesia decreases the likelihood of spontaneous delivery (Evidence level A).*

Epidural block increases the odds of vacuum or forceps delivery, but there is still an ongoing debate whether epidural analgesia affects cesarean section rates. Many studies have noted an association with an increased likelihood of cesarean delivery, but results are heavily practice-based. The crux of the discussion is whether the differences in cesarean rates observed are due to the epidural itself or to other differences between women who receive epidural analgesia and women who do not. One pair of systematic reviewers simply concludes that there is no effect, because no statistically significant differences were found.[48] The latest Cochrane meta-analysis, however, showed a 42% increase in the relative risk of cesarean section for fetal distress in the epidural group, with a confidence interval very close to statistical significance (RR = 1.42; 95% CI 0.99–2.03), but failed to detect an increase in cesareans for dystocia.[44] The Boston group found a strong association with increased overall cesarean rates, but stated that the available data were insufficient to reach definitive conclusions.[46] What is clear, though, is that epidural block prolongs first-stage labor, but this can be prevented by proper use of oxytocin.[49] A critical look at the external validity of the randomized trials[50] suggests that cesarean rates need not be increased by epidural analgesia, provided labor is augmented with appropriately high doses of oxytocin as advocated in Chapter 17.

It should be noted that the conclusions of the cited systematic reviews were based on mixed parity data. For nulliparous labors, the findings might be quite different. Clearly, there is an urgent need for more research. Moreover, faced with the virtual ban on VBAC, each possible additional cesarean delivery in first labor related to epidural should actually be multiplied by two, because of the routine repeat cesareans in next pregnancies. For now, the overall conclusion must be that existing evidence does not rule out a causal relationship between epidural analgesia in labor and cesarean delivery, especially in inappropriately augmented nulliparous labors.

> *Epidural analgesia associated with low-dose oxytocin augmentation increases the odds of cesarean.*

Drugs used for epidural block include local anesthetics and opiates. Several trials comparing low and standard doses have failed to find differences in cesarean odds. Readers are encouraged to consult the systematic review by Lieberman and O'Donoghue, which is in our view the most balanced treatise to date on unintended effects of epidural analgesia during labor.[46]

20.2.6 Economic costs

The incremental expected cost to society of providing routine epidural analgesia in labor is substantial. On top of direct expenses, which have been calculated to be approximately USD 338 per patient in 1998 values,[51] the cost must be taken into account of increased neonatal admission rates, surgical repairs of third- and fourth-degree lacerations, and possibly increased cesarean rates in the index labors plus the related repeat surgery in following pregnancies.

> *The direct and indirect economic costs of epidural analgesia in labor are substantial.*

20.2.7 Prejudicing nursing labor support

An important issue that has attracted much less attention so far than it should have is the impact of epidural analgesia on nursing and caregiving procedures. Use of epidural involves a complex cascade of technical nursing duties. It is typically recommended that maternal blood pressure be assessed frequently, as often as every 2–5 minutes during the first 30 minutes and every 15 minutes thereafter with stabilization, and then continued frequently throughout the remainder of labor.[52] IV fluid loads must be adjusted to blood pressure readings. Continuous electronic fetal monitoring is another standard component of intrapartal care with epidurals. Normal supportive care may be severely jeopardized when nurses are immersed in these technical activities. On many maternity centers with high epidural rates, the ability to provide quality nursing care for all women, including those who do not choose epidural analgesia, becomes a major concern. Nurse work-sampling studies in centers with high epidural rates revealed that actual labor support activities were minimal compared with time spent on other unit-level activities.[53–55] Continuous and supportive nursing activities enhance a woman's sense of control and satisfaction with her childbirth experience and are implicated in decreased cesarean delivery rates (Chapter 16). It seems, unfortunately, that many maternity centers have already reached the point at which the labor support role must be rediscovered, and that nurses and other birth attendants must be newly trained in this important task.

> *Use of epidural involves a complex cascade of technical monitoring duties, increasing the workloads of nurses and midwives, and distracting their attention from their labor support role.*

20.2.8 General considerations

Clearly, there is an urgent need to define a joint nursing/midwifery and medical approach to epidural analgesia, heeding the following considerations advanced by O'Driscoll *et al.*:[2]

- Epidural analgesia has an invaluable contribution to make to nulliparous labor, but, equally importantly, the relative contribution to labor in parous women is much less.
- Epidural service should be available 24/7, but:
  - A prelabor commitment to epidural analgesia should not be made.
  - An epidural should never be given until a diagnosis of labor is firmly established.
  - An epidural should never be used as a substitute for supportive care.
  - An epidural should never be used as a substitute for corrective action if labor is slow.
  - An epidural should never be used as a cover for prolonged labor.

The fundamental distinction between nulliparous labor and parous labor is the continuous thread through the pages of this manual and this issue is of particular importance in the context of epidural analgesia. High use of epidural analgesia

in parous women stems from the mistaken belief that a valid comparison can be drawn between a first and a subsequent labor.[2] A woman who has had an unpleasant first experience, during which she may or may not have had epidural analgesia, frequently seeks a prior commitment on the next occasion because she fears that prolongation of labor is likely to be repeated. However, there are no grounds for this assumption. Obstetricians would serve the interests of a parous woman best were they to address her fears with a clear explanation of the essential differences between a first and a second birth (Chapter 13). Moreover, especially if her first labor ended with a cesarean delivery, epidural analgesia acts to increase the risk of a ruptured uterus, because pain has an important warning function in this regard. Indeed, epidural analgesia has emerged as an important factor in the late recognition of this calamity and this late recognition effectively slashed the number of trials of labors after cesarean (Chapter 2).

> *Epidural analgesia in parous labor should be approached with specific reservations.*

A readily available epidural service is a prerequisite to high-quality maternity care, but so is individualization of its use. The fundamental objection against a prelabor commitment was explained in the previous chapter (section 19.4.2): a promise prior to the event confirms a tacit premise that the natural pain of labor will be an intolerable experience. There are two other reasons why an expectant approach to epidural should be practiced. Firstly, the reaction of each individual to the actual experience of first labor can scarcely be foretold, perhaps least of all by the woman herself; and secondly, the duration of first labor cannot be predicted.

> *Epidural analgesia should not be used on a routine basis.*

20.2.9 Timing of epidural block

Appropriate timing is critical. In some maternity centers an epidural is sometimes given even before a firm diagnosis of labor is established. The result may be that, after much confusion, a cesarean section is eventually performed on a woman who was not in labor. This consideration should preclude the use of epidural during priming/induction with prostaglandins before a firm commitment to delivery is established.

> *Timing of beginning and ending epidural analgesia is critical for expert labor management.*

Sometimes an epidural is given too late, when the cervix is close to full dilatation. The result is that the beneficial effects in the first stage are more than offset by the adverse effects in the second stage, the beginning of which is fully obscured by epidural analgesia (Chapter 11). It is for this reason that we advise discontinuation of epidural medication once full dilatation is to be expected within an hour. Commencement of active pushing is best delayed until the natural expulsion reflex is activated or no longer suppressed (Chapter 9, section 9.3.2).[56]

20.2.10 Improper use

In too many maternity centers epidural analgesia is used as a palliative measure when labor is prolonged, as if duration of labor in itself were not important provided the mother suffers no pain. This is a serious misconception. Numerous risks increase strongly with prolonged labor, including fetal distress, aspiration of meconium, intrauterine infection, neonatal sepsis, instrumental or cesarean delivery, birth injuries, perineal damage, cesarean section-related complications, and so forth. Moreover, an epidural does not prevent the uterus from exhaustion after an extended duration of labor, leading to a refractory uterus resistant to aug-

mentation or to the uterus reacting with hypertonia between contractions, which further compromises fetal well-being (Chapter 8). Epidural analgesia is pain management, not a therapeutic treatment for labor disorders. There is only one exception: cervical edema in a panicked woman who bears down prematurely long before full dilatation has been reached (Chapter 21).

> *Epidural analgesia is pain relief, not therapy for a prolonged labor.*

Good maternity care requires an overall plan and mutual respect between physicians, midwives, and nurses. Doctors in particular should admit that the standards of care in labor are determined almost entirely by the efforts of well-motivated nurses and midwives. An obstetrician who appears critical of a nurse/midwife simply because occasionally a woman complains during a post-delivery visit that she had not had timely and adequate pain relief strongly undermines the team spirit between caregivers, with detrimental overall consequences. O'Driscoll *et al.* drily observed: "Doctors are seldom present to witness the particular circumstances, and it is all too easy to pose as being more humane, after the event. No personal commitment is required for this mode of behavior."[2]

20.2.11 Case selection for epidural

Pain management should always be individualized and discussed in the context of all other aspects of labor care and modalities of pain relief. In our hospital (P.R., A.F.), fewer than 10% of all parturient women request epidural analgesia. Subject to the above reservations, there are three broad categories of patients who derive most benefit from epidural analgesia:

1. Nulliparas who are so disturbed at the very prospect of labor that they are already unduly upset at the point of admission. Their number is very limited thanks to adequate prelabor preparation (Chapter 19).

2. Nulliparas who, despite an initial appearance of composure, become unduly upset soon afterward. Their number is very limited thanks to the high level of nursing support (Chapter 16).
3. Nulliparas who are transferred too late from home, in an attempt to retrieve their battered composure. Their number is closely related to the duration of labor as tolerated by midwives working out-of-hospital (Chapter 26).

20.2.12 Informed consent

Women's preferences and choices should be honored. That is to presume that the above information about the trade-offs of epidural analgesia in labor has been provided without any pressure for or against. Antenatal visits to the birth educator, as explained in the previous chapter, ensure that each woman, as she approaches childbirth, has access to all relevant information and becomes familiar with all pain-related issues and options, including epidural analgesia. Giving information once labor has already started is much too late to acquire valid informed consent, which the anesthetist will justifiably demand when summoned to place the epidural catheter. Women should be informed well in advance and have access to this information again during labor, as part of an open and respectful informed consent process oriented toward women rather than toward professional liability concerns.[1]

> *Women should be informed about all the evidence based pros and cons of epidural analgesia, well in advance of childbirth.*

20.3 Summary

- Pain management should always be considered in the context of all other aspects of labor support and good labor management.
- A far more critical approach to the whole question of pharmacological pain relief is highly desirable.

- The pain-relieving effect of opiates is so dubious, and the list of adverse effects and dangers is so formidable, that the best advice should be to ban them from the labor and delivery room completely.
- Various aspects of the use of epidural analgesia deserve far more serious consideration than they usually get.
- Epidural analgesia has an invaluable contribution to make to nulliparous labor, but, equally importantly, the relative contribution to labor in parous women is much less.
- Epidural analgesia should not be used on a routine basis and never as a cover for prolonged labor or as a substitute for intensive nursing care and support.

REFERENCES

1. Caton D, Corry MP, Frigoletto FD, *et al.* The nature and management of labor pain: Executive summary. *Am J Obstet Gynecol* 2002; 186: S1–15.
2. O'Driscoll K, Meagher D, Robson M. *Active Management of Labour*, 4th edn. New York: Mosby; 2003.
3. Hawkins JL, Beaty BR. Update on obstetric anesthesia practices in the US. *Anesthesiology* 1999; 91: A1060.
4. Chamberlain G, Wraight A, Steer P. *Pain and Its Relief in Childbirth. The results of a National Survey Conducted by the National Birthday Trust.* Edinburgh: Churchill Livingstone; 1993.
5. Bricker L, Lavender T. Parenteral opioids for labor pain relief: A systematic review. *Am J Obstet Gynecol* 2002; 186: S94–109.
6. De Kornfield D, Pearson JW, Lasagna L. Methotrimeprazine in the treatment of labor pain. *N Engl J Med* 1964; 270: 391–4.
7. Paech M. Newer techniques of labor analgesia. *Anesthesiol Clin North America* 2003; 21(1): 1–17.
8. Nimmo WS, Wilson J, Prescott LF. Narcotic analgesics and delayed gastric emptying during labour. *Lancet* 1975; 1: 890–3.
9. Box D, Cochran D. Safe reduction in the administration of naloxone to newborn infants. Royal College of Paediatricians and Child Health, Fourth Spring Meeting, York, UK, April 10–13, 2000. *Arch Dis Child* 2000; 82(Suppl 1): A31.

10. Caldwell J, Wakile LA, Notarianni LJ, *et al.* Maternal and neonatal disposition of pethidine in childbirth – a study using quantitative gas chromatography–mass spectrometry. *Life Sci* 1978; 22(7): 589–96.

11. Wiener PC, Hogg MI, Rosen M. Neonatal respiration, feeding and neurobehavioural state. Effects of intrapartum bupivacaine, pethidine and pethidine reversed by naloxone. *Anaesthesia* 1979; 34(10): 996–1004.

12. Schnider SM, Moya F. Effects of Meperidine on the newborn infant. *Am J Obstet Gynecol* 1964; 89: 1009–15.

13. Brice JE, Moreland TA, Walker CH. Effects of pethidine and its antagonists on the newborn. *Arch Dis Child* 1979; 54(5): 356–61.

14. Rooth G, Lysikiewicz A, Huch R, Huch A. Some effects of maternal pethidine administration on the newborn. *Br J Obstet Gynaecol* 1983; 90(1): 28–33.

15. Kron RE, Stein M, Goddard KE. Newborn sucking behaviour affected by obstetric medication. *Paediatrics* 1966; 37: 1012–16.

16. Hodgkinson R, Bhatt M, Wang CN. Double-blind comparison of the neurobehaviour of neonates following the administration of different doses of meperidine to the mother. *Can Anaesth Soc J* 1978; 25(5): 405–11.

17. Belsey EM, Rosenblatt DB, Lieberman BA, *et al.* The influence of maternal analgesia on neonatal behaviour: I. Pethidine. *Br J Obstet Gynaecol* 1981; 88(4): 398–406.

18. Righard L, Alade MO. Effect of delivery room routines on success of first breast-feed. *Lancet* 1990; 336(8723): 1105–7.

19. Nissen E, Lilja G, Matthiesen AS, *et al.* Effects of maternal pethidine on infants' developing breast feeding behaviour. *Acta Paediatr* 1995; 84(2): 140–5.

20. Matthews MK. The relationship between maternal labour analgesia and delay in the initiation of breastfeeding in healthy neonates in the early neonatal period. *Midwifery* 1989; 5: 3–10.

21. Crowell MK, Hill PD, Humenick SS. Relationship between obstetric analgesia and time of effective breast feeding. *J Nurse Midwifery* 1994; 39(3): 150–6.

22. Bonta BW, Gagliardi JV, Williams V, Warshaw JB. Naloxone reversal of mild neurobehavioral depression in normal newborn infants after routine obstetric analgesia. *J Pediatr* 1979; 94(1): 102–5.

23. Welles B, Belfrage P, de Chateau P. Effects of naloxone on newborn infant behavior after maternal analgesia with pethidine during labor. *Acta Obstet Gynecol Scand* 1984; 63(7): 617–19.

24. Wiener PC, Wallace S. Effects of naloxone on pethidine-induced neonatal depression. *Br Med J* 1980; 280 (6209): 252.

25. Jacobson B, Eklund G, Hamberger L, *et al.* Perinatal origin of adult self-destructive behavior. *Acta Psychiatr Scand* 1987; 76: 364–71.

26. Jacobson B, Nyberg K, Eklund G, Bygdeman M, Rydberg U. Obstetric pain medication and eventual adult amphetamine addiction in offspring. *Acta Obstet Gynecol Scand* 1988; 67: 677–82.

27. Jacobson B, Nyberg K, Gronbladh L, *et al.* Opiate addiction in adult offspring through possible imprinting after obstetric treatment. *BMJ* 1990; 301 (6760): 1067–70.

28. Nyberg K, Buka SL, Lipsitt LP. Perinatal medication as a potential risk factor for adult drug abuse in a North American cohort. *Epidemiology* 2000; 11: 715–16.

29. Thurlow JA, Laxton CH, Dick A, *et al.* Remifentanil by patient-controlled analgesia compared with intramuscular meperidine for pain relief in labour. *Br J Anaesth* 2002; 88(3): 374–8.

30. Evron S, Glezerman M, Sadan O, *et al.* Remifentanil: a novel systematic analgetic for labor pain. *Anesth Analg* 2005; 100(1): 233–8.

31. Blair JM, Dobson GT, Hill DA, *et al.* Patient controlled analgesia for labour: a comparison of remifentanil with pethidine. *Anaesthesia* 2005; 60(1): 22–7.

32. Volikas I, Male D. A comparison of pethidine and remifentanil patient-controlled analgesia in labour. *Int J Obstet Anesth* 2001; 10(2): 86–90.

33. Volmanen P, Akural EI, Raudaskoski T, Alahuhta S. Remifentanil in obstetric analgesia: a dose-finding study. *Anesth Analg* 2002; 94(4): 913–17.

34. Kan RE, Hughes SC, Rosen MA, *et al.* Intravenous remifentanil: placental transfer, maternal and neonatal effects. *Anesthesiology* 1998; 88(6): 1467–74.

35. Mattingly JE, D'Alessio J, Ramanathan J. Effects of obstetric analgesics and anesthetics on the neonate: a review. *Paediatr Drugs* 2003; 5(9): 615–27.

36. Alran S, Sibony O, Oury JF, *et al.* Differences in management and results in term-delivery in nine European referral hospitals: a descriptive study. *Eur J Obstet Gynecol Reprod Biol* 2002; 103: 4–13.

37. Marmor TR, Krol DM. Labor pain management in the United States: Understanding patterns and the issue of choice. *Am J Obstet Gynecol* 2002; 186: S173–80.

38. Blomberg RG, Olsson SS. The lumbar epidural space in patients examined with epiduroscopy. *Anesth Analg* 1998; 68: 157–60.

39. Althaus J, Wax J. Analgesia and anesthesia in labor. *Obstet Gynecol Clin N Am* 2005; 32: 231–44.

40. Kemmerly JR, Lambard WW, Russell RC. Epidural anesthesia performed during labor by obstetricians: outcome analysis. *Prim Care Update Ob Gyns* 1998; 5(4): 197.

41. Cunningham FG, Leveno KJ, Bloom SL, *et al.* Obstetric Anesthesia. In: *Williams Obstetrics*, 22nd edn. New York: McGraw-Hill; 2005: 484.

42. American College of Obstetricians and Gynecologists: Obstetric analgesia and anesthesia. *Practice Bulletin* 36, July 2002.

43. Sharma SK, Sidawi JE, Ramin SM, *et al.* Cesarean delivery: A randomized trial of epidural versus patient-controlled meperidine analgesia during labor. *Anesthesiology* 1997; 87: 487–94.

44. Anim-Somuah M, Smyth R, Howell C. Epidural versus non-epidural or no analgesia in labour. *Cochrane Database Syst Rev* 2005; (4): CD000331.

45. Mayberry LJ, Clemmens D, De A. Epidural analgesia side-effects, co-interventions, and care of women during childbirth: A systematic review. *Am J Obstet Gynecol* 2002; 186: S81–93.

46. Lieberman E, O'Donoghue C. Unintended effects of epidural analgesia during labor: A systematic review. *Am J Obstet Gynecol* 2002; 186: S31–68.

47. Breen T, Shapiro T, Glass B, Foster-Payne D, Oriol N. Epidural anesthesia for labor in an ambulatory patient. *Anesth Analg* 1993; 77: 919–24.

48. Leighton BL, Halpern SH. The effects of epidural analgesia on labor, maternal, and neonatal outcomes: A systematic review. *Am J Obstet Gynecol* 2002; 186: S69–77.

49. Impey L, MacQuillan K, Robson MS. Epidural analgesia need not increase operative delivery rates. *Am J Obstet Gynecol* 2000; 182: 358–63.

50. Kotaska AJ, Klein MC, Liston RM. Epidural analgesia associated with low-dose oxytocin augmentation increases cesarean births: A critical look at the external validity of randomized trials. *Am J Obstet Gynecol* 2006; 194: 809–14.

51. Huang C, Macario A. Economic considerations related to providing adequate pain relief for women in labour: comparison of epidural and intravenous analgesia. *Pharmacoeconomics* 2002; 20(5): 305–18.

52. Cunningham FG, Leveno KJ, Bloom SL, *et al.* Chapter 19: Obstetric Anesthesia. In: *Williams Obstetrics*, 22nd edn. New York: McGraw-Hill; 2005: 483.

53. Cagnon AJ, Waghorn K. Supportive care by maternity nurses: a work sampling study in an intrapartum unit. *Birth* 1996; 23: 1–6.

54. McNiven P, Hodnett E, O'Brian-Pallas LL. Supporting women in labor: a work sampling of the activities of labor and delivery nurses. *Birth* 1992; 19: 3–9.

55. Gale J, Fothergill-Bourbonnais F, Chamberlain M. Measuring nursing support during childbirth. *MCN Am J Matern Child Nurs* 2001; 26: 264–71.

56. Fraser WD, Marcoux S, Krauss I, *et al.* Multicenter, randomized, controlled trial of delayed pushing for nulliparous women in the second stage of labor with continuous epidural analgesia: the PEOPLE (Pushing Early or Pushing Late with Epidural) Study Group. *Am J Obstet Gynecol* 2000; 182(5): 1165–72.

21

Dynamic dystocia unraveled

Dystocia, or failure to progress, is the most frequent indication for operative delivery reported in obstetric databases (Chapter 2). However, this ill-defined classification does not provide any clues for improvement of birth care, so the main purpose of these databases is defeated. Dystocia is not a diagnosis but a symptom and a common pathway of a wide variety of problems encountered in labor. Failure to unravel this complex of birth disorders and subject the separate problems to detailed analysis and diagnosis renders a structured policy for the reduction of excessive operative delivery rates virtually impossible. Interventions should be based on a diagnosis rather than on a symptom. Only a precise diagnosis allows for preemptive measures and specific, causally directed treatment. Diagnosis is the most important single issue in responsible labor care and is critical for meaningful audit of procedures and outcomes (Chapter 27). Cause and effect need to be explored if progress in treatment is to be made.

> *Dystocia, or abnormal progress of labor, is a symptom not a diagnosis.*

The discussion is intentionally limited to labor disorders with a single, normal fetus in vertex presentation; twins, breeches, and abnormal fetal lies such as compound and transverse presentation are not included because these are primary abnormal situations and direct causes of fetal obstruction and related jeopardy. With a vertex presentation, however, there are essentially two main groups of dystocia:

1. Mechanical birth disorders, which involve unfavorable fetopelvic relationships (*passenger–passage*).
2. Dynamic birth disorders, which involve insufficient uterine force in relation to resistance (*the powers*).

Since fetal and pelvic sizes have not changed in recent decades, dynamic dystocia must account for the increasing rates of cesarean delivery seen in recent years. This obvious conclusion is rarely appreciated by conventional birth professionals. One of the many outstanding lessons we have learned from O'Driscoll is that ensuring adequate uterine force not only shortens labor but has the additional effect of isolating mechanical dystocia or obstructed labor as a separate clinical entity that is actually far less prevalent than generally assumed (Chapter 22).

21.1 The spectrum of dynamic labor disorders

Dynamic labor disorders are specific to first births and may arise at various times during labor as distinct clinical types with distinct physical causes. Each type, however, always has one common feature, and that is insufficient force. This is proven time and again by the observation that progress of labor can – almost without exception – be restored with amniotomy and oxytocin, provided these measures are undertaken in time before the myometrium itself becomes exhausted (refractory uterus).

> *Dynamic dystocia is heterogeneous in its manifestation and causation. Cause and effect need to be explored if progress in handling dystocia is to be made.*

Primary ineffective uterine action corresponds with a disorder in the retraction phase, whereas secondary arrest of labor corresponds to a disorder in the wedging phase or in the expulsion stage (Chapter 9). The refractory uterus and hypertonic dystocia are separate and clearly distinct clinical entities within the syndrome of dynamic dystocia (summarized in Table 21.1).

21.2 Primary ineffective labor

Typically, dysfunctional labor presents as a persistent pattern of slow dilatation from the very onset (Fig. 21.1). It is the most common yet least appreciated complication of first labor, occurring in about 25% of all nulliparas. Slow progress is almost exclusively confined to nulliparas in whom the cervix is dilated less than 3 cm at the onset of labor. What many professionals typically take for latent labor is actually primary ineffective labor (Chapters 9, 11). The fallacious concept of the latent phase explains why this condition is often not recognized as a true labor disorder (Chapter 14). This leads to inept (non-)management in slow early labor whereby treatment is started too late and only after the fact. If not treated properly, such a prolonged early labor is strongly associated with adverse labor outcomes.[1,2]

Slow progress in the retraction phase is a purely dynamic problem that originates in suboptimal transformation of the myometrium and/or the cervix, with insufficient uterine force in relation to the cervical resistance as a result (Chapter 8). When judged only by the painfulness and the manual assessment of uterine tone, the uterus appears to

Table 21.1. Distinct types of dynamic dystocia

Clinical manifestation	Physical diagnosis	Fundamental causes
1. Primary ineffective labor	– Insufficient uterine force in relation to cervical resistance	– Suboptimal myometrial and cervical transformation – Adrenergic stress response
2. Secondary protraction or arrest	– Disturbance in the wedging action	– Insufficient transmission of uterine force onto the cervix – True mechanical obstruction (rare)
3. No pushing reflex at full dilatation	– Insufficient descent upon full dilatation	– Insufficient uterine force
4. Arrested expulsion	– Lack of descent, rotation and/or extension	– Insufficient uterine force – Maternal exhaustion – Pushing too early – Ineffective pushing technique
5. Refractory uterus	– Failure to respond to oxytocin – Uterine spastic hypertonia	– Induction – Loss of oxytocin receptors – Exhausted, acidified uterus
6. Hypertonic dystocia	– Uncoordinated contractions – Insufficient uterine relaxation – Fetal distress	– Cytokines production as a result of intrauterine meconium, blood, or pus

contract vigorously, but the contractions are insufficiently coordinated and therefore fail to produce sufficient force on the cervix. Undoubtedly, an adrenergic stress response plays an additional role in many cases (Chapter 7). This is why primary dysfunctional labor occurs more frequently since hospitals have replaced the trusted environment of the woman's home, although this

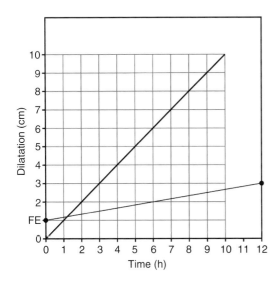

Figure 21.1. Example of untreated primary ineffective labor. FE = full effacement.

consequence is hardly ever recognized by clinicians.

It is of the utmost importance to appreciate that primary, slow progress is specific to first labor; it does not occur in multiparas, except as an iatrogenic result of induction (owing to absent or incomplete prelabor cervical and myometrial transformation) or as a residual result of negative conditioning from inadequate support at the first birth (emotional trauma → adrenergic stress response). Primary ineffective labor has nothing to do with unfavorable fetopelvic relations or fetal obstruction (Chapters 9, 22).

> *Primary ineffective uterine action presents as a persistent pattern of slow dilatation from the very onset of labor. This common problem is specific to first labor.*

21.2.1 Prevalent non-management

Failure to confirm an early diagnosis of labor results in failure to recognize primary ineffective labor (Chapter 14). Hesitant and insecure birth attendants do not dare declare a woman who has regular contractions and a fully effaced cervix to be in labor. Such muddling indecision circumvents diagnosis and blocks rational conduct. Other care providers, who rightly accept labor, are reluctant to rupture the membranes in the alleged "latent phase" and use loose, inaccurate criteria for normal labor such as painful and "strong" contractions on palpation instead of progress. This misapprehension leaves them one step behind from the outset if labor is too slow. Traditional midwives trust nature as long as possible and some primarily resort to herbal tea, foot massage, and the bathtub when labor gets tough. Such dilly-dallying is typically paired with refraining from "disruptive" vaginal examinations to assess progress, let alone rupturing the membranes. At first glance all this seems woman-friendly but it is a waste of time and energy. Four hours or more is much too long to discover that labor has hardly progressed. At the end of the day, the slowly progressing mother pays with a cesarean or instrument-assisted delivery. The alleged maximum chance for a "natural" birth, thanks to endless patience, actually denies the woman a fair chance of a spontaneous delivery.

21.2.2 Early recognition and correction

Slow progress should lead to early diagnosis and prompt treatment, long before the woman begins drifting toward prolonged labor and exhaustion. The uterus and cervix of a woman in labor are so predictably responsive to stimulation with amniotomy (Fig. 21.2) and oxytocin (Fig. 21.3) that, whenever the rate of dilatation does not accelerate sharply after such treatment, the diagnosis of labor is almost certainly wrong. "Such cases are commonplace in practices where little attention is paid to the diagnosis of labor."[3]

> *Primary ineffective uterine action is by far the most frequent and most underrated complication of first labor. It should be resolved with early diagnosis and prompt treatment.*

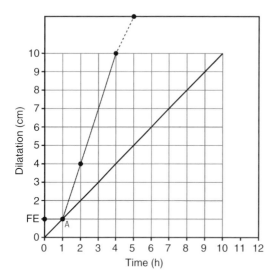

Figure 21.2. Early recognition and treatment of primary ineffective labor. A = amniotomy.

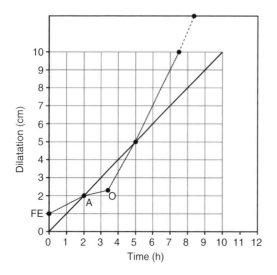

Figure 21.3. Primary ineffective labor corrected by amniotomy (A) and oxytocin treatment (O).

21.2.3 Appropriate management

Strict diagnosis and sticking to the effect criterion are far more constructive and preventive. Early

augmentation of slow labor is safe and effective (Chapter 17). Amniotomy enhances the production and release of PGE_2 in the cervix and the myometrium. In many cases this measure alone will normalize labor (Fig. 21.2) and, if not, additional oxytocin will almost certainly accomplish this (Fig. 21.3). The moment labor begins spontaneously, oxytocin receptors are widespread and the binding of oxytocin to those receptors enhances the production and release of PGE_2 in the myometrium – precisely where it must act. In sluggish early labor the formation of the uterine conduction system is not yet adequate or complete (Chapter 8), but oxytocin quickly overcomes this. Initially ineffective contractions are greatly improved by early stimulation through quick completion of formation of the myometrial gap junctions. Now uterine contractions become orchestrated and thus efficient (Chapter 8). The effect is a normal dilatation rate (Fig. 21.3).

21.2.4 Proactive support of labor

Good obstetrics is not confined to technical measures for early detection and correction of slow labor. The overall plan for conduct and care during pregnancy and labor is specifically directed to the prevention of this common birth disorder:

- The functional transformation of the cervix and myometrium is given the maximum chance. Thus, the spontaneous onset of labor is awaited. Labor is induced only on the relatively rare occasion of a strong medical necessity (Chapter 23).
- "Black cloud psychology" (Chapter 4) resulting in stimulation of adrenergic stress responses must be carefully avoided. Therefore, discouraging terms such as "trial of labor" should be deleted from our vocabulary and a confident attitude and positive motivation for normal birth should continually be nurtured.
- All women are well prepared for labor and policies are consistent, clear, and rigidly enforced.
- Every effort should be made to ensure that the birth environment is nonstressful and empowering, affords privacy, communicates respect, and is not characterized by routine measures and

interventions that add stress and risks without clear benefit.

- Personal attention and continuous support are guaranteed for the entirety of labor (Chapter 16).

> Proactive support of labor *implies much more than just acceleration of early-presenting slow progress.*

Empathetic care is a prerequisite, but the care provider cannot simply and meekly share the woman's ordeal. Indeed, clinical vigilance and measures to assure normality are equally import-ant. That is why:

- The diagnosis of labor is objectively verified and the caregiver should pledge that the mother-to-be will hold her baby in her arms within 12 hours. A latent phase of labor is denied (Chapter 11).
- Throughout labor the utmost effort toward clarity is maintained. Nothing is as demoralizing for the parturient woman as ongoing pain without a useful effect and no end in sight. Thus, regular assessments of progress are made and the expected time of delivery is communicated.
- Progress of less than 1 cm/h is corrected within one or at the most two hours in order to avoid unnecessary exhaustion of both the mother and her uterus.
- The first measure is amniotomy. If adequate progress is not achieved within one hour, oxytocin therapy is started (Chapter 15).
- As long as these measures are taken in time, nulliparas almost invariably respond with a spectacular improvement in labor.
- This policy does not lead to more frequent use of oxytocin but rather to better timed use (Chapter 17). In fact, the majority of women cared for in this way do not receive oxytocin at all.

21.3 Secondary protraction and arrest of dilatation

Much less frequently – in about 10% of first labors – dilatation slows down after having smoothly

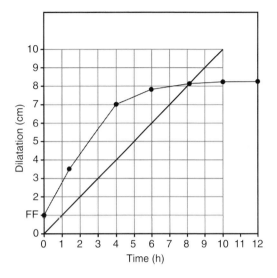

Figure 21.4. Untreated secondary protraction and arrest of dilatation.

attained the initial 7–8 cm. Secondary protraction or arrest disorder is readily and instantly evident when a partogram is kept (Fig. 21.4).

The underlying physical problem is inadequate wedging action (Chapter 9). The fundamental causes of this are insufficient uterine force to pro-voke descent and/or unfavorable fetopelvic pro-portions, or a combination of these two. Secondary arrest in dilatation is indeed suggestive of fetal obstruction (Chapter 22), but relatively insufficient uterine force is still the more likely cause in first labors. This is proven time and again through the restoration of progress by amniotomy and oxytocin in most cases, provided adequate doses are used (Chapter 17) and treatment is started in time to avoid uterine exhaustion (Fig. 21.5).

21.3.1 Classic misapprehensions

A systematic approach to the understanding and treatment of secondary arrest in first labor has been inhibited by the persistent mechanistic view of childbirth. This view maintains the tenacious misconception that stimulation of the uterus can

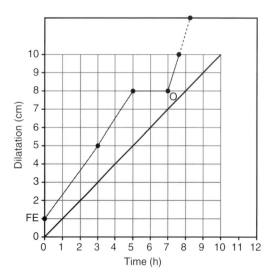

Figure 21.5. Successful treatment of secondary arrest in nulliparous labor. O=oxytocin, membranes ruptured spontaneously.

result in serious injury to both mother and child when there is the faintest possibility of cephalopelvic disproportion. "As cephalopelvic disproportion can never, strictly speaking, be wholly excluded until labor has come to a successful conclusion, this caveat effectively ensures that oxytocin is not used to its potential effect for fear of dire consequences."[3] As labor cannot be brought to a successful conclusion without improvement in uterine action, this gives rise to a classic therapeutic deadlock and overdiagnosis of cephalopelvic disproportion (Chapter 22).

> *In most cases, secondary arrest is a dynamic birth disorder and must be treated as such with amniotomy and oxytocin. There is one overriding reservation: multiparity.*

21.3.2 Clinical approach to secondary arrest of dilatation

At all times a clear distinction must be maintained between first labor and parous labor. As a rule,

strong uterine action is the key to normality, but the parous uterus is naturally efficient in this regard, with much less cervical resistance to overcome. Secondary arrest in multiparous labor is therefore highly indicative of mechanical obstruction.[4] The main causes are fetal macrosomia or malposition of the fetal head (occiput posterior, deflexion attitude, or asynclitism). As multiparas are vulnerable to uterine rupture, late augmentation is not without risk for both mother and child. For this reason we allow augmentation of parous labor only in exceptional cases in which fetal malposition is explicitly excluded and uterine contractions are too infrequent and/or too weak. This must be definitively proven by the absence of molding, the absence of caput succedaneum, and the absence of extreme hyperflexion.

> *The most common cause of secondary protraction and arrest disorders in nulliparous labor is insufficient uterine force, whereas in multiparas it is mechanical obstruction caused by malposition.*

In contrast, the possibility of a mechanical obstruction is not considered in first labors before uterine force is optimized by the judicious use of oxytocin (Chapter 17). In most cases augmentation of uterine force results in molding and formation of caput succedaneum, which improves the application of the fetus's head to the dilatational ring. This restores the wedging action and thus progress (Fig. 21.5). In addition, optimized uterine force may correct a possible asynclitism and the additional hyperflexion of the fetal head will also afford an easier descent. It is important to remember that the force of (augmented) contractions poses no threat to the fetus and that nulliparas are virtually immune to uterine rupture. It is only when progress fails to respond to these measures that we resort to a cesarean section (Fig. 21.6). For every nullipara, assurance of forceful uterine contractions has the effect of isolating true fetal obstruction or fetopelvic

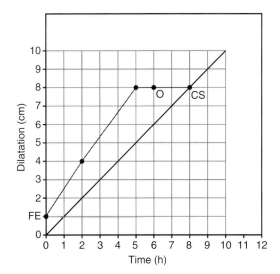

Figure 21.6. Secondary arrest of first labor due to mechanical obstruction. O = oxytocin; CS = cesarean section.

disproportion as a distinct clinical problem (Chapter 22).

> *The cause of secondary protraction in first labor must not be ascribed to cephalopelvic disproportion until oxytocin has been given for a restricted period to ensure forceful uterine contractions.*

21.3.3 Cervical edema versus maximal cervical relaxation

In some cases secondary arrest coincides with or may result from cervical edema. This cervical thickening is typically asymmetrical and localized to the anterior lip of the cervix. This may occur with back labor, in ill-prepared and uncoachable women, or in a protracted, insufficiently supported labor. When the woman is panicked, she pushes long before her cervix attains full dilatation and the natural bearing down reflex is activated. Her attempt to speed up her labor has the opposite effect as a result. It is typically too late to clearly

explain the situation to her and instruct her not to push. Often, the only remaining options are attempts to massage away the edema or to perform a cesarean section. Prompt correction of slow progress, good coaching, and effective pain relief with epidural block should have prevented this problem at a much earlier stage.

Cervical edema should not be confused with a symmetrically, maximally dilated cervix that hangs loosely and to which the high-station fetal head no longer applies pressure during contractions (*maximal cervical relaxation*). This rare phenomenon is clinical proof of mechanical obstruction (Chapter 22).

> *Cervical edema originates in poor labor attendance and inept labor management, whereas maximal cervical relaxation indicates mechanical birth obstruction.*

21.4 Secondary arrest at full dilatation

Occasionally progress of labor halts for the first time at complete dilatation (Fig. 21.7). This becomes manifest when the fetal head fails to descend and the mother shows no inclination to push despite the achievement of full dilatation. The caput remains above 0-station and, hence, the reflex to push is not activated. By definition the active expulsion stage has not yet begun in this situation (Chapter 10) and the woman should not be encouraged to bear down. It is a disorder of the first stage of labor. Attempts at expulsion in the absence of the physiological reflex to push are generally ineffective, a waste of maternal energy, and virtually senseless. It must be noted that epidural analgesia obscures proper diagnosis.

> *An epidural infusion should be stopped in time to avoid confusion about whether the epidural has blocked the pushing reflex or the woman is still in the first stage of her labor.*

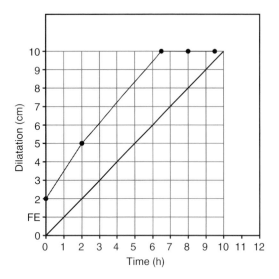

Figure 21.7. Secondary arrest at full dilatation.

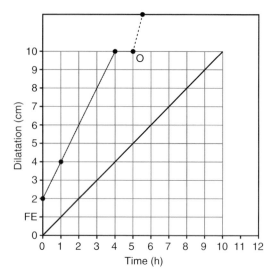

Figure 21.8. Oxytocin (O) treatment for secondary arrest at full dilatation in nulliparous labor.

21.4.1 Mechanistic fallacies

Some of the most serious misunderstandings in conventional obstetrics arise from the incorrect proposition that the expulsion stage begins at full dilatation (Chapters 9, 11). This assumption causes professionals to instruct women to push prematurely in the absence of the physiological reflex to do so, and this often results in premature maternal exhaustion and instrument-assisted delivery.

Such is the dominance of the mechanistic view of birth that many obstetricians even regard full dilatation as the natural line of demarcation between abdominal and vaginal delivery (Chapter 11). This is a serious misapprehension that could lead to the use of a forceps or vacuum extractor simply because the cervix no longer presents an obstacle. In this situation the woman is still in the first stage of her labor and the head of the fetus is still high and in the transverse or oblique diameter of the pelvis. Delivery will entail forced traction and a difficult rotation, and although the cervix is fully dilated the vagina and pelvic floor are not. Thus, the maneuver is associated with an unacceptable risk of severe injuries to both mother and child. In

such a case, mother and baby would have been much better off were full dilatation not achieved at all. Evidently, the use of forceps or ventouse in first-stage labor cannot be defended in any circumstances. The supposedly safe alternative in conventional obstetrics is a cesarean delivery and, indeed, the decrease in instrumental deliveries in many hospitals has coincided with increasing cesarean rates. In first labors, however, oxytocin is a much better alternative (Fig. 21.8).

> *Secondary arrest at full dilatation is a disorder of the first stage of labor.*

21.4.2 Expert management

Since the absence of the pushing reflex at full dilatation is a disorder of the first stage of labor, it should be handled in a manner identical to that described in section 21.3.2. Nulliparas should receive oxytocin, which can be given with confidence that no harm can befall mother or baby.

Generally progress is quickly restored (Fig. 21.8). If one hour of oxytocin treatment does not induce descent to the level where the pushing reflex is activated (at least 0-station), a cesarean delivery for proven mechanical birth obstruction is warranted. One might start a trial of pushing in the absence of the natural urge to do so in the mostly vain hope that the fetal head will descend, but the temptation to attempt delivery by traction from 0-station or higher should be resisted.[5] Once again, the fundamental difference between nulliparas and multiparas must be constantly kept in mind: as a rule of thumb, oxytocin in secondary labor arrest is disallowed in multiparas. Cesarean delivery is the only safe option in arrested parous labor.

21.5 Failed expulsion in nulliparas

The natural second stage of labor begins only when the irresistible pushing reflex is activated after the attainment of full dilatation by the impact of the fetal head on the levator ani muscle, rectum, and pelvic floor (Chapter 11). At this point vaginal delivery is virtually assured and should the need arise a forceps or vacuum extractor can be used safely. Apart from extremely exceptional women with a selective narrow outlet of the bony pelvis – in whom an otherwise uncomplicated instrumental extraction is no more possible than a spontaneous birth – pelvic dimensions no longer play any obstructive role during expulsion (Chapters 9, 11). Having reached the true expulsion stage, as redefined in Chapter 10, the largest diameter of the head (biparietal plane) has passed well through the pelvic inlet and the entire head is at least in the midpelvis. From this point on, the woman only has to overpower soft-tissue resistance. This, admittedly, requires a lot of force in a first labor. Failure to overcome the soft-tissue resistance is a dynamic problem, not an expression of mechanical obstruction. It should be treated with oxytocin.

There is no principal time constraint for the expulsion stage unless a woman fails to achieve any further progress after one hour of pushing. Too few

Table 21.2. Causes of arrested expulsion

1. Maternal exhaustion
2. Pushing too early
3. Ineffective pushing technique
4. Insufficient uterine force

birth attendants seem to appreciate that a baby who can be safely born by instrumental traction can also be pushed out, provided the woman has sufficient reserves of energy. If scrutinized, there are four, primarily iatrogenic, factors involved in failed expulsion (Table 21.2).

21.5.1 Maternal exhaustion

Failure to accomplish expulsion by the woman's own efforts is often related to the antecedent events, because the mother is emotionally drained and physically exhausted after too long a first stage of labor and is now unable or unwilling to push. An instrumental delivery then seems the only solution, but this circumstance should have been anticipated and prevented much earlier. In current conventional practice an instrumental vaginal delivery is performed in 20–30% of all nulliparas who eventually achieve full dilatation (Chapter 2). *Proactive support of labor* – provided it is employed in all its components – effectively diminishes this inappropriate instrumental delivery rate (Chapter 29).

> *Failing expulsion in first labor is a dynamic birth disorder.*

21.5.2 Pushing too early

The prevalent misconception that the expulsion stage begins at full dilatation is a direct cause of many iatrogenic expulsion arrests. All too often women are instructed to push too early and thereby lose too much strength too soon. Impatience on the part of the birth attendants at full dilatation (especially at night) in awaiting the start of the actual pushing reflex to occur, or the vain hope of speeding up the conclusion of the woman's labor, may play a role. In fact, one should have acted much earlier. Pushing before the onset of the natural pushing reflex is generally ineffective and counterproductive in its effect: instrumental delivery rates rocket sky-high.

> *Too often energy and resolve are wasted by encouraging women to push before the true reflexive urge to do so has occurred.*

When the fetal head reaches the level of the ischial spines (0-station) the irrepressible urge to push gradually arises. There is nothing wrong with the woman pushing instinctively at the top of each contraction. At this stage, however, it is contrary to her natural instincts and thus wrong policy to encourage the woman to push for the whole contraction with all her might. Not until the caput reaches the pelvic floor (meaning that it is visible at the pelvic floor when the labia are spread) is the natural, irrepressible urge to push from the beginning of each contraction activated. The woman will not fail to show this herself. The sudden pressure on her pelvic floor is an overwhelming and often cataclysmic sensation that marks the transition from her passive role in the first stage of labor to an active role in the expulsion stage (Chapter 11). The wise birth attendant makes the most of this natural process and keeps a close eye on the woman. From this moment forward, all reserves of strength must be gathered. With adequate coaching and expert conduct of labor, expulsion takes nulliparas about 30 minutes on average and in multiparas substantially less.

It is worth noting that in vaginal breech deliveries women are wisely instructed not to give way to their pushing reflex for as long as possible so as to effect deep descent and internal rotation of the breech, after which they can push with all their might. Indeed, the delay in active pushing helps in a smooth and safe spontaneous expulsion. Strangely, this physiological fact is often forgotten

with cephalic presentations, where women are encouraged to push even before the onset of the physiological reflex to do so.

> *With expert labor management and adequate coaching, expulsion takes nulliparas about 35 minutes on average and in multiparas substantially less.*

21.5.3 Ineffective pushing techniques

In many places pregnant women are being prepared for labor by independent birth instructors who teach them how to push, for instance in the upright position, sitting on a birthing stool, or squatting supported by a specialized pillow, only to find that such facilities are not available. Similarly, the prelabor instructions on how to breathe and push often do not correspond with the instructions given by the birth attendants in the delivery room. Confusion resulting from mismatches between prelabor training and actual practice strongly undermines the effectiveness of the woman's efforts in delivering her baby. To reiterate: prelabor education that corresponds with actual practice is critical (Chapter 19). Furthermore, faulty pushing techniques are not infrequently the result of thoughtless care providers who allow three or more onlookers, position the woman with her legs in stirrups, and place an intern or student-midwife astride between her legs facing her vulva closely. Can this be the setting in which caregivers expect women to push best? Women's natural embarrassment, conditioned prudishness, and their natural desire to maintain personal cleanliness generally tend to override the pushing reflex. Measures with the declared purpose of stimulating the pushing reflex, such as applying pressure on the rectum using fingers placed in the vagina, as well as stretching the perineum, are painful, woman-unfriendly, and often counterproductive. Additional encouragement including making comparisons to "pooping" (literally heard in many delivery rooms) will not improve the woman's pushing technique. For didactic sport, every birth attendant should at least once during their training strip down, put their legs in stirrups, and have strangers offer the same "encouraging" words.

> *Faulty maternal pushing techniques are often iatrogenic in origin.*

21.5.4 Insufficient uterine force at expulsion

In spite of or because of the management of labor up to the second stage, the expulsive force can be insufficient to effect the cardinal movements of the fetal head and conquer the resistance of the pelvic floor. The assumption that a delayed rotation is the cause of stagnation – which must be manually corrected and/or resolved by rotational forceps or vacuum extraction – is a misconception of the mechanistic perspective (Chapter 10). The truth is that internal rotation and deflexion of the fetal head originate from force. That is why oxytocin is the first measure in nulliparas and an instrument-assisted delivery should be the last resort. Maximization of uterine force can still bring about the cardinal movements, resulting in a spontaneous delivery. If not, it at least ensures that the caput is as deep as possible and that its position is more favorable for facilitating a safe instrumental delivery. The higher the level at which instrumental extraction begins, the greater the risk of fetal and maternal trauma.

21.6 Failing expulsion in multiparas

The overriding proposition that arrested multiparous labor originates in fetal obstruction remains valid at all times including the expulsion stage. After a properly managed first stage, failing expulsion is exceedingly rare in multiparas. Less maternal force is required because the soft birth canal has already been stretched at the previous birth. Failed parous expulsion mostly results from instructions to push while the true expulsion stage has not yet been reached.

If the head is unusually molded or if there is an extensive caput formation, or both (the so-called "pharaoh head"), full engagement might not have taken place even though the head appears to be at 0-station. This pitfall can be circumvented through combined vaginal and suprapubic palpation or ultrasound examination. The fetal head can then still be felt or seen above the pelvic inlet, indicating that it is not yet entirely in the pelvis. A decelerative partogram should alert that this might occur. Problematic obstruction should be anticipated. When, after secondary delay, the parous woman reaches complete dilatation, efforts at expulsion are still likely to fail. In these circumstances an attempt at forced vaginal extraction poses inexcusable risks of maternal and fetal injury. If one succeeds in delivering the fetal head safely, severe shoulder dystocia will almost certainly follow. In conclusion: instrumental delivery for arrested parous labor must be judged as malpractice in most cases. The only exception is a frightened multipara (with a traumatic first experience that should have been avoided) who now hardly dares to push while the fetal head can be easily delivered by outlet forceps or vacuum extractor.

> *The use of forceps or vacuum to resolve obstructed* parous *birth is dangerous for both mother and child.*

21.7 The refractory or unresponsive uterus

Ineffective uterine action is common in the inexperienced nullipara and this condition – regardless of when it occurs – can almost always be resolved with amniotomy and oxytocin provided labor augmentation is started in a timely fashion and oxytocin is properly dosed. Two clinical conditions wherein the uterus often fails to respond properly to oxytocin must be recognized:
1. Augmentation that is performed too late
2. Induction of labor

21.7.1 Delayed augmentation

Picture the legs of a marathon runner who hits the proverbial "wall" and collapses as a result of either lack of strength or muscle cramp. The exhausted myometrium reacts similarly. Over an extended period, lactic acid accumulates and the uterus loses its ability to respond to oxytocin stimulation or it reacts with hypertonia during the contraction intervals. Added to this, prolonged labor may result in myometrial desensitization through a significant reduction in both oxytocin-binding sites and oxytocin receptor mRNA (Chapter 8). The result is decreased uterine responsiveness (oxytocin-resistant dystocia). This is the exhausted, refractory uterus, a common but mostly unrecognized complication in conventional obstetrics, where the decision to accelerate slow labor is often postponed for too long. Incidentally, postpartum hemorrhage also occurs more often in women with a depleted uterus.

When labor is augmented at too late a stage the response to oxytocin treatment is also much less safe. If the uterus reacts like any overburdened muscle full of lactic acid – with tetanic spasms – the result is insufficient uterine relaxation between the contractions, leading to fetal distress. The longer the uterus has run ineffectively, the smaller the therapeutic range of oxytocin.

The exhausted, refractory myometrium

An exhausted uterus fails to respond properly to oxytocin or may react with hypertonia in the inter-contraction intervals, leading to fetal distress.

The term refractory uterus actually refers to a preventable and thus iatrogenic complication as it results from unfounded tolerance of long labor. Clinical stalemate, whereby late stimulation fails to restore progress or results in fetal distress, is a frequent indication for cesarean delivery that could have been prevented by timely and far less intrusive measures. The root of the problem – a depleted uterus that has now become oxytocin resistant – is seldom appreciated and it is this lack of under-standing as well as the general use of too-low doses (Chapter 17) that feeds the unfounded skepticism surrounding oxytocin as therapy for dysfunctional labor. Clearly, *proactive support of labor* prevents this dynamic and iatrogenic problem.

21.7.2 Induction

The second cause of an unresponsive uterus – induction – is even more obtrusively iatrogenic. Unsuccessful induction must be recognized as the dynamic and iatrogenic disorder that it is and should be recorded as "failed induction," not as "dystocia." Exact diagnosis and continuous audit of all procedures are the key ingredients of quality management programs aimed at lowering cesarean rates (Chapter 27).

Origins of a refractory or unresponsive uterus

1. *Exhausted uterus (preventable and thus iatrogenic)*
2. *Induction (downright iatrogenic)*

21.8 Augmentation versus induction

A great deal of confusion exists regarding the true nature of labor induction and labor augmentation. Because both procedures begin with artificial rupture of the membranes followed by oxytocin administration, doctors, nurses, and mothers may be confused and wrongly believe that induction and augmentation are somehow extensions of the same procedure, merging imperceptibly into each other. Nothing could be farther from the truth. This misconception is as logical as drawing the conclusion that watering the flower garden is the same as extinguishing a fire because both actions use water and hose.

There should be no confusion between acceleration and induction of labor, as they concern two fundamentally different procedures with overall opposite effects.

21.8.1 The fundamental difference

Once labor begins spontaneously, oxytocin receptors are abundant and the cervix and myometrium have transformed at least to the point that the physiological circle is complete: contractions → *myometrial gap junctions* → electrical myometrial orchestration → effect on the cervix → prostaglandin release → contractions, and so forth (Chapter 8). The already laboring but ineffective nulliparous uterus reacts in a predictably favorable fashion to amniotomy and oxytocin. Augmentation of labor improves a physiological process that has already begun spontaneously.

In contrast, induction interrupts the natural course of pregnancy and the biological uterine transformation is not yet complete and activation of the myometrium has, by definition, not yet occurred. Electrical cell-to-cell coupling in the myometrium has not yet begun and the number of oxytocin receptors may be low (Chapter 8). This explains why the induced uterus usually reacts unpredictably to oxytocin: either with poorly coordinated, inefficient contractions or with disorganized hypertonia. At the same time the cervix is not yet optimally transformed, which means that the cumulative force the uterus has to exert to effect dilatation is always more than would be necessary if one had waited for the spontaneous onset of labor. The intended effect – progress in dilatation – is extremely varied with inductions: mostly progress is much too slow and not infrequently is even entirely absent. Induction sets in motion effects that are the exact opposite of those of augmentation of spontaneous labor in nearly every respect (Chapter 23).

> *Induction creates slow and difficult labor, whereas augmentation corrects slow and difficult labor.*

21.9 Hypertonic uterine dysfunction

Uterine dysfunction – by far the most common cause of abnormal first labor – is subdivided in the majority of textbooks into two distinct types: hypotonic and hypertonic inertia. This classic subdivision is based on intrauterine pressure measurements and is typically coupled with the warning that while oxytocin could be useful in the former case, it could be detrimental in the latter. In reality, however, as long as slow progress is the only problem this assertion lacks any rational or factual basis. What is more, reliance on pressure measurements may lead to therapeutic impasse because birth attendants are tempted to wait despite minimal progress simply because of "adequate Montevideo units." However, contractions building up pressure may very well be ineffective (Chapter 8) and effectiveness of labor is usually established by timely and properly dosed oxytocin administration. Progressive dilatation is the only parameter that counts for the indication and evaluation of the treatment of slow progress and pressure readings are not needed and should be omitted. Pressure is not the measure.

> **Dynamic dystocia**
>
> *Intrauterine pressure gauges should not be used routinely in augmented labor. Progress in cervical dilatation is the sole measure of uterine efficiency and effectiveness.*

In fact, signs of imminent fetal hypoxia are the only contraindication for oxytocin and the only indication for monitoring intrauterine pressure (Chapter 24). If the fetus cannot tolerate the contractions that are required for normal progress, a cesarean delivery is the only rational and safe solution. Waiting will benefit neither the fetus nor the mother. As always, decisive management is mandatory. Hypertonic dystocia is a separate clinical entity altogether.

21.9.1 Hypertonic or uncoordinated dystocia

In pathological circumstances, chorioamnionitis, meconium, or free intrauterine blood may randomly excite the myometrium cells to the extent that the electrical orchestration and consequently the efficiency and effectiveness of the contractions are lost (Chapter 8). Progress halts and hypertonia between contractions further compromises fetal oxygenation, creating a dangerous and vicious circle involving dystocia and fetal distress. This is true hypertonic or uncoordinated dystocia. Whether intrauterine infection is the cause or the result of dysfunctional labor is a typical chicken-or-egg riddle that cannot be answered in conventional practices where long labors are tolerated.

The sequence of events will become evident when the rules of *proactive support of labor* are applied. Clearly, the chances of meconium and/or infection will increase with an extended duration of labor as more vaginal examinations are performed and intrauterine catheters are used. This typically happens with induction and ill-managed, out of control labors. A preventable or iatrogenic component is then not difficult to identify. The proper measures must primarily address the underlying problems with amnion-infusion, antibiotics, tocolytics, etc. (Chapter 24). However, owing to the practical dilemma in which the uterus cannot be stimulated safely but progress remains minimal, a cesarean delivery is often the only feasible solution. As always, decisive action is required in these circumstances. As in the case of an unresponsive uterus due to induction, this dynamic birth complication can also occur in multiparas.

Hypertonic dystocia

This term is reserved for a singular clinical entity in which meconium, blood, or pus disturbs uterine coordination, leading to a vicious circle of uterine dysfunction and fetal compromise.

As may happen with all overburdened muscles loaded with lactic acid, an exhausted uterus after too long a labor can also react with spasms. This is difficult if not impossible to distinguish from the hypertonic dystocia resulting from beginning infection. This diagnostic problem is circumvented by adherence to the policies of *proactive support of*

labor because this approach effectively prevents prolonged labor, uterine exhaustion, and intra-uterine infection.

21.10 Final diagnosis for audit purposes

Dystocia – or equivalent labels such as "failure to progress" or "dysfunctional labor" – is heterogeneous in its causation and manifestation, and the term thus represents a pseudo-diagnosis. The terms should no longer be used without further explanation. Instead of simply attributing the indication for an operative delivery to "dystocia," the precise nature and causal diagnosis of the birth disorder at hand (as listed in Table 21.1) should be assessed. Cause and effect need to be explored before the conduct and care of labor can be improved with any semblance of a rational basis. What is more, only detailed and causal diagnoses allow for meaningful audit of all procedures and outcomes of childbirth. Continual audit of all procedures is another essential component of *proactive support of labor* (Chapter 27).

Detailed diagnosis is the most important single issue in responsible labor care and is critical for meaningful audit. Cause and effect need to be explored if progress is to be made.

21.11 Summary

- Dynamic dystocia is common in first labors but rare in subsequent labors because the parous uterus is highly efficient and has much less resistance to overcome.
- Dynamic dystocia is heterogeneous in its causation and manifestation. Failure to unravel this complex of birth disorders and subject the separate problems to detailed analysis and diagnosis renders a structured policy for the reduction of operative delivery rates virtually impossible.

- Dynamic dystocia is specific to first labor and may occur at various points as distinct clinical types with distinctively different causes.
- Primary ineffective labor presents as a persistent pattern of slow dilatation from the very onset and corresponds to a disorder in the retraction phase of labor. This situation should be handled with early diagnosis and prompt correction, long before the woman begins drifting toward a long labor and exhaustion.
- Secondary arrest at 7–8 cm corresponds to a disturbance in the wedging phase of first-stage labor. This may be indicative of fetal obstruction, but insufficient uterine force is still the more likely explanation in first labors. Progress is usually restored through oxytocin, which can be administered safely without inflicting harm on mother or baby. This is certainly not so in multiparous labor.
- Secondary arrest at full dilatation in nulliparous labor is a dynamic birth disorder of the first stage that should be treated with labor augmentation.
- As a rule, failed expulsion in first labor is a dynamic birth disorder, due to maternal exhaustion and/or premature pushing before the onset of the natural reflex to do so. Several iatrogenic factors play a role in ineffective pushing techniques.
- The exhausted, refractory uterus is a common but insufficiently appreciated labor disorder that can be effectively prevented by following the policies of *proactive support of labor*.
- The unresponsive uterus during induction is an iatrogenic problem.
- Hypertonic dystocia is a separate clinical condition in which meconium, blood, or pus disturbs uterine coordination, which results in a dangerous and vicious cycle of uterine dysfunction and fetal distress.

REFERENCES

1. Chelmow D, Kilpatrick SJ, Laros RK Jr. Maternal and neonatal outcome after prolonged latent phase. *Obstet Gynecol* 1993; 81(4): 486–91.
2. Enkin M, Keirse MJNC, Neilson J, *et al.* Prolonged labor. In: *A Guide to Effective Care in Pregnancy and Childbirth*, 3rd edn. Oxford: Oxford University Press; 2000.
3. O'Driscoll K, Meagher D, Robson M. *Active Management of Labour*, 4th edn. Mosby; 2003.
4. Norwitz ER, Robinson JN, Repke JT. Labor and delivery. In: Gabbe SG, Neibyl JR, Simpson JL, eds. *Obstetrics: Normal and Problem Pregnancies*, 4th edn. Philadelphia: Churchill Livingston; 2002: 353–94.
5. American College of Obstetricians and Gynecologists: Operative Vaginal Delivery. *Practice bulletin* No. 17, June 2000.

22

Mechanical birth obstruction

The concept of *proactive support of labor* is specifically designed to prevent, diagnose, and treat labor disorders that arise in initially normal cases. The subject is therefore strictly confined to women carrying a single fetus in the cephalic presentation. Multiple pregnancies, breeches, and obstetric rarities such as hydrocephaly, transverse lies, and shoulder and compound presentations are all explicitly excluded. These are primary abnormal situations that are strongly associated with fetal trauma and, in multiparas, occasionally even with rupture of the uterus. For the approach of deviating fetal presentations and twins the standard textbooks are recommended, which usually discuss these obstetric abnormalities at length while hardly ever addressing a systematic approach to labor protraction in common cases with cephalic presentation. Limitation of the subject to cephalic presentation is fundamental because obstruction of the fetal head in itself bears no risk for trauma, provided temptation to force an instrumental delivery is resisted. In cephalic presentations, fetal and maternal injuries are almost exclusively associated with operative interventions.

> It is imperative to ensure that breech or other malpresentation, relevant fetal malformation, and twins have all been excluded from the outset, before the rules of proactive support are engaged.

22.1 Definition

Assuming the diagnosis of labor to be correct, the onset to be spontaneous, and efficient uterine contractions to be assured, there remains but one reason why labor may continue to stagnate: obstruction. Obstruction of the fetal head may be caused either by disparity between the absolute size of the head and the pelvic capacity – generally referred to as "cephalopelvic disproportion" (CPD) – or by its clinical analog: malposition of the head including occiput posterior, deflexion attitude, or severe asynclitism. This chapter discusses CPD and fetal head malposition under one heading – "mechanical birth obstruction" – as their clinical picture and clinical approach are virtually identical.

> The term mechanical dystocia, or obstructed labor, refers to obstruction of the fetal head such as to preclude safe vaginal delivery. Causative factors are fetal size, pelvic capacity, and malposition of the fetal head.

22.2 Diagnosis

A thorough understanding of the dynamics and mechanics of birth in cephalic presentation, as discussed in Section 2, is critical for rational and responsible obstetrics. Now it is abundantly clear that the clinical diagnosis "mechanical birth disorder" is a diagnosis by exclusion. Only by assuring – from the very beginning – adequate forces of labor, can obstruction be isolated as a separate clinical entity and diagnosed with a reasonable degree of certainty. The ratio between the dimensions of the pelvis and the fetal head plays a role in labor progress only during the wedging phase of first-stage labor (Chapter 9). Therefore, disparity between passage and passenger can only be diagnosed by definitive arrest at 7–8 cm dilatation in the presence of strong contractions, not earlier. The presence of strong contractions must of course be established by the appearance of substantial caput succedaneum and molding. The only reliable test for birth obstruction is labor itself. If the proposed diagnostic criteria are strictly applied, birth obstruction is a plausible diagnosis in less than 1% of all births. Mechanical birth disorders are no longer common since the elimination of rickets.

> **Diagnosis of Mechanical Labor Disorder**
>
> *Secondary arrest of cervical dilatation and descent in first-stage labor in the presence of strong contractions, demonstrated by substantial molding and sizable caput succedaneum.*

22.3 Common fallacies

General failure to appreciate the fundamental distinction between first and subsequent labors and between cephalic presentations and abnormal lies has prevented progress in rational labor management for a very long time. In addition to this, the onset of the expulsion stage of labor is generally erroneously defined as full dilatation (Section 2). These omissions and obsolete definitions account for the widespread persistence of mechanistic misunderstandings and explain many of the prevalent errors in labor management. Several examples were given earlier, but there are more.

22.3.1 Unfounded concerns

There may have been good reasons for the preoccupation with the mechanics of birth when rickets was a common disease, but this situation no longer exists. Nonetheless, in the collective memory of many obstetricians, obstructed labor is still widely regarded as a situation dangerous to both mother and child.[1,2] To those it may come as a surprise to learn that an extensive search in Medline/PubMed yields zero evidence for either contention if the subject is confined to first labors with cephalic presentation. Obstruction of the fetal head bears no fetal risks; long-term follow-up of 5- to 6-year old infants delivered after prolonged secondary labor arrest disorders does not show an increase in the risk of neurological abnormalities.[3] Clearly, birth obstruction can be safely diagnosed by assuring optimal uterine force, provided the vertex presents and fetal status is monitored as carefully as in any labor (Chapter 24). Uterine rupture is a calamity that befalls parous women only, whereas the nulliparous uterus is virtually rupture-proof. Severe fetal and maternal trauma is associated almost exclusively with forcible traction, regardless of parity.

> *The power of contractions poses no threat to the fetus, even in obstructed labor. In first labors, mechanical birth disorders can be safely diagnosed by assuring optimal uterine force.*

22.3.2 Poorly defined concept of CPD

The classic concept of cephalopelvic disproportion originally described obstructed labors occurring as a result of pelvic contracture or deformity, which is a permanent condition. By inference, once CPD was diagnosed, future vaginal birth was deemed impossible. But CPD or contracted pelvis proves to be a very unreliable diagnosis: two-thirds or more of women diagnosed as having this disorder and therefore delivered by cesarean section deliver equally large or even larger babies vaginally in their next pregnancy, if given the chance.[4] Clearly, CPD or its equivalent, "contracted pelvis," is generally over-diagnosed. The main reason is underdiagnosis and undertreatment of dynamic labor disorders (Chapter 21). Although labor augmentation is extensively performed in many hospitals, oxytocin is usually used too late and in too low a dose (Chapter 17).

> ### Overdiagnosis
>
> *CPD or contracted pelvis is a tenuous diagnosis frequently abused as an excuse for a cesarean delivery in women who did not get a fair chance to prove the functional capacity of their pelvis.*

The second reason for overdiagnosis of CPD is that obstructed labor is not associated simply with contracted pelvis or excessive fetal size. Unfavorable position of the head – persistent occiput posterior, asynclitism, deflexion – more often obstructs passage of the head through the birth canal.[5] Obviously, CPD is ill-defined and in most cases the concept of CPD does not cover the accepted clinical significance of contracted pelvis and permanent impossibility of birth. As strict definition and reliable diagnosis are critical for rational and responsible obstetrics, preference should be given to the more neutral and more accurate terms "mechanical birth disorder" or "obstructed labor."

22.3.3 Elusive prelabor prediction

By definition, mechanical birth disorders or obstructed labor can only be diagnosed during labor. This terminology also serves to eliminate the widespread but mistaken practice of diagnosing "CPD" even before labor has begun. In reality, selection of a fetal size threshold to predict birth obstruction remains elusive, despite advanced sonographic fetometry.[6] This is because of the inaccuracy of the method and because most cases of diagnosed disproportion occur in fetuses whose weight is well within the range of the general obstetric population. Efforts to predict CPD on the

basis of fetal head circumference have proved equally disappointing, in part because malposition of the fetal head is an additional causative factor. This also explains why sophisticated imaging techniques, including computed tomography (CT) and magnetic resonance imaging (MRI), are unable to predict obstructed labor reliably.[7] The only reliable test is labor itself.

> *Neither fetal size estimation nor radiological assessment of pelvic dimensions are particularly accurate in predicting the outcome of labor (Evidence level A).*

A floating, non-engaged fetal head in late pregnancy is also not predictive of birth obstruction. In black nulliparous women, in whom such non-engagement commonly occurs, it is slightly associated with longer labors, but not with operative delivery or increased maternal or fetal morbidity.[8] Not even women with short stature need be regarded with suspicion, since smaller mothers usually give birth to smaller babies. This observation is as important in countries with immigrants from Asia and Africa as it is in the third world; western doctors tend to place undue emphasis on short stature without directing equal attention to low birthweight. A floating fetal head in late pregnancy is no reason for pelvimetry or fetometry. It is imperative, however, to exclude placenta previa or occasionally occurring obstructive cysts and myomas in the lesser pelvis.

> *The only reliable test for disparity between the fetal head and the pelvis is labor itself.*

22.3.4 Self-fulfilling prophecies

Although induction is widely practiced for suspected fetal macrosomia ("to prevent the child from getting even bigger"), there is no evidence whatsoever to support such a policy. Rather the reverse is true, because induction of labor mainly induces dynamic labor disorders. In a meta-analysis of studies in women with suspected fetal macrosomia, neonatal outcomes were similar but cesarean rates were twice as high in women whose labor was induced as in those followed with expectant management (16.6% vs. 8.4%).[9] Through circular logic, however, faulty policies tend to create their own justification; after induction, uterine contractions are often inefficient and thus ineffective. The failing labor is then wrongly attributed to the anticipated birth obstruction. Such fallacies explain the stubborn persistence of fundamental mistakes in practice. Hard evidence, instead, shows that reliable prediction of mechanical birth obstruction is simply not possible. Labor induction or a prelabor cesarean delivery for fetal macrosomia are therefore unfounded and unjustified policies. "These strategies represent classical examples of a clinical situation where application of the generally laudable principle of prevention becomes counterproductive in its effects."[10]

> "All efforts to anticipate birth obstruction are not only misguided, they result in a rate of intervention grossly in excess of the true prevalence of fetopelvic disparity"[10] (Evidence level A).

22.4 Expert policy and diagnosis in first labors

Birth obstruction is a diagnosis by experiment and the appropriate clinical approach is therefore purely pragmatic. According to the principles of *proactive support of labor* no consideration whatsoever is given to the possibility of fetopelvic disproportion in the course of routine antenatal care in normal pregnancies with a normal cephalic presentation. The pelvic size should never be assessed, either by clinical means or by radiographic pelvimetry or MRI. Fetal weight in the upper league should never be estimated, either by palpation or by sonographic fetometry. All refer-

ence to fetal macrosomia should be either avoided or put into perspective. For a woman carrying an undeniably big baby it is better stressed that her baby is fine and that she is built normally and in perfect condition to deliver her child normally. Cautionary notes should never be written in the patient's chart by senior staff, because such reservations place an unbearable burden of responsibility on the midwives and junior doctors who actually attend the labor. Pessimistic anticipations tend to self-fulfillment. For similar reasons, the discouraging term "trial of labor" should never be used; a "trial of labor" often fails simply because the outcome is prejudiced beforehand. Induction of labor is contraindicated rather than indicated and the spontaneous onset of labor is therefore patiently awaited. A positive state of mind is intentionally nurtured and confidence is consciously radiated, as "all is well."

> *Negative predictions are carefully avoided because they generally tend to self-fulfillment.*

The possibility of a mechanical obstruction is first considered only when initially normal labor ceases to progress secondarily, but such a diagnosis should never be entertained seriously until efficient uterine force has been established. This usually requires oxytocin in first labors, which can be given in the sure knowledge that oxytocin treatment does not cause rupture of the nulliparous uterus or trauma to the child. Unfounded reservations originate in failure to draw a clear distinction between nulliparous and parous labor. Malposition (occiput posterior, asynclitism, deflexion) is usually transient when uterine force is adequate.[11] Only if progression fails to recover, despite judicious stimulation and, crucially, adequate uterine force has been proven by substantial caput succedaneum formation and molding, can a mechanical birth obstruction be diagnosed. A cesarean delivery is then the only rational and safe option.

> A diagnosis of head obstruction is considered only after efficient uterine contractions have been established. In first labors this usually requires the use of oxytocin.

22.5 Mechanical birth disorders in parous labors

Women who have previously given birth vaginally – be it spontaneously or by an atraumatic instrumental delivery – should experience few problems in the subsequent delivery. These multiparas have previously provided proof of adequate pelvic capacity and have efficient uterine contractions by nature, provided the onset of labor is spontaneous. Consequently, extreme caution is warranted if initially normal progress slows down. Secondary protraction of parous labor is extremely suspicious for birth obstruction. The causes are either persistent malposition of the fetal head or a child substantially bigger than the previous one. Uterine contractions usually remain vigorous, whereas occasional decline of contractions should first of all be regarded as a sign of a physiological protection mechanism preventing the lower segment of the uterus from overstretching. As obstruction carries a risk of uterine rupture, augmentation of parous labor is allowed only in exceptional cases when obstruction has explicitly been ruled out on the basis of the following compulsory assessments:
- There is no caput succedaneum.
- There is no molding.
- There is no extreme hyperflexion.
- Malposition of the fetal head has been excluded.

> Multiparas
>
> Secondary stagnation of parous labor is a mechanical problem until proven otherwise. Parous labor may therefore be augmented with oxytocin only under strict conditions.

Again, birth obstruction is diagnosed by exclusion of dynamic disorders. The latter, however, are exceedingly rare in parous labor, provided the onset is spontaneous, membranes are broken, and the woman feels in control. Occasionally, contractions may decline owing to stress-related sympathetic arousal caused, for example, by an unnerving clinical environment or undue concerns about fetal condition, often unfounded (Chapter 24). Temporary decline of contractions is almost invariably seen after a stressful ambulance drive that is occasionally needed because of unforeseen complications in home deliveries. When a state of undue stress is patent, comforting measures and professional reassurance should be used to try to reestablish a parasympathetic atmosphere of calmness, composure, and confidence. On top of this, careful use of oxytocin may be warranted. On the other hand, there is an absolute bar on the use of oxytocin in parous labor whenever birth obstruction cannot be rigidly excluded on the basis of the reservations mentioned above, which then leaves cesarean delivery as the only safe option.

22.6 Pitfalls and common mistakes

It is not birth obstruction that carries the dangers for mother and child but mainly the obstetrician who neglects the significance of parity, disregards proper definitions, and misconstrues full dilatation as the deciding demarcation line between abdominal and vaginal operative delivery.

22.6.1 "Functionally full dilatation" – a misnomer

True labor obstruction is caused by either absolute CPD or malposition of the fetal head. Obstruction becomes manifest in the wedging phase of first-stage labor only, not earlier and not later (Chapter 9). Although at times full dilatation may be reached, in particular if membranes are intact, the true second stage of labor will never be reached because the obstructed fetal head fails to descend and the pushing reflex is not activated (Chapter 11). The phenomenon of "maximal cervical relaxation" may be observed, marked by a remaining cervical ring that does not tighten any further during contractions (Chapter 21). At times this phenomenon first becomes manifest by retrogression to 8 cm after the membranes are broken at full dilatation.

"Maximal cervical relaxation" should never be construed as "functionally full dilatation." This term is a treacherous misnomer used by some obstetricians to justify an irresponsible attempt to demonstrate their manual dexterity with forceps or vacuum extractor in spite of incomplete dilatation and a high station. Such a high instrumental delivery involves difficult rotation and forcible traction and is almost inevitably traumatic in its effect. Even if extraction of the head might succeed, a severe shoulder dystocia will follow in most cases.

> *True birth obstruction is a disorder specific to first-stage labor and should never be resolved by vaginal operative delivery.*

22.6.2 Unexpectedly high instrumental delivery

Although high and rotational forceps delivery is now hardly ever practiced, the tendency to attempt vacuum deliveries at stations higher than is usually attempted with forceps is worrying.[12] Prerequisite for any instrumental delivery is that the head is fully engaged,[13] but extensive caput succedaneum formation and molding sometimes make reliable determination of the station and rotation of the fetal head problematic. When difficulties in station and rotation assignment occur, a supposedly "low-forceps" or "low vacuum extraction" might actually be a more difficult and potentially traumatic mid-pelvic operation. Such a delivery entails rotation and forced traction and these maneuvers are strongly associated with severe injuries to both mother and child.[14–17] Evidently, in such cases mother and baby would have fared much better had full dilatation not been achieved at all. True

birth obstruction should have been recognized through proper first-stage labor management and use of the partogram. True birth obstruction should never be resolved by vaginal operative delivery.

> **Instrumental delivery**
>
> *Station and rotation are the most important discriminators of risks for both mother and child. True birth obstruction precludes safe vaginal operative delivery.*

22.6.3 Occiput posterior in first stage labor

At the onset of labor 15% of fetuses present in the occiput posterior position.[18] On the basis of old radiographic studies this position is still widely construed as a sign of a narrow forepelvis.[19] In reality, however, occiput posterior is predominantly associated with anterior placentation.[20] In most cases with occiput posterior position in first-stage labor the mechanism of expulsion is identical to that observed in transverse or anterior varieties, except that the head has to rotate through a larger angle. With adequate driving force 85–90% of cases rotate to the anterior position as soon as the occiput reaches the pelvic floor.[19,21] Labor is not lengthened appreciably in these cases.

For these reasons the clinical approach should be no different from that in any labor with cephalic presentation: no attention should be paid to posterior position, either at antenatal clinics or in the delivery room, as long as progress proves satisfactory. As with fetal macrosomia, the greater the emphasis, the more likely it is that difficulties will follow. "Anxious doctors tend to create their own problems under these headings."[10] Oxytocin can safely be used in first labors with occiput posterior.

> *The great majority of cases with initially occiput posterior position undergo spontaneous anterior rotation during expulsion, most often followed by uncomplicated delivery.*

To avoid creating the impression that occiput posterior may have an adverse effect on the course and outcome of labor, no record is kept in first-stage labor. In reality, forward rotation during expulsion is incomplete (transverse position) or does not take place at all (persistent occiput posterior) in only 10–15% of cases presenting with occiput posterior in first-stage labor.[5,21] Predisposing factors are poor contractions, maternal exhaustion, and epidural analgesia, which suppresses reflex action, diminishing abdominal muscular pushing.[22] These dynamic factors are the commonest contributors to failed expulsion and should have been anticipated and prevented by expert labor management and discontinuation of epidural block when approaching full dilatation (Chapter 20).

22.6.4 Deflexion attitude and asynclitism

As in cases with occiput posterior position, no consideration should be given to asynclitism and deflexion attitudes of the fetal head (sinciput and brow presentation) as long as progress in dilatation is normal. In most cases these positions (attitudes) are transient when uterine contractions are strong. In two-thirds of cases deflexion of the fetal head spontaneously converts to occiput or face presentation, thus allowing spontaneous passage through the pelvis.[21] When this conversion does not occur, dilatation and descent will definitely arrest. Persistent malposition is now put on permanent record as the valid indication for the inevitable cesarean delivery.

> *Asynclitism and brow presentation are usually transient.*

22.7 Failed expulsion

Proper understanding of the nature and sequence of cardinal movements of the fetal head during expulsion, as discussed in detail in Chapter 10, is crucial for proper second-stage labor management.

It prevents common mechanistic misinterpretations in cases of failing expulsion.

22.7.1 Importance of correct definitions

Whenever the pelvic inlet does not match the dimensions of the entering head – owing to absolute disproportion or faulty attitude (persistent brow presentation) – engagement cannot take place and the true expulsion stage will not be reached. Labor obstructed by anatomical disparity typically jams in the wedging phase of first-stage labor (Chapter 9) and cesarean delivery is the only safe exit strategy. As there are still too many obstetricians who incorrectly equate full dilatation with the point of no return in labor, we redefined the onset of true second-stage labor as the moment the irresistible pushing reflex is fully activated after full dilatation has been reached (Chapter 11). Whenever the true expulsion stage is established, the head is, by definition, fully engaged and a vaginal delivery is almost a certainty. A woman's bearing down while the fetal head is still above 0-station should always be looked upon with the gravest suspicion (see "cervical edema," Chapter 21).

Since the entire fetal head is in the pelvis when reflex action is activated (Chapter 10), and because isolated constriction of the bony pelvic outlet is extremely rare, the normal capacity of the bony pelvis to allow passage of the fetal head is virtually assured when the true expulsion stage of labor begins. The only physical resistance remaining at this stage of labor comes from the soft pelvic tissues which, admittedly, may require tremendous effort to surmount. It must be concluded that in almost every case in which true second-stage labor arrest occurs, the predominant cause is dynamic in origin, not mechanical obstruction. When expulsion fails, the composite force of uterine contractions and reflex action of voluntary muscles is apparently not equal to the task. Prevention and treatment of failed expulsion were therefore discussed in more detail under the heading "dynamic labor disorders," where they predominantly belong (Chapter 21).

> *True birth obstruction is a disorder of first-stage labor, not of the second stage. Protraction and arrest of active expulsion is predominantly a dynamic and not a mechanical disorder.*

22.7.2 Transverse arrest

The term transverse arrest is widely misinterpreted as a mechanical problem that could and should be resolved by manual or instrumental rotation. This misapprehension originates in a misunderstanding of the physics of expulsion. In particular, the station at which rotation normally takes place is generally underestimated. In the majority of labors the fetal head is still in the transverse or oblique position when true second-stage labor begins. With ongoing descent, internal rotation of the fetal head normally occurs at the pelvic floor, not earlier (Chapter 10).

Transverse arrest usually occurs at a higher station and is typical of first labors. It results from insufficient driving force and not, as the term seems to imply, from mechanical obstruction. Persistent transverse position should therefore be treated with oxytocin first and not with manual or instrumental rotation followed by extraction. Optimizing uterine force may still bring about anterior rotation and spontaneous birth of the head by further extension. Vacuum delivery should be regarded as the last resort and is permissible only under the strict condition that the head is well past 0-station. Vacuum delivery still allows "spontaneous" rotation. Rotational forceps should never be used nor should attempts be made at manual correction by displacing the head upward for this purpose. Such maneuvers no longer have any place in contemporary obstetrics.

> *"Transverse arrest" is not the cause of delay, but rather the result.[10] The term should be discarded, because it is a misnomer based on a misunderstanding of the natural process of descent and rotation.*

22.7.3 Occiput posterior in second-stage labor

In approximately 5% of all vertex presentations the fetus is eventually delivered with occiput posterior. In about one-third of these cases the occiput persisted in the posterior position in which it started, and in the other two-thirds the head was in the anterior position in first-stage labor.[18] It should be noted that so-called "faulty" rotation to occiput posterior is actually the normal birth mechanism when the head remains in the "neutral" position (sinciput or "military" attitude: neither flexed nor extended) (Chapter 10). In these cases the posterior occiput makes a relatively wide curve and experiences more resistance from the pelvic soft tissues. That is why expulsion with occiput posterior is usually prolonged. If the composite expulsive forces are not equal to the task, the first measure is oxytocin in first labors, even at this late stage. An episiotomy at the moment of crowning is both helpful and prudent. In most cases with sinciput position, delivery is spontaneous with occiput posterior.

If the woman does not manage to conclude birth herself, operative assistance is indicated. The route of operative delivery depends on the station of descent. If the pelvic floor has been reached – meaning that the scalp is visible at the introitus without separating the labia – an outlet forceps or vacuum delivery is permissible, but forceps should never be used to rotate[13,14] because it is traumatic and in conflict with the natural birth mechanism with posterior rotation in case of sinciput position. Because assisted birth in occiput posterior is associated with a 7-fold increase in anal sphincter disruption,[23] a precautionary mediolateral episiotomy is indicated. When expulsion fails with the fetal head positioned in occiput posterior above the pelvic floor, cesarean delivery is indicated.

> Occiput posterior position at expulsion
>
> *The mode of operative delivery depends on station of descent. Safe vaginal instrumental delivery requires descent to the pelvic floor at least and instrumental rotation should not be performed.*

22.8 Obstetric rarities

Discussions on the mechanics of birth and related birth disorders are often confused and frustrated by the introduction of exceptional cases. A short comment on obstetric curiosities makes sense here.

22.8.1 Brow presentation

Persistent brow presentation makes birth a mechanical impossibility unless the fetal head is small (premature infants) or the pelvis is unusually large. However, persistent brow presentation is extremely rare (incidence 1:10 000).[19] Brow presentation in early labor is commonly unstable and often converts to an occiput or a face presentation in the first stage of labor.[11,21] In both circumstances the fetus can be delivered smoothly through the normal vaginal route.

22.8.2 Pelvic deformity

Anatomical deformity of the bony pelvis is equally rare since the elimination of rickets. It usually originates in a limp from early childhood (poliomyelitis) or from injury in a road traffic accident. Fractures of the pubic rami may compromise the birth canal by malunion or callus formation.[24] Identification of women at risk for pelvic deformity presents no problem since they declare themselves by their gait and their medical history. Only in these cases is assessment of the pelvis indicated and, exceptionally, might a prelabor cesarean delivery for reasons of deviant pelvic architecture be justified.

> *Exceptional women with pelvic deformity declare themselves by their gait and/or their history of pelvic fracture.*

22.9 Shoulder dystocia

After delivery of the fetal head, sometimes there are mechanical problems with the delivery of the shoulders resulting from a size discrepancy between the fetal shoulders and the pelvic inlet. The incidence varies between 0.6% and 1.4% depending on the criteria used for diagnosis.[25] Despite its infrequent occurrence, shoulder dystocia continues to represent a subject of immense importance because it may occur without prediction. All birth care providers, including those who only attend "low-risk" pregnancies, must be prepared to deal with this obstetric emergency. Severe shoulder dystocia may require intrusive manual interventions strongly associated with fetal trauma, including permanently disabling brachial plexus injuries, bone fractures, severe hypoxic morbidity, and even perinatal death.[26] Maternal injuries include fourth-degree lacerations extending into the rectum and permanent psychological trauma.

22.9.1 Unpredictability

Maternal risk factors – multiparity, obesity, diabetes – all exert their effects because of the association with increased birth weight.[27] Despite this, a prophylactic cesarean delivery for fetal macrosomia is hardly ever appropriate.[25] Such a policy does not eliminate the problem because half of the newborns with shoulder dystocia weigh less than 4000 g[5,27] and, even if the birth weight of an infant is more than 4000 g, shoulder dystocia complicates only 3% of the deliveries.[28,29] Rouse and Owen convincingly argued that a policy of prophylactic cesarean for identified macrosomia involves "a Faustian bargain" because it would require more than 1000 cesarean deliveries and millions of dollars to avert a single permanent brachial plexus injury.[30] On the basis of the available evidence, ACOG concluded that performing cesarean deliveries for all women suspected of carrying a macrosomic infant is not appropriate, except possibly for estimated fetal weights over 5000 g in nondiabetic women and over 4500 g in those with diabetes.[25] A more realistic approach to the problem, in our view, is recognition of intrapartum harbingers of shoulder dystocia: secondary protraction of labor and difficult instrumental delivery of a macrosomic infant.[28,29,31–33]

22.9.2 Intrapartum warning signs

Evident warning signs are protraction of the wedging phase of first-stage labor followed by a prolonged expulsion stage despite strong contractions (manifested by caput succedaneum and molding), particularly but not necessarily in conjunction with fetal macrosomia.[28–33] These warning signs are the more ominous if occurring in parous labors. In those circumstances the obstetrician on duty should be called into the delivery room in time for stand-by assistance in case shoulder dystocia should occur. The only rational preventive measure is an absolute bar on instrumental deliveries in parous labor for failure to progress. If instrumental traction is needed for the conclusion of parous birth, shoulder dystocia almost certainly follows.

> *In general, undue attention is given to prelabor identification of risk factors for shoulder dystocia, whereas clearly identifiable warning signs in late labor are too often neglected.*

22.9.3 Preparedness

Regardless of parity, after a normal progress of dilatation and a smooth delivery of the head the risk of traumatic shoulder dystocia is small, but not absent. That is why all health care providers who attend vaginal deliveries must be able to handle this obstetric emergency. Thorough knowledge of the composite actions and maneuvers required for the alleviation of shoulder dystocia as atraumatically as possible is important, not only for obstetric residents and attending house staff but also for midwives, nurse-midwives, and family practitioners attending home births. Periodic institutional shoulder dystocia "drills" should be performed, not only to coordinate a teamwork approach to this obstetric emergency but to provide an opportunity to practice the maneuvers on a regular basis.[34]

22.10 Final classification for meaningful audit

From the foregoing analyses it is evident that the great majority of dystocia cases that are currently resolved by cesarean delivery actually involve dynamic birth disorders that can be prevented or corrected in a timely manner in most cases. Where a proper labor management protocol is followed and strict definitions are used, birth obstruction occurs far less frequently than generally assumed and recorded in obstetric databases. Mechanical labor obstruction, if properly defined, occurs in only about 1% of all term pregnancies (Chapter 29).

While the evidence and common sense dictate that "dystocia" should not be anticipated ante partum, a detailed and causal diagnosis of each labor disorder is critical for meaningful medical audit and ongoing education of all care providers involved in childbirth. All operative deliveries for "dystocia" should therefore be formally reviewed at the daily morning report on the basis of all the evidence available (Chapter 27). First a differential diagnosis between dynamic and mechanical dystocia is made (Chapter 21). If, in retrospect, dynamic factors for protraction of labor have been convincingly excluded, a formal decision on the cause of obstruction is made: either malposition of the fetal head or true CPD. This final diagnosis is officially recorded in the institutional files as well as in the patient's chart because the definitive conclusion may imply consequences for the next pregnancy and route of delivery. Where rigorous standards of diagnosis are applied, true CPD is exceedingly rare, occurring in fewer than 0.5% of all pregnancies.[10] Birth obstruction attributable to malposition of the fetal head occurs in another 0.5% of all pregnancies (Chapter 29). Well-defined mechanical birth obstruction is a relatively rare disorder indeed.

> *Formal review and detailed diagnosis of every case of "dystocia" is crucial for meaningful medical audit of procedures and outcomes, and for ongoing education of all care providers involved in childbirth.*

22.11 Summary

- Failure to appreciate the fundamental distinctions between spontaneous labor and induction, between first and subsequent labors, and between cephalic presentations and abnormal fetal lies has prevented progress in rational labor management for a very long time.
- Obstruction of the fetal head, referred to as "mechanical dystocia," may be caused either by cephalopelvic disproportion or by its clinical analog: malposition of the fetal head.
- Mechanical dystocia should never be anticipated in late pregnancy. The only reliable test for the mechanical impossibility of birth is labor itself.
- Mechanical birth obstruction is diagnosed by exclusion of dynamic labor disorders. The possibility of birth obstruction is considered only after efficient uterine force has been assured for a limited period of time. In first labors this diagnosis usually requires use of oxytocin.
- It is not birth obstruction that introduces hazards for mother and child but the obstetrician who neglects the significance of parity, disregards appropriate first-stage labor management, and misconstrues full dilatation as the demarcation line between abdominal and vaginal delivery.
- Proper diagnosis is only possible after rational first-stage labor management. Detailed analysis of dystocia and proper causal diagnosis prevent obstetricians from undertaking undue cesarean deliveries because of overdiagnosis of CPD. Equally importantly, it also prevents forced and severely traumatic instrumental vaginal deliveries in cases of true birth obstruction.

REFERENCES

1. Stewart KS, Philpott RH. Fetal response to cephalopelvic disproportion. *Br J Obstet Gynaecol* 1980; 87(8): 641–9.
2. Miller DA, Goodwin TM, Gherman RB, *et al.* Intrapartum rupture of the unscarred uterus. *Obstet Gynecol* 1997; 89: 671–3.
3. Rosen M, Debanne S, Thompson K, *et al.* Abnormal labor and infant brain damage. *Obstet Gynecol* 1992; 80: 961–5.
4. Brill Y, Windrim R. Vaginal birth after cesarean section: review of antenatal predictors of success. *J Obstet Gynaecol Can* 2003; 25: 275–86.
5. Cunningham FG, Leveno KJ, Bloom SL, *et al.* Chapter 20: Dystocia: abnormal labor. In: *Williams Obstetrics*, 22nd edn. New York: McGraw-Hill; 2005: 495–524.
6. American College of Obstetricians and Gynecologists. *Guidelines for diagnostic imaging during pregnancy*. Committee Opinion No. 158. September 1995.
7. Pattinson RC. Pelvimetry for fetal cephalic presentations at term. *Cochrane Database Syst Rev* 2000; (2): CD000161.
8. Enkin M, Keirse MJNC, Neilson J, *et al.* Prolonged labor. In: *A Guide to Effective Care in Pregnancy and Childbirth*, 3rd edn. Oxford: Oxford University Press; 2000.
9. Sanchez-Ramos K, Bernstein S, Kaunitz AM. Expectant management versus labor induction for suspected fetal macrosomia: a systematic review. *Obstet Gynecol* 2002; 100: 997–1002.
10. O'Driscoll K, Meagher D, Robson M. *Active Management of Labour*, 4th edn. Mosby; 2003.
11. Cruikshank DP, White CA. Obstetric malpresentations: twenty years' experience. *Am J Obstet Gynecol* 1973; 116: 1097–104.
12. Broekhuizen FF, Washington JM, Johnson F, *et al.* Vacuum extraction versus forceps delivery: Indications and complications, 1979 to 1984. *Obstet Gynecol* 1987; 69: 338–42.
13. American College of Obstetricians and Gynecologists: Operative Vaginal Delivery. *Practice bulletin* No. 17, June 2000.
14. American Academy of Pediatrics and the American College of Obstetricians and Gynecologists. *Guidelines for Perinatal Care*, 5th edn. Washington DC: AAP and ACOG; 2002.
15. Menticoglou SM, Perlman M, Manning FA. High cervical spinal cord injury in neonates delivered with forceps: Report of 15 cases. *Obstet Gynecol* 1995; 86: 589–94.
16. Towner D, Castro MA, Eby-Wilkens E, *et al.* Effect of mode of delivery in nulliparous women on neonatal intracranial injury. *N Engl J Med* 1999; 341: 1709–14.
17. Hagadorn-Freathy AS, Yeomans ER, Hankins GDV. Validation of the 1988 ACOG forceps classification system. *Obstet Gynecol* 1991; 77: 356–60.

18. Gardberg M, Laakkonen E, Salevaara M. Intrapartum sonography and persistent occiput posterior position: a study of 408 deliveries. *Obstet Gynecol* 1998; 91: 746–9.

19. Cunningham FG, Leveno KJ, Bloom SL, *et al.* Normal Labor and Delivery. In: *Williams Obstetrics*, 22nd edn. New York: McGraw-Hill; 2005: 407–441.

20. Gardberg M, Tupparainen M. Anterior placental location predisposes for occiput posterior presentation near term. *Acta Obstet Gynecol Scand* 1994; 73: 151–2.

21. Cruikshank DP, Cruikshank JE. Face and brow presentations: a review. *Clin Obstet Gynecol* 1981; 24(2): 333–51.

22. Sizer AR, Nirmal DM. Occipitoposterior position: associated factors and obstetric outcome in nulliparas. *Obstet Gynecol* 2000; 96: 749–52.

23. Fitzpatrick M, McQuillan K, O'Herlihy C. Influence of persistent occiput posterior position on delivery outcome. *Obstet Gynecol* 2001; 98(6): 1027–31.

24. Speer DP, Peltier LF. Pelvic fractures and pregnancy. *J Trauma* 1972; 12: 474–80.

25. American College of Obstetricians and Gynecologists. Shoulder Dystocia. *Practice bulletin* No. 40, November 2002.

26. Gherman RB, Ouzounian JG, Goodwin TM. Obstetric maneuvers for shoulder dystocia and associated fetal morbidity. *Am J Obstet Gynecol* 1998; 178: 1126–30.

27. Gherman RB. Shoulder dystocia: Prevention and management. *Obstet Gynecol Clin N Am* 2005; 32: 297–305.

28. Acker DB, Sachs BP, Friedman EA. Risk factors for shoulder dystocia. *Obstet Gynecol* 1985; 66: 762–8.

29. Geary M, McParland P, Johnson H, *et al.* Shoulder dystocia: is it predictable? *Eur J Obstet Gynecol Reprod Biol* 1995; 62: 15–18.

30. Rouse DJ, Owen J. Prophylactic cesarean delivery for fetal macrosomia diagnosed by means of ultrasonography; a Faustian bargain? *Am J Obstet Gynecol* 1999; 181: 332–8.

31. Baskett TF, Allen AC. Perinatal implications of shoulder dystocia. *Obstet Gynecol* 1995; 86: 14–17.

32. Nocon JJ, McKenzie DK, Thomas LJ, *et al.* Shoulder dystocia: An analysis of risks and obstetric maneuvers. *Am J Obstet Gynecol* 1993; 168: 1732–9.

33. Iffy L, Varadi V, Jakobovits A. Common intrapartum denominators of shoulder dystocia related birth injuries. *Zentralbl Gynakol* 1994; 116: 33–7.

34. Hernandez C, Wendell GD. Shoulder dystocia. In Pitkin RM, ed. *Clinical Obstetrics and Gynecology*, vol XXXIII. Hagerstown, PA: Lippincott; 1990: 526.

23

Curtailed use of induction

As documented in nearly all previous chapters, induction of labor provokes the exact opposite of *proactive support of labor*. For this reason we strongly advise against this procedure. In spite of this clear stand, the subject must be discussed because the widespread popularity of induction of labor shows that several adverse aspects of this intervention are severely underestimated by many obstetricians and patients: direct iatrogenic harm, indirect negative effects on others, educative drawbacks, and detrimental effects on maternity care as a whole. This chapter is written mainly to promote self-reflection by those well-intending colleagues who practice liberal induction policies.

23.1 Iatrogenic harm

There can be no doubt that elective induction for convenience of the practitioner or the patient is becoming more prevalent. Induction rates up to 30% are now accepted as normal practice despite the fact that all controlled studies on elective induction, in search of the health consequences, came up with the same answer: more co-interventions, more prolonged labors, more need of analgesia, more intrauterine infections, and above all, a staggering increase in cesarean and vaginal operative delivery rates, especially in nulliparas but also in parous women.[1–10] Most of these studies reported that labor induction results in at least a 2- to 3-fold risk for cesarean delivery. This trend appears to be unchanged even when the cervix is judged to be "favorable" for induction.[11,12]

Induction of labor

The duration of labor is prolonged; physical and emotional stress soar; the workload of nurses and midwives is increased disproportionately; there is a greater demand for analgesia; the chance of chorioamnionitis increases; and operative delivery rates rocket (Evidence level B).

Surgical excess due to elective induction is present in all studies regardless of the method of induction (prostaglandins or amniotomy plus oxytocin). This illustrates that in many cases of induction – even when the cervix is presumed to be "ripe" – the myometrium is poorly prepared for labor, with consequent dynamic labor disorders (Chapter 8). Yeast *et al.*[12] found a 70% increase in cesarean rate in nulliparous women induced with a "favorable cervix" (RR 1.7; 95% CI 1.4–2.0), which clearly proves that it takes more than "cervical ripeness" to prepare the uterus for birth, viz. myometrial transformation (Chapter 8). The lack of prelabor myometrial transformation prevents a normal, smooth labor and delivery in induced women. As a result, induction is one of the main contributors to women's dissatisfaction with labor and the high overall cesarean delivery rates. Given this evidence, induction of labor without a strong medical indication cannot be justified in any circumstances. One effective way to reduce requests for elective induction is to provide the above evidence-based information and then ask the woman to sign informed consent. Most women will abandon their request.

> *Induction of labor without a strong medical indication cannot be justified in any circumstances.*

23.1.1 Misinterpretation of statistics

One of many unfortunate consequences of uncritical extrapolation of statistical information from survey studies is an almost unbridled expansion of indications to induce labor. Post-term pregnancy and hypertension are the two most common examples, accounting for about 80% of reported inductions. In some countries the official guideline even dictates 41 weeks as the gestational age at which induction is justified or indicated.[13] Menticoglou and Hall, however, convincingly pointed out that the basis of these guidelines is a "nonsensus consensus," because "adversity odds are significantly overestimated, normalcy odds are even more significantly underestimated, and both logic and behavior are warped as a result."[14] These authors presented an elegant, comprehensive and compelling plea against routine or "ritual" induction at 41 weeks as a "rescue from normalcy ... that does more harm than good." However, as long as such guidelines are not withdrawn, doctors tend to stick to them for fear of medicolegal implications. The potential harmful effects of (ill-grounded) official guidelines in a medicolegal context have been illustrated in various situations.[15–17]

> *For most "indications" labor induction does not save children, but does inflict harm on mothers.*

Hypertension is another example. Statistically, there is an association with perinatal and even maternal mortality. Against this background, induction of labor is too often undertaken on a rule-of-thumb basis without serious attempts to select the individuals who are genuinely in need of delivery: those with strictly defined preeclampsia. Mild gestational hypertension in late pregnancy is a completely different and much less dangerous gestosis than preeclampsia. In patients with term gestational hypertension, Gofton *et al.* found no differences in fetal outcome or hypertension-related maternal morbidity between women whose labor was induced and those managed expectantly, but they confirmed a significantly higher cesarean delivery rate in the induced group (21.6% vs. 13.8%).[18] Evidently, the treatment with induction is far more dangerous than the disease.

Induction is also widely employed for suspected fetal macrosomia, but neither is this practice supported by evidence. On the contrary, in a recent meta-analysis of observational studies in women with suspected fetal macrosomia, neonatal outcome was similar but cesarean rates were twice as high in cases treated with induction compared with those followed with expectant management (16.6% vs. 8.4%).[19] In conclusion:

> *Given the evidence, induction of labor should be rigorously restricted to a select number of individuals in whom the indication is genuine and conditions seem to be favorable.*

23.2 Limitation of cervix scores

The failure rate of induction is related partly to the preinduction cervical state. However, assessment of the cervix is highly subjective and even experienced examiners may differ in their appraisal of cervical suitability for induction. So-called cervix scores – the classic Bishop score is most used – suggest a level of precision that does not exist. Recent studies[20–22] have suggested transvaginal ultrasound for the assessment of "inducibility," but there is no evidence that sonography performs any better in this respect than digital examination. More importantly, all attempts to assess "inducibility" completely disregard the critical requirement for effective labor, and that is myometrial transformation with the formation of CAPs and precursors of myometrial gap junctions (Chapter 8). The absence of myometrial readiness for labor explains the cesarean delivery odds after induction, even in women with a supposedly "favorable cervix." Moreover, Bishop based his recommendations purely on multiparas and wrote: "Owing to the unpredictability in the nullipara, even in the presence of apparently favorable circumstances, induction of labor brings little advantage for either obstetrician or patient."[23] Bishop would turn in his grave if he knew that currently tens of thousands of nulliparous women are induced on a daily basis because of a "favorable Bishop score."

> *Nulliparous women whose labor is induced with a "favorable" cervical score have a 70% increased chance of cesarean delivery (Evidence level B).*

23.3 Hazards of cervical priming

Amniotomy followed by oxytocin is the classic method of labor induction, requiring at least some cervical maturation to the extent that the membranes can be artificially ruptured. Following the clinical introduction of prostaglandins, however, this physical barrier to induction could be circumvented and the state of affairs around induction became even more confusing. Prostaglandins are claimed to improve the readiness of the cervix for induction ("inducibility") through "priming" of the cervix. The effect is that now prostaglandins are used for preinduction "priming" or for the induction procedure itself. In practice, these procedures merge imperceptibly into each other and most patients do not realize the difference. Prostaglandins almost invariably induce uterine contractility, but often ineffectively because the myometrium is not ready for labor (Chapter 8). The result is a disastrous false start (Chapter 14).

Cervical priming is not a trivial intervention. The risks involved are not limited to those related to priming itself – false expectations, unrest, uterine irritability, discomfort, and uterine hypertonia and related fetal distress – but include all the risks associated with induction of labor including exploding cesarean rates.[24,25] Prysak and Castronova reported a 3-fold higher cesarean delivery rate in women who underwent cervical priming compared with case-controls with spontaneous onset of labor (RR 3.06; 95% CI 1.46–6.4).[26] On the other hand, if induction of effective labor is easily achieved, labor was most likely to start spontaneously within a very short period of time anyhow. The gain? . . . zero!

> *"The laxity, or otherwise, of the indications for priming/induction determines the magnitude of the iatrogenic problems created by these forms of medical interventions in each hospital."[27]*

The greatest hazard of cervical priming is erosion of its indication. The technical ease of the procedure may result in unnecessary priming/induction of labor in women for whom an artificial ending of pregnancy would not otherwise have been contemplated. The result is that even women with an "unfavorable" cervix are now easily exposed to cervical priming, sometimes for several days in a row, without the prospect of any advantage to themselves or their babies. An exploratory trial of priming/induction, "just to see what happens," is frequently undertaken but is utterly imprudent. The allegation that "no harm is done if labor is not achieved because the membranes are left intact" is invalid: expectations are raised that are difficult to undo. Disappointment, agitation, or a full-blown and iatrogenic false start may be the result (Chapter 14) and the membranes might rupture without establishing labor. All these effects may occur after even a single administration of prostaglandins. Although frequently done, repeated priming for days in a row is an utterly reprehensible practice: it drives women (and nursing staff) nuts.

> *The greatest hazard of prostaglandins is erosion of the indication for their use.*

23.4 Indirect adverse effects

Liberal indications for priming/induction not only carry risks for the women in question but also frustrate the whole obstetrical practice and preclude the development of integrated patterns of thought about labor in the associated caregivers.

23.4.1 Effect on others

Inductions make disproportionate claims on the delivery room staff. The nurses need to take care of women for prolonged periods who are not in labor, or who are experiencing the burden of a false start, or who have an iatrogenic long labor with increased demands for analgesia. This nursing staff attention can only be made available at the expense of other women who are spontaneously in labor. "It is a strange paradoxical reality in many labor and delivery units that women who are not in labor receive more attention from staff and for a longer time than women who are in labor."[27]

> *The procedure and effects of priming/induction make a disproportionate claim on the labor room staff to the detriment of care of women who are spontaneously in labor.*

23.4.2 Educative drawbacks

A normal reaction to the misfortune of others is to trivialize one's own role by looking for external causes, and doctors are very human in this regard. Many a cesarean delivery to resolve a failed induction is performed under pseudo-diagnoses such as "dystocia" or "cephalopelvic disproportion." The reality, however, is that surgery was the only way out of a situation caused by the doctor himself or herself and that often on dubious grounds that would not in themselves have justified a cesarean section. The turmoil surrounding the surgical conclusion of an induced labor easily conceals the reality that the need for this intervention should be attributed to the procedure of priming and/or induction itself, which caused ineffective long labor and/or uterine hypertonia with fetal distress. Natural reluctance to acknowledge the plain truth that the problem is doctor-caused is destructive in a training situation where aspiring obstetricians are malconditioned by the liberal induction practices of their superiors. When obstetric training is largely based on experience with inductions, the critical importance of the diagnosis of onset of spontaneous labor remains completely obscure to aspiring specialists. In addition, long labors are wrongly considered normal and a convenient epidural as an indispensable component of modern obstetrics. Nulliparous labor and delivery are no longer followed from beginning to end, and thanks to fragmented involvement it has become nearly impossible for young doctors to gain insight and overview. Personal involvement and continuous commitment are increasingly seen as impossible ideals from times past before the labor act that disallows duty shifts of more than 12 hours was passed. The fundamental difference between induction and augmentation is hardly recognized or not realized at all, so that the possibilities and limitations of oxytocin in these different situations are completely misjudged. Mechanical birth obstruction cannot reliably be discerned from iatrogenic dynamic labor disorders after induction, resulting in a sharp overdiagnosis of CPD (Chapter 22). In conclusion: liberal induction practices operate at virtual loggerheads with responsible obstetric training. Certainly, residents and fellows develop dexterity with forceps, vacuum extractor, and scalpel, but they remain mostly lacking in fundamental insight into the physiology of spontaneous labor and in logical patterns of thought about integrated care for normal labor by which operative deliveries can largely be prevented.

> Induction of labor and obstetric training
>
> *The acquisition of professional skills and confidence is frequently built on a constant repetition of the same mistakes.*

23.5 Methods of labor induction

To date, investigators have concentrated almost exclusively on the evaluation of diverse techniques of labor induction rather than on the more important question of when an induction is preferable over watchful expectation until the spontaneous onset of labor. The efforts spent on these comparative studies are disproportionate to their value. All induction methods have their (hidden) drawbacks and hazards despite other claims in glossy brochures of manufacturers. As the renowned and esteemed godfathers of evidence-based obstetrics conclude: "The most important decision to be made when considering the induction of labor is whether or not the induction is justified, rather than how it is to be achieved. . . . There is too little evidence to allow any judgment about whether prostaglandins are more safe for the babies or the mother than amniotomy plus oxytocin, or to claim superiority of any of the various prostaglandins or method of administration."[28] Since the concept of *proactive support* primarily concerns labor and delivery after spontaneous onset, a detailed evaluation of the diverse induction methods is not relevant and, hence, not included in this manual.

> *"There is little purpose in assessing the relative merits of different ways of achieving elective delivery if there is no need for elective delivery in the first place."*[28]

23.6 Balancing the trade-offs

On balance, the direct and indirect drawbacks of priming/induction are so numerous and impres-

sive and the individual advantages so dubious, that women's well-being and the maternity service as a whole were best served with a "virtual embargo on this procedure."[27] As an embargo is hardly a practical suggestion, we propose the formulation of strict guidelines to guard indications for priming/induction and we advise continual and relevant audit of outcomes as well (Chapter 27).

23.6.1 Firmness clauses

- An induction should always be seen as the lesser of two evils. Even with a "favorable" cervix, induction remains a calculated risk, especially in nulliparas. This gamble is only justified if the pathological condition for which the termination of labor is considered is so serious that a cesarean section is justified if induction proves to be impossible.
- The indication should be made without prior cervical assessment. Only after the decision to end pregnancy is made, should inducibility be assessed and the choice between induction and cesarean delivery made. This clause prevents relaxation of indication and undue use of prostaglandins.
- The indication for priming/induction must be indisputable and unanimously carried by the obstetric staff. The indication for each individual case has to be discussed at the daily plenary staff session. This is the most effective clause for reducing the currently inappropriate priming/induction rates (Chapter 27). There are hardly any emergency indications for priming/induction that cannot wait until the next morning.
- To prevent any false expectations and associated confusion, residents are forbidden even to suggest priming/induction to patients without prior consultation with the responsible senior staff.
- To impress on all caregivers involved that this is no physiological labor, all inductions are preferably performed in the same delivery room (induction room) and all additional interventions and labor outcomes should be registered separately (Chapter 27).

Leading firmness clause

On balance, the pathological condition for which the termination of labor is considered must be so serious that a cesarean delivery is justified if induction proves impossible.

23.6.2 Continual audit

The suggestion that cesarean delivery after induction was inherent in the problem for which labor was being induced is mostly untenable: most pregnancy complications regarded as indications for induction do not in themselves constitute causes of labor disorders, except perhaps postmaturity beyond 42 weeks (meconium). One of the most important boosts to quality improvement is continual evaluation of each labor procedure and its outcome by plenary staff review (Chapter 27). The aim of induction is to effectuate a vaginal delivery, and each cesarean delivery after priming/induction should therefore be classified as a "failed induction." This is no accusation that the policy was wrong – that is to presume that the indication for induction was valid – just logic and clarity of thought.

Each cesarean delivery after priming/induction is put on permanent record as a "failed induction."

If the will is there, inductions can responsibly be limited to 10–15% of all nulliparas and even less in multiparas without any detriment to fetal outcomes (Chapter 29). It mainly concerns patients postmature beyond 42 weeks (or earlier in case of anhydramnion or nonreassuring antenatal CTG) and patients with prolonged prelabor ruptured membranes, preeclampsia, insulin-dependent diabetes, blood type isoimmunization, and so forth.

23.6.3 Food for thought

It should be noted that most diagnoses of so-called "fetal compromise" are extremely nebulous and ill-defined, while the impaired placental circulation of the truly endangered fetus disallows a safe labor and vaginal delivery. It is astonishing, on consideration, how many presumed "compromised" fetuses are actually exposed to the extra hazards of priming-related uterine hypertonia, and often even without continuous fetal surveillance in the antenatal ward. Besides, the fetus that does tolerate induced contractions without problems by definition has an excellent placental circulatory reserve capacity (Chapter 8). So where is or was the need for induction? Current clinical practice is often incomprehensible indeed.

23.7 Summary

- There should be no confusion between induction of labor and acceleration of spontaneously begun labor.
- *Proactive support* specifically excludes labor induction because induction has extremely negative effects on women's childbirth experience and on the outcome of labor.
- Cervical priming is also by no means a trivial intervention and should be considered as an implicit part of induction: priming is induction.
- Priming/induction artificially prolongs the physical and emotional burden of childbirth.
- Priming/induction dramatically increases the need for pain relief measures.
- Priming/induction increases the incidence of fetal distress due to iatrogenic uterine hypertonia.
- Priming/induction causes cesarean and instrumental delivery rates to rocket owing to iatrogenic dynamic labor disorders.
- The nursing resource implications of priming/induction are staggering. All staff are occupied with non-laboring patients to the detriment of the care of patients who are really in labor.
- Liberal induction policies frustrate proper education and training in labor and delivery skills.
- The crucial diagnosis of onset of labor is hopelessly obscured by priming/induction.

- After labor induction a reliable distinction between (iatrogenic) dynamic labor disorders and genuine mechanical birth obstruction is virtually impossible.
- When the fundamental distinction between use of oxytocin for induction and for augmentation remains undervalued, the therapeutic range of oxytocin in these different situations continues to be completely misjudged.
- Because priming/induction brings about the exact opposite of *proactive support of labor*, we plead for well-defined firmness clauses and for continual audit of all outcomes.
- The indication to end pregnancy should be so firm that a prelabor cesarean delivery is medically justified if labor induction appears to be impossible.
- The critical decision to be made when considering induction of labor is whether the induction is justified rather than how it is to be achieved.
- For factual and meaningful audit a failed induction should be recorded as a "failed induction."

REFERENCES

1. Seyb ST, Berka RJ, Socol ML, Doodley SL. Risk of cesarean delivery with elective induction of labor at term in nulliparous women. *Obstet Gynecol* 1999; 94: 600–7.
2. Macer JA, Macer CL, Chan LS. Elective induction versus spontaneous labor: a retrospective study of complications and outcome. *Am J Obstet Gynecol* 1992; 166: 1690–6.
3. Cammu H, Marten G, Ruyssinck G, Amy JJ. Outcome after elective induction in nulliparous women: a matched cohort study. *Am J Obstet Gynecol* 2002; 186: 240–4.
4. Luthy DA, Malmgren JA, Zingheim RW. Increased Cesarean section rates associated with elective induction in nulliparous women; the physician effect. *Am J Obstet Gynecol* 2004; 191: 1511–15.
5. Dublin S, Lydon-Rochelle M, Kaplan RC, Watts DH, Critchlow CW. Maternal and fetal outcomes after induction without an identified indication. *Am J Obstet Gynecol* 2000; 18: 986–94.
6. Van Gemund N, Hardeman A, Scherjon SA, Kanhai HH. Intervention rates after elective induction of labor compared to labor with a spontaneous onset: a matched cohort study. *Gynecol Obstet Invest* 2003; 56(3): 133–8.
7. Maslow AS, Sweeny AL. Elective induction of labor as a risk factor for cesarean delivery among low-risk women at term. *Obstet Gynecol* 2000; 95: 917–22.
8. Smith KM, Hoffman MK, Scicione A. Elective induction of labor in nulliparous women increases the risk of cesarean section. *Obstet Gynecol* 2003; 101: S45.
9. Kauffman K, Bailit J, Grobman W. Elective induction: an analysis of economic and health consequences. *Am J Obstet Gynecol* 2001; 185: S209.
10. Vahratian A, Zhang J, Troendle JF, *et al.* Labor progression and risk of cesarean delivery in electively induced nulliparas. *Obstet Gynecol* 2005; 105: 698–704.
11. Hamar B, Mann S, Greenberg P, *et al.* Low-risk inductions of labor and cesarean delivery for nulliparous and parous women at term. *Am J Obstet Gynecol* 2001; 185: S215.
12. Yeast JD, Jones A, Poskin M. Induction of labor and the relationship to cesarean delivery; a review of 7001 consecutive inductions. *Am J Obstet Gynecol* 1999; 180: 628–33.
13. Maternal-Fetal Medicine Committee of the Society of Obstetricians and Gynecologists of Canada. Post-term pregnancy (Committee Opinion). *SOGC Clinical Practice Guidelines*, No 15; 1997.
14. Menticoglou SM, Hall PF. Routine induction of labour at 41 weeks gestation: nonsensus consensus. *Br J Obstet Gynaecol* 2002; 109: 485–91.
15. McIntyre KM. Medicolegal implications of consensus statements. *Chest* 1995; 108: S502–5.
16. Hyams AL, Brandenburg JA, Lipsitz SR, Shapiro DW, Brennen TA. Practice guidelines and malpractice litigation: a two-way street. *Ann Intern Med* 1995; 122: 440–5.
17. Hirshfeld EB. Should practice parameters be the standard of care in malpractice litigation? *JAMA* 1991; 266: 2886–91.
18. Gofton EN, Capewell V, Natale R, Gratton RJ. Obstetrical intervention rates and maternal and neonatal outcomes of women with gestational hypertension. *Am J Obstet Gynecol* 2001; 185: 789–803.
19. Sanchez-Ramos K, Bernstein S, Kaunitz AM. Expectant management versus labor induction for suspected fetal macrosomia: a systematic review. *Obstet Gynecol* 2002; 100: 997–1002.

20. Gonen R, Degani S, Ron A. Prediction of successful induction of labor: comparison of transvaginal ultrasonography and the Bishop score. *Eur J Ultrasound* 1998; 3: 183–7.

21. Ware V, Raynor BD. Transvaginal ultrasonographic cervical measurement as a predictor of successful labor induction. *Am J Obstet Gynecol* 2000; 182: 1030–2.

22. Gabriel R, Darnaud T, Chalot F, *et al.* Transvaginal sonography of the uterine cervix prior to labor induction. *Ultrasound Obstet Gynecol* 2002; 19: 254–7.

23. Bishop EH. Elective induction of labor. *Obstet Gynecol* 1955; 5: 519–27.

24. Vahratian A, Zhang J, Troendle JF, Sciscione AC, Hoffman MK. Labor progression and risk of cesarean delivery in electively induced multiparous women. *Obstet Gynecol* 2005; 105(4): 698–704.

25. Enkin M, Keirse MJNC, Neilson J, *et al.* Preparing for the induction of labor. In: *A Guide to Effective Care in Pregnancy and Childbirth*, 3rd edn. Oxford: Oxford University Press; 2000.

26. Prysak M, Castronova FC. Elective induction versus spontaneous delivery: a case-control analysis of safety and efficacy. *Obstet Gynecol* 1998; 92: 47–52.

27. O'Driscoll K, Meagher D, Robson M. *Active Management of Labour*, 4th edn. Mosby; 2003.

28. Enkin M, Keirse MJNC, Neilson J, *et al.* Methods of inducing labor. In: *A Guide to Effective Care in Pregnancy and Childbirth*, 3rd edn. Oxford: Oxford University Press; 2000.

24

Intrapartum care of the fetus

Although the great majority of fetuses fare well during labor and delivery, for some babies birth can be a hazardous journey. Risks to the fetus include infection, trauma, and asphyxia (hypoxia leading to acidemia). The chance of perinatal infection is directly related to the duration of ruptured membranes, and proactive steps taken to ensure short labor largely prevent this complication. Trauma is to be avoided at all costs and trauma is least likely to occur when women deliver their babies by their own efforts. Clearly, both mother and child benefit from normal, short labor and spontaneous delivery as promoted in this manual. The present chapter focuses on the prevention, timely detection, and expert treatment of intrapartum fetal hypoxia.

> *Promotion of normal, short labor largely prevents perinatal infection, trauma, and asphyxia.*

The desire to prevent fetal hypoxic injury has led to the development and introduction of electronic fetal heart rate monitoring (cardiotocography or CTG). Initially, it was used primarily in high-risk patients, but gradually electronic fetal surveillance came to be used in nearly all hospital births. Its benefits, however, fall short of the initially high expectations that CTG could reveal all about fetal condition during labor. In fact, electronic fetal monitoring is a good method for screening for umbilical cord compression, fetal hypoxia, and acidosis, but the main drawback is its high false-positive rate. This often results in superfluous interventions, rescuing babies from physiological events and needlessly inflicting harm on mothers.

24.1 Leading clinical concepts

Care of the fetus should be aimed at guarding fetal well-being without sliding into medical excess that adds risks to mothers and babies. Reduction of unnecessary interventions for erroneous suspicions of fetal distress requires knowledge and integrated concepts of normal birth and of the fetus's abilities to cope with the exigencies of normal labor and delivery (Chapter 8). Good clinical practice is governed by rational patterns of thought and action and by awareness of the fundamental differences between screening and diagnosis, taking into account the possibilities and limitations of fetal assessment techniques. In addition, rational clinical concepts focus on the causes of fetal problems, if they occur, because identification of the causes of fetal distress allows preventive and corrective measures. Basically, intrapartum threats to fetal oxygenation include:

- Insufficient placental reserves (extremely rare)
- Umbilical cord compression (very frequent)
- Impaired uteroplacental blood flow (hypotension and uterine hypertonia in abnormal labor)

24.1.1 Placental circulatory competence

Overall intrapartum care of the fetus is based on the leading premise that the fetus that thrived in pregnancy and enters labor in good condition is equipped by nature with placental circulatory reserve capacity to cope with normal labor contractions (Chapter 8). If the fetus has been perceptibly active during the past 24 hours and if the amniotic fluid is clear and, most importantly, if the fetal heart rate is not affected by contractions in early labor, it can confidently be concluded that placental reserve capacity is adequate and that the fetus can withstand normal labor contractions. In fact, early labor contractions are the ultimate test for fetoplacental competence.

> *The fetus that tolerates early contractions of labor without any problems has adequate placental reserve capacity to sustain it through the pressures and stress of a* normal *labor and delivery.*

Reassuring findings in early labor therefore signify that preexisting placental failure is virtually excluded as the cause of fetal compromise whenever troubles develop later. The cause of later-occurring oxygenation problems should therefore be sought primarily elsewhere, beginning with umbilical cord compression. A less frequent but equally dangerous threat to the normal fetus involves impaired uteroplacental blood flow, mostly due to uterine hypertonia in the intervals between contractions (abnormal labor). Another cause of reduced uteroplacental blood flow is maternal hypotension, which is mostly related to epidural analgesia (Chapter 20).

24.1.2 Normal labor

Since the basic contention is that normal placental reserves are sufficient to sustain the fetus through normal labor, it is necessary to have a clear understanding of what normal labor means: spontaneously begun and over and done with within 12 hours. If adequate placental circulatory reserve capacity has been assessed at the outset, the only remaining risks for the fetus are brought about either by abnormal labor (induction, unnecessarily prolonged labor, infection, presence of meconium) or by accidental cord compression, which can happen in any normal labor.

24.1.3 Normal fetal stress and coping ability

Fetal oxygenation is entirely dependent on the free-floating umbilical cord; as a result, blood flow is constantly in jeopardy. Inevitably, most fetuses have experienced brief but recurrent periods of hypoxia due to cord compression during normal gestation. The incidence and risks of cord compression are greatest during uterine contractions. The frequency and inevitability of transient cord occlusion have provided the fetus with physiological regulation mechanisms and buffer capacities as a means of coping with brief periods of hypoxia.[1] Many characteristics or "abnormalities" of fetal heart rate tracings during labor therefore reflect physiological responses to stress rather than pathological signs of fetal distress. The challenge is to distinguish normal fetal stress from abnormal fetal distress.

> *The fetus has adequate survival strategies to cope with the physiological stress of brief periods of hypoxia due to cord compression in normal labor.*

24.1.4 Umbilical cord compression

Cord compression is the most prevalent and practically the only fetal problem in *normal* labor. It can be detected by the typical variable decelerations on the CTG characterized by transient series of decelerations in heart rate that vary in duration, intensity, and relation to uterine contraction. It should be noted that the umbilical blood vessels of growth-retarded fetuses are more susceptible to compression because dysmature cords contain less Wharton's jelly.

Occasional cord compression can be identified in about 40% of all fetuses in the retraction phase, increasing to 83% by the end of the wedging phase of first-stage labor.[2] This high prevalence attests to the physiological nature of these events. In second-stage labor, fetal heart rate decelerations are virtually ubiquitous and these can be attributed to cord compression and fetal head compression. In fact, more than 98% of all fetuses respond to second-stage labor contractions with heart rate decelerations.[2] In conclusion: virtually no intrapartum fetal heart rate tracing is "normal" as judged by antepartum criteria of normalcy. This explains the difficulty in assessing intrapartum fetal well-being on the basis of CTG alone and emphasizes the importance of additional diagnostics.

> *Umbilical cord compression is the most prevalent threat to fetal well-being that can happen in any normal labor and delivery.*

Although short periods of umbilical cord compression do not pose a real threat to the healthy fetus, serious asphyxia can develop during frequent and prolonged interruption of the cord circulation. Whether and how quickly harm is inflicted on the child depends on:

- The frequency and duration of cord occlusion
- The recovery time between the contractions, which is needed for the supplementation of oxygen and the removal of waste products of anaerobic glycolysis
- The fetal buffer reserves
- The duration of labor

> *Fetal well-being is highly dependent on expert labor management ensuring normal, short labor.*

24.1.5 Abnormal labor

The second threat to fetal oxygenation after cord compression is impaired uteroplacental blood flow. This results from insufficient uterine relaxation in the intervals between contractions, which in turn results from (1) labor induction, or (2) a needlessly exhausted uterus, loaded with lactic acid (refractory uterus), or (3) disorganized uterine action due to

infection, meconium, or intrauterine blood (see also "Fetal Oxygenation during Labor" in Chapter 8 and "Hypertonic Uterine Dysfunction" in Chapter 21).

> *Abnormal labor jeopardizes uteroplacental blood flow.*

The rules and proactive steps dictated by the concept of *proactive support of labor* largely eliminate these hazards and leave umbilical cord compression as practically the only unpreventable threat to the healthy fetus during *normal* labor and delivery. Vigilant surveillance to detect these cord accidents in time remains mandatory in any labor and delivery.

24.1.6 Fetal distress

Dangerous fetal acidemia is exceptional in normal labor and, if it occurs, fetal condition usually deteriorates gradually. Sudden placental abruption is the obvious but exceedingly rare exception. Assuming "fetal distress" can be defined as hypoxia leading to acidemia, the term is still too broad and vague to be applied with any precision to clinical situations. Uncertainty about the diagnosis "fetal distress" based on fetal heart rate tracings has led to the use of such descriptions as *reassuring* or *nonreassuring* CTG.[3] These patterns during labor are dynamic, in that they can rapidly change from reassuring to nonreassuring and vice versa. Partly because of liability concerns, an operative delivery is commonly performed when the obstetrician loses confidence or cannot assuage doubts about fetal condition. It should be recognized, however, that this clinical judgment, if based purely on fetal heart rate tracings, is highly subjective and inevitably subject to gross imperfection.[3] This is apparent from the disappointing observation that the rate of cerebral palsy has not decreased since the widespread use of continuous electronic fetal monitoring and the associated overuse of cesarean sections.[4,5] To reduce unnecessary operative delivery because of erroneous suspicions of acidosis, it is imperative that fetal heart rate monitoring is supplemented with (serial) fetal scalp blood samplings to assess fetal pH and acid–base buffer reserves (see section 24.3 on "Intrapartum Diagnosis"). Additional diagnosis of the cause of accidental fetal compromise offers opportunities for causal treatment and corrective measures.

> *The clinical diagnosis "fetal distress" based on fetal heart rate tracings needs refinement, qualification, and quantification by fetal blood sampling.*

Brief and transient periods of fetal hypoxia are normal during labor and delivery and the fetus has physiological reserves as a competent strategy for survival. For brain damage to occur, the fetus must be exposed to much more than brief periods of hypoxia: it takes profound and prolonged fetal hypoxia with barely sublethal metabolic acidosis of pH <7.0 and base deficit ≥12.[6] Fortunately, such cases are rare[7–9] and they can be detected in time and thus prevented in nearly every case.

24.1.7 Meconium

Passage of meconium is a separate issue and a complicating factor. It has traditionally been regarded as a warning sign of placental failure and fetal compromise.[10] However, the appearance of meconium during labor does not in itself indicate fetal distress, as it is often associated with healthy fetuses. Amniotic fluid is contaminated with meconium in about 20% of pregnancies at term, and it is now recognized that in the majority of cases meconium indicates a normally maturing gastrointestinal tract, or that it occurs as the result of vagal stimulation from umbilical cord compression.[11,12] In currently prevailing opinion, passage of meconium during labor in most cases represents a sign of physiological reaction to sensory input, a part of the autonomic stress response rather than a marker of fetal distress.[11]

Nevertheless, passage of meconium during labor is always a reason for extra clinical vigilance and often for additional diagnostic measures.

> *In most cases meconium represents a sign of fetal physiological responses rather than a marker of fetal distress.*

The true clinical significance of passage of meconium is its potentially detrimental impact upon myometrial efficiency and the fetal airways when inhaled. Meconium contains bile acids and salts that render it very corrosive. This may lead to a chemical inflammation reaction that, as in cases of bacterial chorioamnionitis, may severely disorganize myometrial electrical coordination (Chapter 8). This may result in poor efficiency and thus poor effectiveness of the contractions, compounded by insufficient uterine relaxation during the contraction intervals. A vicious cycle of fetal distress and dysfunctional labor may ensue ("hypertonic dystocia," see Chapter 21).

Added to this, meconium constitutes a direct environmental hazard for the fetus. The presence of thick meconium in the fetal nasopharynx obstructs the airways at birth, resulting in acute neonatal hypoxia. Deep inhalation of meconium may lead to chemical inflammation of pulmonary tissues and in severe cases chemical pneumonitis may progress to persistent pulmonary hypertension, other neonatal morbidity, and even death. Importantly, aspiration of meconium may already occur before birth as a result of fetal gasping triggered by fetal acidemia. There is accumulating evidence that many neonates with a severe meconium aspiration syndrome have already suffered chronic hypoxia before birth.[13–16] Evidently, both intrauterine fetal gasping triggered by fetal acidemia and inhalation at the first breaths after delivery may lead to meconium aspiration syndrome, which is still a major cause of severe long-term neurological morbidity and neonatal mortality in term infants.[12]

> *Meconium may lead to a vicious cycle of dys-*
> *functional labor and fetal distress. In addition,*
> *meconium is an environmental hazard for the*
> *fetus that may lead to meconium aspiration*
> *syndrome.*

Not every passage of meconium has the same clinical significance, however. There is a world of difference between a mild discoloration of a normal amount of amniotic fluid and undiluted, thick meconium with umbilical cord, membranes, and even decidua colored green through the entire depth when exposed subsequently at cesarean section. We have therefore adopted the proposal of O'Driscoll to distinguish three grades of meconium. Since the grade of meconium dictates further clinical measures (section 24.2.5), all cases of meconium and its grade must be reported to the obstetrician who is ultimately responsible for labor management and the fetal outcome.

> Meconium grading
>
> *Grade 1: Normal amount of amniotic fluid,*
> *lightly stained with diluted, thin meconium*
> *Grade 2: A reasonable amount of amniotic*
> *fluid with a heavy suspension of fresh meconium*
> *Grade 3: No amniotic fluid and thick meco-*
> *nium that resembles thick, green pea soup*

24.1.8 Screening versus diagnosis

Electronic fetal surveillance has now become widely regarded as the standard of intrapartum care. However, the diagnostic imperfection of intrapartum CTG and diagnostic laxity – apparent from general underuse of fetal scalp blood sampling – inevitably lead to many superfluous operative deliveries. To take full advantage of intrapartum fetal surveillance without introducing unintended risks, a strict distinction must be made between screening for potential fetal compromise and diagnosis of fetal distress and its cause:

- Screening requires techniques with as high a sensitivity as possible to miss as few as possible cases. By definition, false-positive rates are high. Because labor progresses over time, screening procedures must be repeated periodically. This is called fetal monitoring.
- Diagnosis, on the other hand, requires techniques with a high specificity to determine the cases of true fetal distress and the causes thereof. Ideally, false-positive rates are low.

> *Screening/monitoring techniques for fetal com-*
> *promise require high sensitivity, whereas diag-*
> *nosis of fetal distress requires techniques with*
> *high specificity.*

Screening techniques for fetal compromise in labor include fetal heart rate monitoring, and amniotomy to assess the amount of amniotic fluid and meconium passage. A positive screening result constitutes a warning sign that calls for further diagnostic tests. Operative interventions should be based on a clear diagnosis instead of a shady screening symptom.

Diagnosis of fetal distress is based on sophisticated interpretation of fetal heart rate tracings supplemented by analysis of fetal blood gas and reserves. These fetal assessments in combination with interpretation of the partogram, intrauterine pressure readings, and other clinical characteristics of labor will help to establish a plausible diagnosis of the cause of fetal compromise. In fact, a causal diagnosis of fetal distress can be made in nearly every case, often allowing causal treatment and corrective measures.

24.2 Practice 1: Intrapartum screening/ monitoring

Proactive support of labor is a concept specifically designed for childbirth of healthy women after a normal and uneventful pregnancy. Responsible care of both mother and fetus is based on the clinical concepts and considerations discussed above. Like rational care for mothers, rational fetal care also requires an overall plan characterized by consistency in thoughts and actions.

24.2.1 Fetoplacental assessment at the onset of labor

Since the leading concept is that a healthy fetus with a normally functioning placenta can smoothly sustain normal labor, it is imperative to assess that the fetus is healthy at the outset and that labor is and remains normal. Good intrapartum care of the fetus therefore begins with:

1. Verification that pregnancy was uneventful
2. Confirmation that the fetoplacental starting condition in early labor is good
3. An overall plan to promote normal labor

The first question is answered during the antenatal visits. The second issue must be addressed at the onset of any labor in order to identify cases of fetoplacental compromise that have escaped detection in late pregnancy, before the additional stress of labor can cause an already precarious balance to deteriorate abruptly. The necessity of proper fetoplacental assessment at the onset of labor dictates:

- Explicit inquiry about recent fetal movements
- Inspection of amniotic fluid (if membranes are broken)
- A thorough check of fetal heart rate in relation to contractions, either by auscultation or by CTG.

Reassuring findings at the onset of labor attest to adequate placental circulatory reserve capacity (Chapter 8). If fetoplacental competence has been established, the only remaining risks for the fetus are brought about either by abnormal labor (induction, prolonged labor, infection, meconium passage) or by accidental cord compression, which can happen in any normal labor. Guarding fetal well-being during labor therefore further entails:

4. Waiting for the spontaneous onset of labor
5. Ensuring that labor is and remains normal, meaning at least 1 cm/h progression

6. Vigilant surveillance to detect unforeseeable cord accidents in time

The basic tools for these assessments include:

A. Serial fetal heart rate counts or electronic fetal heart rate monitoring
B. Keeping a partogram from the very onset of labor
C. Artificial rupture of membranes whenever labor is too slow, even in the early stage of labor. A latent phase is not recognized (Chapters 9, 11).

> *Reassuring fetal assessments in early labor signify that preexisting placental failure is excluded as the cause of fetal compromise if troubles should develop later. The cause of later fetal problems should therefore primarily be sought elsewhere, beginning with umbilical cord compression.*

24.2.2 Fetal heart rate monitoring

Fetal condition is monitored (= repetitive screening) by assessment of fetal heart rate either by intermittent auscultation or by CTG. Both monitoring techniques are highly sensitive in detecting fetal compromise but poorly specific, implying high rates of false-positive findings. No scientific evidence has identified either of the two methods as the more effective screening method for fetal hypoxia, nor is there any scientific evidence to indicate the frequency or duration of these fetal assessments that ensures optimum results.[17,18]

24.2.3 Fetal monitoring by intermittent auscultation

Counting fetal heart rate was originally performed with a wooden stethoscope (Pinard). Use of a handheld Doppler fetal heart detector has revolutionized this procedure, making it possible to count the fetal heartbeat easily with the woman in any position and allowing heart rate assessments during contractions. There are even waterproof machines for use in baths. Auscultation is a duty performed by the personal nurse. The simplicity of Doppler auscultation is an attractive advantage of its use. Many patients appreciate this non-interventional approach to fetal assessment because it allows free movement and because it implies bedside nursing assessments at defined intervals.

ACOG recommends that auscultation should be performed at the end of a contraction and be repeated every 15–30 minutes during first-stage labor and every 5–15 minutes in second-stage labor.[19] This authority-based guideline (Evidence level D) discourages midwifery practices in which laboring women at home are left unattended for periods of three hours or more (Chapter 5).

A fetal heart rate above 150 or below 110 beats/min for more than five minutes and any slowing by more than 15 beats/min after contractions is regarded as an indication for continuous electronic monitoring.[3] Home births should be transferred to the hospital immediately. On the other hand, obstetricians should acknowledge that electronic fetal monitoring does not yield any additional advantage as long as the auscultated fetal heart rate is normal. Rather the reverse might be true. Despite continued emphasis on continuous electronic monitoring in most hospitals, other institutions have taken positive steps to promote intermittent auscultation not only as an option but also as the most reasonable choice of fetal surveillance in low-risk pregnancies.[20]

> *Both intermittent auscultation and electronic fetal heart rate monitoring are highly sensitive but poorly specific methods for detecting fetal distress.*

24.2.4 Continuous electronic monitoring

Intrapartum CTG is now the most prevalent obstetric procedure in western maternity centers without the benefit of scientific validation. Its role in reducing fetal and neonatal morbidity – and ultimately improving long-term outcomes – remains to be defined. Routine use is nevertheless popular, mainly for its convenience, but when continuous fetal monitoring is practiced while the nurse is elsewhere, all standards of birth care slide down a slippery slope (Chapter 4).

> *Indiscriminate or routine electronic fetal monitoring may create more problems than it prevents.*

For a comprehensive discussion of abnormal intrapartum CTG patterns, readers are referred to the renowned standard books.[21–23] The main problem is that the interpretation regarding clinical consequences is notoriously subjective.[24,25] Fetal heart rate patterns are affected by a variety of physiological and pathological mechanisms and, although specialists can reliably distinguish severely abnormal from normal patterns, this is much more difficult for beginners. They either detect fetal problems where there are none or may be overconfident despite their lack of experience. Even the experts find some patterns difficult to interpret and often disagree about the subsequent clinical decision.[24,25] Such manifest discordance confirms the practical notion that CTG in labor represents primarily a screening method and not a reliable diagnostic test.

A normal fetal heart rate is marked by a baseline of 110–160 beats/min, 6–25 beats/min variability, accelerations present, and no decelerations. Such a reassuring pattern during labor strongly predicts a good neonatal outcome. On the other hand, a nonreassuring fetal heart rate pattern is most often inconclusive and reliable identification of imminent fetal danger therefore requires further diagnostic investigation. Although persistent late decelerations often indicate some degree of fetal hypoxia, fetal reserves are variable and the ability of the fetus to cope over a period of time can be assessed only with (serial) blood sampling to give blood gas and pH estimation.

> Many "abnormalities" of fetal heart rate tra-
> cings reflect physiological responses to normal
> stress rather than pathological signs of fetal
> distress.

> Poor labor progress is a firm indication for
> amniotomy to check the presence and color of
> amniotic fluid. There are no contraindications
> for artificial rupture of membranes during labor
> (Chapter 17).

24.2.5 Detection of meconium and clinical consequences

Information on the presence and color of amniotic fluid is directly obtainable in cases of spontaneously ruptured membranes (about 30% of beginning labors). To confirm or exclude passage of meconium, O'Driscoll advocated artificial rupture of membranes as a screening test for fetal compromise at the onset of all labors, but there is no scientific basis for such a policy. On the other hand, there are no objective contraindications to amniotomy once labor has started, provided delivery is accomplished within a restricted time (Chapter 17). Therefore, the first measure in case of insufficient progress is breaking of the membranes, not in the last place to check whether there is passage of meconium, which can play a causative role in dysfunctional labor. It should be emphasized, however, that clear amniotic fluid at early amniotomy should not be considered a reassuring sign during labor. In a cohort study of 8394 "low-risk" women, meconium was not detected until delivery of the fetal head in 51.5% of cases with intrapartum passage of meconium.[26] Meconium was associated with neonatal acidosis and seizures, but the sensitivity of the intrapartum detection of meconium for these outcomes was very poor. The authors concluded that clear amniotic fluid in labor is an unreliable sign of fetal well-being. Evidently, fetal surveillance remains mandatory if amniotic fluid is clear. On the other hand, manifest passage of meconium is always reason for extra vigilance with regard to both uterine contractile efficiency and fetal condition, and clinical management depends on the grade of meconium.

- **Grade 1 meconium** still allows for a wide margin of discretion. After careful review of all the clinical circumstances, no further action beyond continuous fetal heart rate monitoring is taken in most cases. However, if labor is slow and oxytocin is needed, intrauterine pressure should be monitored to detect hypertonic dystocia at an early stage. In healthy, well-oxygenated newborns, inhaled meconium grade 1 is readily cleared from the lungs by normal physiological mechanisms.

- **Grade 2 meconium** is a strict indication for electronic fetal surveillance including intrauterine pressure readings. Treatment is determined by these monitoring results and the progress of labor. As long as the fetal heart rate pattern is normal, there is no increased likelihood of fetal distress. However, abnormal fetal heart rate patterns in conjunction with grade 2 meconium are a compelling reason for (serial) fetal blood sampling to assess pH and fetal reserves. Poor progress of labor should be augmented as in all other cases, but when the uterus responds with inter-contraction hypertonia or whenever the fetus does not tolerate the contractions needed for normal labor progression, operative delivery should be undertaken. Special attention must be paid to proper airway management immediately after birth, preferably by an experienced pediatrician.

- **Grade 3 meconium** with a fetal heart rate pattern suggestive of hypoxia is a sufficient indication for immediate cesarean delivery, even if the fetal pH is still normal, unless an easy vaginal delivery is imminent. Meconium grade 3 mostly occurs in early labor as a sign of preexisting fetal compromise pointing to placental failure. A smooth labor and delivery are exceptional and the risk of fetal gasping with intrauterine meconium aspiration is maximal when fetal acidemia supervenes. Perinatal mortality is increased 7-fold.[27] Prompt cesarean delivery is therefore warranted.

> *The grade of meconium determines the clinical consequences.*

Failure to recover any amniotic fluid at artificial rupture of membranes is, for reasons of safety, approached as meconium grade 2, although clear amniotic fluid frequently appears at a later stage.

In conclusion: artificial rupture of membranes is a poor fetal screening procedure and it does not render any diagnosis. The appearance of meconium grade 1 or 2 does not in itself indicate fetal distress, just as drainage of clear amniotic fluid does not exclude fetal compromise.

24.3 Practice 2: Intrapartum diagnosis

Detection of the transition from brief and innocent periods of hypoxia to a state of hazardous metabolic acidemia is imperative to prevent fetal brain damage, but identification of "fetal distress" based on fetal heart rate tracings alone is mostly imprecise and controversial. Such a diagnosis requires not only expertise in the recognition of ominous fetal heart rate tracings but also the use of additional and objective assessments of fetal pH and buffer reserves.

> *Intrapartum CTG presents primarily a screening method for fetal distress, but not a reliable diagnostic method.*

24.3.1 Ominous fetal heart rate patterns

Even experts in CTG interpretation disagree so often about the clinical consequences of "abnormal" heart rate tracings that one organizer of a state-of-

the-art workshop compared the experts in attendance with marine iguanas of the Galapagos Islands: "all on the same beach but facing different directions and spitting at one another constantly."[28] Nevertheless, after more than 35 years of research and clinical experience, agreement is finally emerging among experts that some particular combinations of fetal heart rate characteristics can be reliably used to identify true fetal distress, justifying a decision for surgical termination of labor without additional tests.[3] Such ominous CTG patterns are marked by zero beat-to-beat variability in conjunction with severe decelerations and/or persistent baseline rate changes.[29] Fortunately, such severely abnormal tracings are rare. Most abnormal CTG tracings are not as specific for fetal acidemia and interpretation is most often problematic. Therefore, in most cases of CTG patterns intermediate between normal and prelethal, a reliable diagnosis of fetal hypoxia/acidemia requires additional diagnostic tests.

> *Only in exceptional cases is a decision for operative delivery justified solely on the basis of CTG without additional fetal pH and reserve assessments:* zero beat-to-beat variability *in conjunction with variable and/or late decelerations or in conjunction with persistent bradycardia or tachycardia.*

24.3.2 Fetal scalp blood sampling

The pH of fetal capillary scalp blood approaches that of umbilical artery blood, and fetal acidosis assessed by fetal scalp blood sampling is generally accepted as the definitive diagnosis of fetal distress. Zalar and Quilligan[30] recommended the following clinical protocol to confirm fetal distress, which is as yet unchallenged:

- If pH > 7.25, labor is allowed to continue and vigilantly observed.
- If $7.20 \leqslant pH \leqslant 7.25$, blood sampling is repeated within 30 minutes.

- If pH < 7.20 another scalp blood sample is collected immediately, and the mother is prepared for surgery. Operative delivery is performed promptly if the low pH is confirmed. Otherwise, labor is allowed to continue and fetal blood samples are repeated periodically.

Unfortunately, the technique of fetal scalp blood sampling is laborious and its use has accordingly declined substantially, even to the extent that the option for fetal blood sampling is currently no longer available in many labor units.[31,32] A recent review of 392 publications on emergent cesarean delivery for fetal distress identified only 31 publications that even mentioned the use of scalp pH before surgery, and only three of them provided specific information on how frequently it was used.[33]

The objections of inconvenience and technical difficulty are largely circumvented, however, if fetal scalp blood is used for determination of fetal lactate concentration instead of pH and base deficit estimates.[34,35] Kruger and co-workers suggest a lactate concentration of 4.8 mmol/l as a suitable cut-off limit for fetal acidemia.[35] Important advantages of measuring lactate over pH estimates in fetal blood samples include:

- The procedure for measuring fetal lactate is more successful than that for pH and base deficit.
- Much less fetal blood is needed (5 µl versus 35 µl).
- Sampling technique is easier and faster.
- Less dilatation of the cervix is needed.
- Fewer scalp punctures are needed.
- Lactate analysis is more sensitive for predicting either an Apgar score <4 at 5 minutes or moderate to severe hypoxic-ischemic encephalopathy.[35]

Fetal scalp blood lactate

New micro-sampling methods of measuring lactate in the fetal scalp blood are suitable for assessing fetal acid–base reserve in a way that is simpler, cheaper, and more reliable.

Only fetal acidosis is accepted as a definitive test for fetal distress. Therefore, a woman should not be subjected to cesarean section for the indication fetal distress without this confirmation by fetal scalp blood sampling, with the exception of rare cases of clear-cut ominous, decelerative CTG patterns with zero variability as discussed above. In practice the indication for fetal blood sampling is likely to arise most frequently in the presence of abnormal heart rate tracings in combination with grade 2 meconium where cesarean section would have to be performed – often unnecessarily – were the test not available. Clearly, in any labor and delivery unit with the slightest pretence of providing high-quality care, facilities for fetal scalp blood sampling must be present and must be used.

Objective diagnosis of fetal acidosis by fetal scalp blood sampling is the only reliable indication for operative termination of labor for fetal distress.

24.3.3 New techniques

Recognition of the low predictive value of intrapartum CTG for fetal acidemia and the associated overuse of cesarean section as well as widespread reluctance to undertake fetal blood sampling have fuelled interest in the development of other intrapartum assessment techniques.[36] These new methods include fetal pulse oximetry[37] and ST-segment analysis of the fetal electrocardiogram (STAN).[38] Unfortunately, history seems to repeat itself through premature introduction of new technology whose benefit may ultimately be disproved. Both fetal pulse oximetry and STAN have considerable failure rates (10–30%) owing to poor signal quality. More importantly, both techniques may falsely identify fetal jeopardy leading to unnecessary interventions, and both techniques may show falsely reassuring data leading to adverse outcomes.[39–47] With such differing research findings it is difficult to support the introduction of these new techniques in routine obstetric care. Ironically, the rate of emergent cesarean deliveries for fetal distress is actually increasing as new technology is being introduced to decrease its occurrence.[48]

> *If fetal pulse oximetry and/or STAN are to be used, it is important that clinicians be aware of the investigational status of the new technology. Fetal blood sampling remains the golden standard.*

Confidential inquiries into perinatal death in England and Wales indicate that in 60% of labor cases there is a clearly preventable element related to incorrect assessment or underuse of standard fetal surveillance techniques.[49] Other studies exploring the causes of perinatal death and cerebral palsy have similarly suggested rates of 50% and 25%, respectively, of clearly avoidable errors related to common fetal assessment in labor.[50–53] Obviously, there is much more to be gained for mothers and babies by improved use of currently available CTG and fetal blood sampling methods than by trying to implement completely new fetal assessment techniques of dubious reliability.

24.3.4 Causal diagnosis

Management of nonreassuring CTG patterns should be directed by the fetal blood gases and fetal reserves in relation to the expected labor duration on the one hand, and by the cause of fetal compromise on the other. Causal diagnosis of the underlying problem requires expertise in CTG interpretation supplemented by intrauterine pressure readings, analysis of the partogram, blood pressure measurements, a thermometer, and strict adherence to rational clinical concepts.

> Imminent fetal distress
>
> *Appropriate management depends on the pathophysiological cause of fetal compromise.*

Depending on the moment when (imminent) fetal compromise first occurs (at the very beginning of labor, or only later in advanced labor), pre-existing placental failure can be distinguished from the other and far more frequent causes. Umbilical cord compression is the most prevalent fetal problem in normal labor and this can be diagnosed by the typical variable decelerations. Intrauterine pressure monitoring is indispensable for diagnosis of hyperstimulation-related fetal distress, which is typical of labor inductions or unduly delayed augmentation (Chapter 21). Diagnosis of hypertonic dystocia (Chapter 21) is based on the deviating partogram and insufficient uterine relaxation in the intervals between contractions in combination with the appearance of meconium, signs of infection (maternal fever and fetal baseline tachycardia), or abnormal blood loss pointing to incipient (partial) placental abruption. Blood pressure measurement may identify maternal hypotension as the cause of impaired uteroplacental blood flow in cases of epidural analgesia. In fact, in the majority of cases of (imminent) fetal distress, a plausible causal diagnosis can be assessed if only practitioners really put their minds to it. Responsible care of the fetus, like responsible care of mothers, rests on accurate diagnosis.

> *Interventions should be based on a diagnosis, rather than a shady symptom.*

24.4 Practice 3: Interventions

The appearance of abnormal fetal heart rate tracings is not a reason to resort to prompt cesarean delivery, even when mild fetal hypoxia is detected by fetal blood sampling. It is, however, a compelling reason to decide what may be causing the abnormalities and to attempt to eliminate these underlying problems.[54]

> *"Appropriate management for significantly variant fetal heart rate patterns consists of correcting any fetal insult, if possible."*[3]

24.4.1 Causal treatment

The most frequent problem in normal labor is cord compression, diagnosed by the typical variable decelerations. Although clinicians generally remember to change maternal position to remove cord compression, they often forget the potential benefits of amnion-infusion and short-acting tocolysis. Meta-analysis of 12 randomized controlled trials indicates that in the presence of cord compression amnion-infusion is associated with significant reductions in heart rate decelerations (RR = 0.54; 95% CI 0.43–0.68) and cesarean delivery for suspected fetal distress (RR = 0.35; 95% CI 0.24–0.52).[55]

> *In cases of cord compression – the most frequent cause of fetal compromise in normal labor – amnion-infusion effectively reduces the need for cesarean delivery (Evidence level A).*

Maternal hypotension leading to impaired uteroplacental blood flow is almost invariably related to epidural analgesia and must be treated with IV fluid loads and vasopressors (Chapter 20). In case of uterine tachysystole, oxytocin must be discontinued according to the protocol discussed in Chapter 17. It should be emphasized that problematic hyperstimulation leading to fetal distress is mostly iatrogenic, since this is particularly related to labor induction or unduly delayed augmentation.

24.4.2 Intrauterine resuscitation

Whatever the cause of fetal compromise in labor, the contractions invariably aggravate the situation. Conversely, uterine relaxation through short-acting tocolysis invariably improves uteroplacental blood flow and alleviates cord compression in nearly all cases, thus achieving fetal resuscitation.[56] A single bolus of 0.25 mg terbutaline, 0.1 mg fenotorol, or 6.25 mg atosiban effectively inhibits contractions for about 15–20 minutes, restoring adequate fetal oxygenation.

Intrauterine resuscitation avoids heroic but superfluous interventions. Fetal resuscitation creates rest and valuable time in which to take a fetal scalp blood sample and to reflect, preventing panicky reactions – especially in less-experienced young doctors who, it must be admitted, attend most labors outside office hours. Intrauterine resuscitation gives the obstetrician on duty time to come to the delivery room, and further corrective measures often allow labor to continue.

In deteriorating cases, (repeated) fetal resuscitation creates time to prepare the operating theater. Precesarean tocolysis diminishes the need to rush and permits meticulous and thus safer surgery. In second-stage labor, intrauterine resuscitation provides the time to place an outlet forceps carefully or to apply vacuum to the ventouse slowly, facilitating an atraumatic instrumental delivery. In conclusion: short tocolysis is an effective and useful temporizing maneuver in the management of (imminent) intrapartum fetal distress.[3]

Despite the evidence and unequivocal recommendations for intrauterine resuscitation by ACOG, RCOG, and other authoritative institutions, overall compliance with the official guidelines is very poor. A recent review of approximately 400 publications on cesarean delivery for fetal distress found that only three papers reported the use of tocolytics before commencing the surgery, and in these studies tocolytics were used in only 16% of the potential candidates.[33] The conclusion must be that in many obstetric practices there is still much room for improving fetal and maternal outcomes if intrauterine resuscitation is used on a more regular basis.

> *Intrauterine resuscitation is a widely undervalued technique and is therefore used much too infrequently.*

24.4.3 Operative delivery

Whenever fetal reserves – estimated by fetal scalp blood sampling – are judged to be insufficient to withstand further labor, and when the worrying fetal heart rate pattern persists despite conservative management and intrauterine resuscitation, delivery should be expedited. In the second stage of labor, vacuum or forceps delivery may be appropriate; otherwise the option should be cesarean delivery. To permit meaningful audit (Chapters 25, 27) the umbilical cord must be doubly clamped at delivery and an arterial blood sample obtained to determine the neonatal acid–base status.

24.5 Summary

- Fetal risks during labor and delivery include infection, trauma, and asphyxia. These hazards are strongly related to abnormal labor, which in turn is often preventable or plainly iatrogenic in origin.
- The fetus that enters labor in good condition is well-equipped by nature to tolerate the challenge of normal labor.
- Safe care of the fetus therefore dictates a spontaneous onset of labor and a management policy ensuring that labor is and remains normal.
- The dominant threat to fetal oxygenation in normal labor is umbilical cord compression.
- Many characteristics or "abnormalities" of fetal heart rate tracings during labor reflect physiological responses to stress rather than pathological signs of fetal distress.
- Passage of meconium may lead to hypertonic dystocia, characterized by a vicious circle of ineffective labor and fetal distress. In addition, meconium is an environmental hazard for the fetus that may lead to meconium aspiration syndrome. The clinical approach should be determined by the grade of meconium.
- The doctrine "when in doubt, get it out" is all too often put into practice, but it represents a gross oversimplification of a complex set of problems.

- Reduction of unnecessary interventions for erroneous suspicion of fetal distress requires appreciation of the fundamental differences between screening and diagnosis, taking into account the possibilities and limitations of fetal assessment techniques.
- Fetal heart rate monitoring in labor is primarily a screening method for fetal compromise and not a reliable diagnostic test.
- A positive screening test must be followed by further diagnostic investigation to assess fetal blood gases and reserves, and to determine the cause of fetal jeopardy.
- A causal diagnosis often permits corrective action and causal treatment such as amnion-infusion and change of maternal position, instead of prompt artificial delivery.
- Ideally, fetal blood sampling should be used to confirm fetal distress before cesarean section is undertaken.
- Intrauterine resuscitation is an effective but undervalued temporizing maneuver in the management of nonreassuring fetal heart rate tracings, and further corrective measures often allow labor to continue safely.

REFERENCES

1. Rogers MS, Mongelli M, Tsang KH, Wang CC, Law KP. Lipid peroxidation in cord blood at birth: the effect of labour. *Br J Obstet Gynaecol* 1998; 105(7): 739–44.
2. Melchior J, Bernhard N. Incidence and pattern of fetal heart rate alterations during labor. In Kunzel W, ed. *Fetal Heart Rate Monitoring: Clinical Practice and Pathophysiology*. Berlin: Springer; 1985: 73.
3. Cunningham FG, Leveno KJ, Bloom SL, *et al.* Chapter 18: Intrapartum assessment. In: *Williams Obstetrics*, 22nd edn. New York: McGraw-Hill; 2005: 443–71.
4. Nelson KB, Grether JK. Potentially asphyxiating conditions and cerebral palsy in infants of normal birth weight. *Am J Obstet Gynecol* 1998; 179(2): 507–13.
5. Nelson KB. Can we prevent cerebral palsy? *N Engl J Med* 2003; 349: 1765–9.
6. American College of Obstetricians and Gynecologists. *Neonatal Encephalopathy and Cerebral Palsy: Defining*

the Pathogenesis and Pathophysiology. Washington DC: ACOG; 2003.

7. Goldaber KG, Gilstrap LCD, Leveno KJ, Dax JS, Mcintire DD. Pathologic fetal acidemia. *Obstet Gynecol* 1991; 78: 1103–7.

8. Sehdev HM, Stamilio DM, Macones GA, Graham A, Morgan MA. Predictive factors for neonatal morbidity in neonates with an umbilical artery cord pH less than 7.00. *Am J Obstet Gynecol* 1997; 177: 1030–4.

9. Goodwin TM, Belai I, Hernandez P, Durand M, Paul RH. Asphyxial complications in the term newborn with severe umbilical acidemia. *Am J Obstet Gynecol* 1992; 167: 1506–12.

10. Walker J. Foetal anoxia. *J Obstet Gynaecol Br Commonw* 1953; 61: 162.

11. Nathan L, Leveno KJ, Carmody TJ, Kelly MA, Sherman LM. Meconium: a 1990s perspective on an old obstetric hazard. *Obstet Gynecol* 1994; 83: 329–32.

12. Ahanya SN, Lakshmanan J, Morgan BL, Ross MG. Meconium passage in utero: mechanisms, consequences, and management. *Obstet Gynecol Surv* 2005; 60(1): 45–56.

13. Ghidini A, Spong CY. Severe meconium aspiration syndrome is not caused by aspiration of meconium. *Am J Obstet Gynecol* 2001; 185(4): 931–8.

14. Blackwell SC, Moldenhauer J, Hassan SS, *et al.* Meconium aspiration syndrome in term neonates with normal acid-base status at delivery: is it different? *Am J Obstet Gynecol* 2001; 184(7): 1422–5; discussion 1425–6.

15. Dollberg S, Livny S, Mordecheyev N, Mimouni FB. Nucleated red blood cells in meconium aspiration syndrome. *Obstet Gynecol* 2001; 97: 593–6.

16. Jazayeri A, Politz L, Tsibris JCM, Queen T, Spellacy WN. Fetal erythropoietin levels in pregnancies complicated by meconium passage: does meconium suggest fetal hypoxia? *Am J Obstet Gynecol* 2000; 183: 188–90.

17. Thacker SB, Stroup DF, Peterson HB. Efficacy and safety of intrapartum electronic fetal monitoring: an update. *Obstet Gynecol* 1995; 86: 613–20.

18. Alfirevic Z, Devane D, Gyte GM. Continuous cardiotocography (CTG) as a form of electronic fetal monitoring (EFM) for fetal assessment during labor. *Cochrane Database Syst Rev* 2006; 19(3): CD006066.

19. American College of Obstetricians and Gynecologists. *Fetal Heart Rate Patterns: Monitoring, Interpretations, and Management.* Technical Bulletin No 207. July, 1995.

20. Royal College of Obstetricians and Gynaecologists. *The Use of Electronic Fetal Monitoring: The Use and*

Interpretation of Cardiotocography in Intrapartum Surveillance. London: Royal College of Obstetricians and Gynaecologists; 2001.

21. Ingermarsson J, Ingermarsson H, Spencer J. *Fetal Heart Rate Monitoring: A Practical Guide.* Oxford: Oxford University Press; 1993.

22. Freeman RK, Garite TH, Nageotte MP. *Fetal Heart Rate Monitoring*, 3rd edn. Philadelphia: Lipincott Williams & Wilkins; 2003.

23. Murray ML. *Antepartal and intrapartal fetal monitoring*, 3rd edn. Springer; 2007.

24. Keith RD, Beckley S, Garibaldi JM, *et al.* A multicentre comparative study of 17 experts and an intelligent computer system for managing labour using cardiotocogram. *Br J Obstet Gynaecol* 1995; 102: 688–700.

25. Ayres-de-Campos D, Bernardes J, Costa-Pereira A, Pereira-Leite L. Inconsistencies in classification by experts of cardiotocograms and subsequent clinical decision. *Br J Obstet Gynaecol* 1999; 106: 1307–10.

26. Greenwood C, Lalchandini S, MacQuillan K, *et al.* Meconium passed in labor: How reassuring is clear amniotic fluid? *Obstet Gynecol* 2003; 102: 89–93.

27. Grant A. Monitoring the fetus during labour. In: Chalmers I, Keirse MJNC, Enkin M, eds. *Effective Care in Pregnancy and Childbirth*, Vol 2. Oxford: Oxford University Press; 1989.

28. Parer J. NIH sets the terms for fetal heart rate pattern interpretation. *Ob/Gyn News* Sept 1, 1997.

29. National Institute of Child Health and Human Development Research Planning Workshop: Electronic fetal heart rate monitoring: Research guidelines for integration. *Am J Obstet Gynecol* 1997; 177: 1385–90.

30. Zalar RW, Quilligan EJ. The influence of scalp sampling on the cesarean section rate for fetal distress. *Am J Obstet Gynecol* 1979; 135: 239–46.

31. Clark SL, Paul RH. Intrapartum fetal surveillance: the role of fetal scalp blood sampling. *Am J Obstet Gynecol* 1985; 153: 717–20.

32. Goodwin TM, Milner-Masterson L, Paul RH. Elimination of fetal scalp blood sampling on a large clinical service. *Obstet Gynecol* 1994; 83: 971–4.

33. Chauhan SP, Magann EF, Scott JR, *et al.* Emergency cesarean delivery for nonreassuring fetal heart rate tracings: compliance with ACOG guidelines. *J Reprod Med* 2003; 48: 975–81.

34. Westgren M, Kruger K, Ek S, *et al.* Lactate compared with pH analysis at fetal scalp blood sampling: a prospective randomized study. *Br J Obstet Gynaecol* 1998; 105: 29–33.

35. Kruger K, Hallberg B, Blennow M, Kublickas M, Westgren M. Predictive value of fetal scalp blood lactate concentration and pH as markers of neurologic disability. *Am J Obstet Gynecol* 1999; 181: 1072–8.

36. Dildy GA. Intrapartum assessment of the fetus: historical and evidence-based practice. *Obstet Gynecol Clin N Am* 2005; 32: 255–71.

37. Yam J, Chua S, Arulkumaran S. Intrapartum fetal pulse oximetry; Part I. Principles and technical issues; Part II. Clinical application. *Obstet Gynecol Surv* 2000; 55: 163–83.

38. Amer-Wahlin I, Hellsten C, Noren H, *et al.* Cardiotocography only versus cardiotocography plus ST analysis of fetal electrocardiogram for intrapartum fetal monitoring: a Swedish randomized controlled trial. *Lancet* 2001; 358: 534–8.

39. Garite TJ, Dildy GA, McNamara H, *et al.* A multicenter controlled trial of fetal pulse oximetry in the intrapartum management of nonreassuring fetal heart rate patterns. *Am J Obstet Gynecol* 2000; 183: 1049–58.

40. Smith JF, Onstad JH. Assessment of the fetus: intermittent auscultation, electronic fetal heart rate tracing, and fetal pulse oximetry. *Obstet Gynecol Clin N Am* 2005; 32: 245–54.

41. American College of Obstetricians and Gynecologists. Fetal pulse oximetry: ACOG Committee opinion No 258. *Obstet Gynecol* 2001; 98: 523–4.

42. Rijnders RJP, Mol BWJ, Reuwer PJHM, *et al.* Is the correlation between fetal oxygen saturation and blood pH sufficient for the use of fetal pulse oximetry? *J Matern Fetal Neonatal Med* 2002; 11: 80–3.

43. Kwee A, Dekkers A, van Wijk HPJ, van der Hoorn CW, Visser GHA. Occurrence of ST-changes recorded with the STAN S21 monitor during normal and abnormal fetal heart rate patterns during labour. *Eur J Obstet Gynecol Reprod Biol* 2007; 135(1): 28–34.

44. Dervaitis KL, Poole M, Schmidt G, *et al.* ST segment analysis of the fetal electrocardiogram plus electronic fetal heart rate monitoring in labor and its relationship to umbilical cord arterial blood gases. *Am J Obstet Gynecol* 2004; 191(3): 879–84.

45. Westerhuis M, Kwee A, van Ginkel A, *et al.* Limitations of ST analysis in clinical practice: three cases of intrapartum metabolic acidosis. *Br J Obstet Gynaecol* 2007; 114(10): 1194–201.

46. Norén H, Luttkus AK, Stupin JH, *et al.* Fetal scalp pH and ST analysis of the fetal ECG as an adjunct to cardiotocography to predict fetal acidosis in labor – a multi-center, case controlled study. *J Perinat Med* 2007; 35(5): 408–14.

47. Doria V, Papageorghiou AT, Gustafsson A, *et al.* Review of the first 1502 cases of ECG-ST waveform analysis during labour in a teaching hospital. *Br J Obstet Gynaecol* 2007; 114(10): 1202–7.

48. Chauhan SP, Magann EF, Scott JR, *et al.* Cesarean delivery for fetal distress: rate and risk factors. *Obstet Gynecol Surv* 2003; 58: 337–50.

49. *Confidential Enquiry into Stillbirths and Deaths in Infancy.* London: Maternal and Child Research Consortium; 1998.

50. Draper ES, Kurinczuk JJ, Lamming CR, *et al.* A confidential enquiry into cases of neonatal encephalopathy. *Arch Dis Child Fetal Neonatal Ed* 2002; 87(3): 176–80.

51. Papworth S, Cartlidge P. Learning from adverse events – the role of confidential enquiries. *Semin Fetal Neonatal Med* 2005; 10(1): 39–43.

52. Liston R, Crane J, Hamilton E, *et al.* Fetal health surveillance in labour. *J Obstet Gynaecol Can* 2002; 24: 250–76.

53. Rosser J. Confidential Enquiry into Stillbirths and Deaths in Infancy (CESDI). Highlights of the 6th annual report. *Pract Midwife* 1999; 2(9): 18–19.

54. American College of Obstetricians and Gynecologists. *Cesarean Delivery for Nonreassuring Fetal Status.* Criteria set No 33; May, 1998.

55. Hofmeyr GJ. Amnioinfusion for umbilical cord compression in labour. *Cochrane Database Syst Rev* 2000; (2): CD000013.

56. Hendrix NW, Chauhan SP. Cesarean delivery for nonreassuring fetal heart rate tracing. *Obstet Gynecol Clin N Am* 2005; 32: 273–86.

25

Prevention of litigation

Fear of lawsuits brought against obstetricians for not preventing neonatal brain damage or perinatal death continues to raise operative intervention rates, in many cases to no avail. This chapter focuses on medicolegal issues and suggests practical measures to avoid malpractice litigation for disappointing neonatal outcomes without resorting to excessively defensive medicine.

25.1 The specter of cerebral palsy

Few events evoke more fear and apprehension in parents than hearing the pediatric verdict "neonatal brain damage." This label immediately conjures up horrific visions of severely spastic handicap, epileptic seizures, and hopeless mental retardation. Although most neonatal brain disorders are less disabling, they are nevertheless a major source of severe psychological suffering, economic damage, and malpractice litigation, placing accountability in the human endeavor of obstetrics in many cases where none should reasonably be placed. It is now recognized that only a relatively few cases of neonatal brain damage can be attributed to intrapartum asphyxia or trauma, and that most cases of cerebral palsy are not preventable by intrapartum interventions.[1]

> *Advances in perinatal medicine, including the use of fetal monitoring and cesarean delivery, have led to false expectations that doctors should be able to prevent most cases of cerebral palsy.*

Cerebral palsy is a heterogeneous group of pediatric-neurological conditions that are characterized by chronic disorders of movement or posture, frequently accompanied by seizure disorders and cognitive limitation. It is cerebral in origin, arises early in life, and is not the result of progressive disease. Our current understanding that cerebral palsy is heterogeneous in its causation was preceded by over a century of misconceptions linking its cause invariably with perinatal asphyxia. This misunderstanding goes back to 1862 when William Little, a London orthopedist, first described cerebral palsy and concluded that abnormalities of birth caused this condition.[1] Although some notables such as Sigmund Freud (1897) – having observed that difficult birth frequently produced no adverse long-term effects – challenged this view long ago, the birth-injury etiology for cerebral damage dominated debates for more than a hundred years and was generally accepted by science, medicine, and society.[1] The introduction of electronic fetal surveillance techniques in the 1970s consequently led to the expectation that cerebral palsy could now be prevented. This goal, in conjunction with increasing fear of malpractice litigation, contributed to the escalating rate of cesarean deliveries in the 1980s and 1990s without, however, resulting in any significant decline in the rate of cerebral palsy, or in reduction of malpractice lawsuits for that matter.

> *"Cerebral palsy has continually been linked with perinatal asphyxia, but, in reality, most cases of*

> *neonatal brain damage are unrelated to intra-partum events and, therefore, cannot be prevented by operative delivery."[2]*

25.1.1 Myriad causes

It was more than a century after Little's observations that research was begun in earnest to elucidate the etiology of neonatal brain disorders. Roughly 2 in 1000 infants in the industrialized nations are diagnosed with cerebral palsy and prematurity proves to be the most important contributor.[1] Although premature births constitute only a small proportion of all births, approximately half of all children with cerebral palsy are born prematurely.[2]

Conversely, half of the children with cerebral palsy are born at term. Recognized risk factors are (1) evidence of genetic abnormalities such as maternal mental retardation, microcephaly, and congenital malformation; (2) antenatal intoxication; (3) infection; (4) intrauterine growth restriction; and finally (5) perinatal asphyxia.[1,2] Accumulated research data indicate that 70% of all cases of cerebral palsy result from an event prior to the onset of labor.[3] This explains why the recent increase in cesarean deliveries has not diminished the overall incidence of cerebral palsy. Reviewing pooled data from nine industrialized countries, Hankins and Speer concluded that "despite a 5-fold increase in the rate of cesarean section, based in part on the electronically derived diagnosis of fetal distress, cerebral palsy prevalence has remained stable."[4] Consistent conclusions of all systematic studies on this subject have now led to the acceptance – except by plaintiff attorneys – that only a relatively few cerebral palsy cases are caused at the time of birth and that the majority cannot be prevented by operative deliveries.[1–4]

> *Cerebral palsy is heterogeneous in its manifestation and its causation. It is a complex and multifactorial condition caused by genetic, infectious, environmental, and obstetrical factors.*

25.1.2 Hypoxic-ischemic encephalopathy

Nevertheless, some cases of cerebral palsy certainly arise from peripartal asphyxia, which sometimes can indeed be prevented, but not always. These specific cases of cerebral palsy resulting from birth asphyxia are currently labeled "hypoxic-ischemic encephalopathy."

Although "perinatal asphyxia" has been clearly defined, the term is still widely misused in legal courts. Plaintiff attorneys and self-proclaimed "expert witnesses" frequently base the diagnosis on low Apgar scores alone, which may be caused by other factors such as preterm birth, maternal sedation, anesthesia, vigorous suction or intubation, and newborn neurological or cardiorespiratory disease. To clarify the potential role of intrapartum events in causing permanent neurological injuries, a joint task force of the American Academy of Pediatrics and ACOG[5] has developed a precise definition of perinatal asphyxia that includes all three of the following:

- Profound metabolic or mixed acidemia (pH less than 7.0) determined on an umbilical cord arterial blood sample at birth
- Persistent Apgar score of 0 to 3 for longer than 5 minutes
- Evidence of neonatal neurological sequelae such as seizures, coma, or hypotonia; or dysfunction of one or more of the following systems: cardiovascular, gastrointestinal, hematological, pulmonary, or renal.

When these three factors are associated with brain injury, they suggest that perinatal hypoxic-ischemic encephalopathy developed. In fact, their absence in association with brain damage helped to falsify the birth-injury etiology in the majority of cases of cerebral palsy.[3,4]

> *The evidence indicates that fewer than 30 percent of cases of neonatal brain injury are at least partly attributable to intrapartum hypoxic events.*

25.2 Legal liability concerns

The known causes of cerebral palsy account for only a minority of the total cases and even for most of these cases evidence of the preventability of the disorder is lacking. Despite this, lawsuits brought against obstetricians for not preventing neonatal brain damage continue to be a major contributor to the high cost of malpractice insurance and the disruptive consequences of the climate of litigation. The courts often permit unsupported "expert" opinion to supersede the consistent evidence of clinical trials, structured meta-analyses, and population-based time trends.

> *"The practice of contemporary obstetrics continues to be modified in part by societal expectations and correlate legal pressures to optimize outcomes and place accountability in the human endeavor of obstetrics, when none should be reasonably placed."*[6]

Despite excessively defensive medicine in the USA, the average American obstetrician is sued 2.5 times during his or her career and about 75% of obstetricians have been sued at least once. Almost 50% of obstetrical claims are for neurologically impaired infants or stillbirths.[7] About half of the claims are dropped by the plaintiff attorney or found to be without merit. There has been a steady escalation, however, in the value of awards in the USA, with the median award now nearly 1 million dollars, and professional liability insurance premiums have continued to escalate accordingly. The cost of malpractice coverage passed on to patients adds an estimated $350 to annual health care premiums for the average American family, and an increasing number of people in so-called "civilized" western countries are currently uninsured for medical aid as a result.[8] Frustration and fury raised by outrageous payouts have sparked a grassroots tort reform that has been successful in limiting non-economic damages in some European nations and American states.[9] Despite this, the availability

of affordable liability insurance becomes a grave concern in many other states. Contrary to what is alleged by plaintiff attorneys who personally profit from legal procedures and huge settlements, the litigation crisis has resulted in sparse or no obstetric care in some areas.[7] This may very well cause more overall morbidity, pain, suffering, financial costs, and mortality than bad medical outcomes with or without errors in judgment. As always, many a societal system brings its unforeseen misfortunes.

Some obstetricians, especially those who have stopped practicing for liability reasons, protest publicly with bumper stickers stating: "Let lawyers deliver babies." They may take solace in knowing that a study called "On being a happy, healthy, and ethical member of an unhappy, unhealthy, and unethical profession" identified increasing rates of job dissatisfaction and unhappiness among plaintiff lawyers in the USA, and reported that many were planning to leave their profession.[10]

In many western countries the litigation crisis is not as severe and acute as in the USA – where anyone can sue for almost anything, as it seems – because of differences in medical insurance systems, different levels of social security, and fundamental differences in judicial systems. These factors surely modify malpractice litigation as well as obstetrical practices. In countries with a fair social security system – including a safety-net for victims of medical injury or other accidents and misfortunes with or without somebody to blame – people are less likely to be inclined to sue in court for compensation. Unjust claims by avaricious attorneys are more likely to succeed in Anglo-Saxon countries where the care provider has to disprove his or her guilt, whereas in many European countries the plaintiff attorney has to prove guilt in the court of law, which is more difficult to do. What is more, evidence of liability is less easily accepted in the courts of countries where the verdict is in the hands of well-informed, prudent judges and medical peers, rather than lay juries. Of course, judicial systems and other societal environments cannot be changed easily and the medical profession will have to live with that. The good news for the USA is that a broad coalition – consisting of leading politicians, scientists of law, judicial and medical opinion leaders, health officials, university presidents, and heads of thinktanks on both sides of the aisle – has recently taken on important initiatives to try to reform the American system of medical justice.[11] The bad news is that, optimistically, the achievement of results will take years or decades, requiring intensive political lobbying and prolonged public campaigns. Until better times, defensive medicine will continue to raise interventions and costs without improvement in overall neonatal outcome and to the detriment of women's well-being and health. Surely, as long as society does not accept evidence-based and data-driven practice and as long as parents hold obstetricians to the impossible standard of delivering "the perfect baby," the practice of obstetrics is going to be defensive, significantly influenced by the emotions of the unexpected outcome and the disappointment, denial, and anger that are associated with it. "Few areas of medicine amplify these issues as acutely as neurological impairment in children."[6]

25.2.1 Steps to minimize malpractice litigation

The human endeavor of obstetrics is not infallible and it never will be. Some, but surely not all, cases of hypoxic-ischemic encephalopathy result from obstetric errors. If this proves to be the case, obstetricians should take full responsibility and their insurers must pay. To avoid unjust claims and to permit an objective medicolegal judgment, the results of all fetal and maternal assessments as well as all uncommon events and interventions during labor should be well documented. The clinical note should clearly mention the time of onset and the type of nonreassuring CTG, the fetal scalp blood gases, the corrective and resuscitative measures undertaken along with the response, and the time of decision for cesarean delivery and the time of incision. CTG tracings should be kept for second opinion. The best way to counteract unjustly incriminating statements by self-proclaimed CTG

experts in court is to provide hard data on fetal scalp blood pH or lactate during labor as well as umbilical artery blood gases immediately after birth. Evidently, the best way to prevent malpractice litigation is avoidance of errors by sticking to the principles and practice of *proactive support of labor* (Chapter 24).

25.2.2 Preventing errors

Perinatal acidemia, defined as umbilical artery pH less than 7.0 and base deficit of at least 12 at delivery, still occurs in 0.26–1.3% of all births.[12] Fortunately, only a minority of these children develop hypoxic-ischemic encephalopathy. Assuming that ideal intrapartum assessment and intervention protocols can effectively prevent neurological damage, hypoxic-ischemic encephalopathy could be avoided in fewer than 1 per 1000 infants. Expectations that new fetal surveillance techniques could substantially reduce long-term neurological morbidity are therefore unrealistic. Doing more harm than good is a much more probable prospect (Chapter 24).

No doubt there is much more to be gained at the moment by improved use of current technology and by sticking to a systematic approach to labor and fetal surveillance and diagnosis as promoted in this manual. This can be deduced from the previously cited studies of the causes of cerebral palsy indicating at least a 25% rate of possibly avoidable errors related to fetal surveillance. A British confidential inquiry into stillbirths and perinatal deaths identified five leading areas of clinical error.[13] These common errors are, in decreasing rank order:

- Assessment of fetal condition during labor, particularly with regard to the use of fetal heart rate monitoring and under-use of fetal scalp blood sampling
- Recognition of risk during labor
- Management of labor
- Assessment of risk factors before labor
- Management of delivery

These were the leading areas found among 873 deaths during labor of normal babies of weight exceeding 1500 g. Better care would have improved outcome in 52% of cases and might have done in another 25%. Evidently, the interests of patients, doctors, and society as a whole are best served with better education and training in the professional management of labor and responsible care of the fetus during labor and delivery (Chapter 24). We trust this manual might help.

> *Protocol-led labor management and meticulous charting of all events avoid unjustified legal claims.*

25.3 Summary

- Fetal distress during labor and delivery is a topic of great obstetric interest because of the associated infant morbidity (cerebral palsy) and potential medicolegal liability.
- Cerebral palsy, however, is heterogeneous in its manifestation and its causation. Only a minority of cases have their origin in labor and delivery and can thus be prevented by obstetricians.
- For overall births and those within major subgroups defined according to birth weight and gestational age, medicine has not yet succeeded in reducing the frequency of neonatal brain damage. The increase in term cesarean deliveries did not result in any significant decline in the rate of cerebral palsy because this intervention does not address the cause in most cases.
- Defensive obstetrics does more harm than good. Responsible care of the fetus should not imply superfluous interventions that needlessly add risks to mothers.
- Labor-related hypoxic-ischemic encephalopathy and associated medicolegal litigation can be avoided by:
  1. Implementation of a systematic approach to all labors based on rational concepts of care of both mother and fetus that are strongly supported by clinical evidence.
  2. Accurate diagnosis of fetal distress and its underlying cause.
  3. Causally directed corrective and resuscitative intrapartum measures.
  4. Meticulous charting of all details of all labors.
  5. Sticking to the principles and practice of *proactive support of labor.*

REFERENCES

1. Cunningham FG, Leveno KJ, Bloom SL, *et al.* Diseases and injuries of the fetus and newborn. In: *Williams Obstetrics*, 22nd edn. New York: McGraw-Hill; 2005: 649–91.
2. Nelson KB. Can we prevent cerebral palsy? *N Engl J Med* 2003; 349: 1765–9.
3. Goodlin RC. Cerebral palsy linkage concepts need revision. *Am J Obstet Gynecol* 1993; 169(4): 1075–6.
4. Hankins GD, Speer M. Defining the pathogenesis and pathophysiology of neonatal encephalopathy and cerebral palsy. *Obstet Gynecol* 2003; 102: 628–36.
5. ACOG committee opinion. Use and abuse of the Apgar score. Number 174; July 1996. Committee on Obstetric Practice and American Academy of Pediatrics: Committee on Fetus and Newborn. American College of Obstetricians and Gynecologists. *Int J Gynaecol Obstet* 1996; 54(3): 303–5.
6. Smith JF, Onstad JH. Assessment of the fetus: intermittent auscultation, electronic fetal heart rate tracing, and fetal pulse oximetry. *Obstet Gynecol Clin N Am* 2005; 32: 245–54.
7. Lockwood CJ. Confronting the professional liability crisis. *Contemp Ob/Gyn* April 2002: 13.
8. McLellan F. Uninsured people in the USA put a strain on health system. *Lancet* 2003; 361(9361): 938.
9. Mello MM, Studdert DM, Brennan TA. The new medical malpractice crisis. *N Engl J Med* 2003; 348: 2281–4.
10. Schlitz P. On being a happy, healthy, and ethical member of an unhappy, unhealthy, and unethical profession. *Vanderbilt Law Rev* 1999; 52: 871.
11. Howard PK. Is the medical justice system broken? *Obstet Gynecol* 2003; 102: 446–9.
12. Chauhan SP, Magann EF, Scott JR, *et al.* Cesarean delivery for fetal distress: rate and risk factors. *Obstet Gynecol Surv* 2003; 58: 337–50.
13. *Confidential Enquiry into Stillbirths and Deaths in Infancy.* London: Maternal and Child Research Consortium, 1998.

26

Organizational reforms

Proactive support of labor is an integral concept of childbirth consisting of five strongly interdependent components: prelabor education, psychological support, prevention of prolonged labor, constant peer review, and sound organization. It would be naive to expect that full implementation of the system could be achieved overnight. As with all major undertakings in health care and beyond, organization makes all the difference between success and failure. Unlike the situation today, wherein the organization directs the content of offered care, the demands of quality care should direct the organization. Most importantly, frontline birth professionals rather than managers should take the lead in the much-needed reforms.[1,2] Sound organization needs to be considered at three levels:

1. The labor and delivery ward
2. Cooperation between nurses, midwives, and physicians
3. Replacement of provider-centered care by woman-centered care

26.1 The labor and delivery ward

"Many delivery units are so disorganized – unable to cope with additional pressures even though overstaffed for much of the time – that there is no possibility of providing efficient and high-quality care." Nursing services often function in a largely fragmentary manner, usually heavily concentrated in daylight hours. Several doctors come and go, leaving capricious or even contradictory instructions. Residents, midwifes, and nurses are frequently placed in the invidious position of having to apply different methods of care, in exactly the same clinical circumstances, for no reason other than that the names of the obstetricians printed on the chart are different. "The sheer irrationality of this situation is a constant affront to the intelligence of labor room staff."[3] As a result, nurses, midwives, and doctors fail to cooperate closely and some even work in open conflict (Chapter 5). Inevitably, poor corporate spirit and poor organizational standards lead to substandard care.

> *"In terms of care, many labor wards border on the chaotic, because a central plan is missing."*[3]

26.1.1 Staff consensus

Clearly, a delivery unit cannot begin to function properly unless a common goal and strategy of care are agreed on by all care providers: obstetricians, midwives, and nurses alike. This manual may serve as the evidence-based blueprint for such a plan.

Obstetricians are in the prime position to improve the standards of care in labor, simply by agreeing on a common policy and by providing the tools and back-up needed for the nurses and midwives to execute their pivotal tasks. Naturally, an obstetrician, with recognized authority and supported by hospital management, should take the lead.[1] "All colleagues cooperating within the confines of a delivery unit must be called together and each obstetrician must be prepared to surrender a small portion of his or her jealously guarded independence for the sake of the common good."[3] This is the acid test of goodwill on the part of the obstetricians.

The next step is to redefine the working relations between regulated midwives and physicians in a mutually satisfactory manner. The common plan should put an end to the silly animosity that all too often exists between these professional groups. Institutional commitment to high-quality care and low operative delivery rates is a corporate undertaking, requiring determination and team spirit.

> *Staff consensus on a common goal and strategy is the prerequisite of high-quality care in labor.*

Consensus should be reached about a system that is based on nursing and midwifery services with constant medical back-up. Once *proactive support of labor* has been introduced, the nurses and midwives convert most standards into practice, greatly improving care and enhancing the job satisfaction for everybody. With their pivotal roles clearly defined, they will further guard, extend, promote, and carry the system. It is particularly the nurses and midwives in our practice who unremittingly explain the methods and procedures to the ever-rotating undergraduate students and medical residents who, in turn, profit immensely from the clarity now offered. In our experience, these student-midwives and residents spread the system in their future careers and working environments.

26.1.2 Equal service around the clock

All pregnant women – without exception – are entitled to the same high level of care and expertise during labor and delivery, regardless of the hour of the day or the day of the week when birth happens to occur. This fundamental right implies that the same complement of labor room staff, of equal status, should operate day and night; so-called daylight obstetrics is bad obstetrics (Chapter 23).

Furthermore, the labor and delivery unit should be designated an area of intensive nursing support, exclusively for women in labor. Staff attention should not be distracted by other tasks. The labor and delivery ward is not meant to serve as a gynecological first-aid facility, nor for antenatal assessments, external cephalic version of breech presentations, or intensive surveillance of severely ill pregnant women or postoperative patients, etc. A labor and delivery ward should be used exclusively for labor and delivery; patients who are not in labor do not belong there.

> *The delivery ward is an intensive care unit, meant exclusively for women in labor and evenly staffed around the clock, seven days a week.*

26.1.3 Scale

Adequate scale is an obvious advantage in eliminating peaks and troughs in the number of deliveries at different hours of the day and on different days of the week. A volume of 2000 deliveries or more permits a nucleus of highly skilled professional personnel – nurses, midwives, and physicians – to be employed on a whole-time commitment to the delivery unit, so that they are not required to divide their attention and responsibility with antenatal clinics, antenatal wards, or postnatal care. In smaller delivery units, adequate nursing services might be achieved by a flexible system with on-call nurses, on standby to complement the on-site nurse(s) if needed. Regardless of scale, one-on-one nursing support extended to all women in labor is a compulsory quality demand. However, cost-efficiency must co-exist and in the final analysis many small hospitals will need to face the reality that an obstetric unit is not in the best interests of either the patient or the hospital.

> *The welfare of pregnant women should not be influenced by the time at which birth happens to occur.*

26.1.4 Central direction

A delivery unit catering for low-, medium- and high-risk deliveries cannot be directed under a committee system and, therefore, a chain of command must be clearly defined. There should be one obstetrician only in charge at any given time. There is no more room for divided direction in a busy delivery unit than there is in the cockpit of an airplane, so all nurses, midwives, and residents should be subject to the immediate authority of the obstetrician in charge.[3]

Obviously, this obstetrician should have no other obligations and activities during his/her labor ward shift. He/she should review every woman and unborn child in the delivery unit in the company of the attending midwife or resident, at regular intervals, especially late at night and early in the morning. As soon as all attending obstetricians have committed themselves to the common guidelines, medical policies should be consistent around the clock. Any departure from standard policy should always be explicitly approved by the obstetrician in charge and documented.

> *One obstetrician only should be in charge of a delivery unit at any given time.*

26.2 Professional cooperation

With a common strategy of care, the professional roles and responsibilities of nurses, midwives, and physicians can finally be defined. One-on-one nursing is the backbone of the system and, equally importantly, there is no longer place for rivalry or competition between well-trained and legally certified midwives and physicians. Their roles are fully complementary: the midwife's expertise lies in the supervision of health and the prevention and detection of disease, whereas the specialty of the obstetrician is the treatment of disease and the restoration of health. These professional groups should recognize and value their complementary skills and work together for the common good.

> *Optimal care can only occur when nurses, midwives, and obstetricians acknowledge their specific roles and their complementary skills.*

26.2.1 Nursing services

Good nursing service does not mean a group of nurses caring for an equivalent number of patients on a collective basis. Hard evidence shows that a woman's childbirth experience largely depends on the quality of the relationship established with the nurse assigned to her personally.[4] The attention of each nurse should therefore be confined to one patient in labor only. In contrast to common perception, larger scale favors personal attention and human compassion in labor, provided that the full system of *proactive support of labor* is adopted *in all its components*. Labor room nurses are selected for their supportive skills and their ability to cope with the variable reactions of laboring women. Although their priorities are set on the supportive role and the bedside monitoring of maternal and fetal well-being, all nurses should also be trained and authorized to site IV lines, administer IV medication on the request of midwives and doctors, and so on. It goes without saying that nurses, like all other professionals, must be able to function in emergency situations. Labor room nurses do not perform vaginal examinations or deliveries. In medical terms they are subject to the authority of the midwives and doctors. However, in terms of labor support and women's satisfaction nurses play the most important and most difficult role. Doctors and midwives should openly acknowledge this and show the much-needed respect for what these labor room nurses do.

> *The key to high-quality care in labor is specialist nursing attention on a one-on-one basis.*

26.2.2 Midwifery services

A risk assessment should be made in the antenatal clinics and again at admission, formally assigning the care of each parturient either to the midwifery service or to the medical-specialist staff. In more than 75% of all women the pregnancy proceeds uneventfully and the supervision of their childbirth can be safely assigned to the midwives, who now supervise all labors according to the principles and guidelines of *proactive support of labor*. There is no place any longer for unfounded midwifery philosophies of wait and see. The midwife is authorized to admit the patient on the basis of a strict diagnosis of labor (Chapter 14) and she guards and ensures normal progression (Chapter 15). As most complications of labor arise in initially normal cases that are not proactively supervised, the midwives must be vested with the authority and the tools required to conduct labor properly, on their own authority, including correction of slow labor according to protocol (Chapter 17). As long as no other problems occur, midwives can and should take full professional responsibility for (augmented) normal labor and delivery. To reiterate: *proactive support of labor* does not medicalize birth. Rather, it ensures normality of the birth process and this is the focus of midwifery care. Ideally, the availability of home-like delivery rooms devoid of redundant technical equipment should emphasize this midwifery assignment. Essential provisions and allowances for women-friendly labor rooms were summarized in Chapters 16 and 18.

> *Midwives play the pivotal role in the supervision of normal labor, including augmentation if needed.*

26.2.3 The role of the obstetrician

The obstetrician in charge focuses primarily on the high-risk patients who are not an issue in this manual. However, in terms of absolute numbers most problems in labor arise in completely normal women initially assigned to the midwives. The obstetrician therefore no longer remains off-stage, "awaiting the occasional summons to perform an emergency operation in a belated attempt to retrieve a situation which could have been anticipated at a much earlier stage."[3] Instead, he or she is continually present and tries to help the midwives and residents prevent such emergencies by regular review of all parturients, regardless of prior risk assessment. It is the obstetrician in charge who will account for the outcome at daily peer review (Chapter 27). All obstetricians should be at pains to ensure that policies are executed through constant education on the spot of new residents, midwives, and nurses.

> *The obstetrician in charge must be instantly available on the premises at all times.*

26.2.4 Responsibilities and liability

For an individual patient there exists no such thing as divided responsibility. "A bland institutional declaration to the general effect is meaningless both in medical and in legal terms."[3] Therefore, each individual woman in labor must know exactly who is directly responsible for her well-being: which midwife or which specialist (or authorized senior resident). Although low-risk care may be (partly) delegated to student-midwives and high-risk labors to residents, the attending midwife and the supervising obstetrician, respectively, bear ultimate responsibility and liability and must be known to the patient by name and face.

Whenever the midwife decides that the limits of her authority are reached, the obstetrician takes over responsibility. There is no place for equivocation on this issue; whenever the consulted obstetrician decides to further delegate the supervision of the compromised labor to the midwife or a resident, it goes without saying that the obstetrician remains ultimately accountable whenever a mishap might occur. Apart from liability concerns, experience shows that all professionals and patients benefit greatly from intensive cooperation between physicians and midwives based on mutual confidence and respect. Such a congenial working environment can only exist when a common birth-plan is adopted and when specific tasks and responsibilities are clearly defined.

> *Full responsibility for low-risk labors can and should be assigned to well-trained, certified midwives.*

26.2.5 Sound economics

The system favors efficient use of the expensive labor and delivery unit because all women now give birth within 12 hours. Investment in one-on-one nursing is cost-effective since the reduction in surgical delivery rates greatly reduces overall hospital expenditure. It equally reduces postoperative care, freeing nurses from the postnatal ward to be employed on the labor ward. The costs of liability claims and insurances will undoubtedly decrease as mistakes will diminish and medical negligence actions will belong to the past. Sound organization not only improves all standards of care but equally enhances job satisfaction of staff, reducing the all too common high rates of sick leave and extremely costly burnout. There is no doubt that the system pays for itself.

> *Good childbirth practice corresponds with good working conditions for staff and sound economics as well. All three issues make good sense.*

26.3 Grassroots system reforms

The proposals touch the very heart of current obstetric services as they segregate the persons who perform antenatal care from those who provide intrapartum care, a trend seen in most practices in recent decades. The advantages in quality of care should outweigh the potential off-sets for both patients and caregivers. In particular, con-

cerns about the inherent disruption of patient–practitioner relationships must be discussed. Physicians, midwives, and patients will have to adapt to many changes, but fortunately recent sociocultural developments lead and pave the way.

26.3.1 Traditional patient–doctor relationships

Traditionally, babies are delivered by the practitioner who provides their mothers with prenatal care. This provider-centered practice model combines an office practice and a hospital practice. That system locks obstetricians into an unending cycle of office visits, hospital rounds, surgeries, deliveries, more office visits, evening rounds, late-night telephone calls, and more deliveries in the middle of the night. The obstetrician ends up driving across town several times a day to see women at different hospitals, leaving other patients waiting at the office, while he or she frequently cannot make it to the labor room in time to deliver the baby. Continuity in patient–doctor relationships is cherished in name, but continuous and personal care in labor is factually non-existent.

Even worse, the combination of grueling working hours and demands of personal commitment encourages practitioners to induce labor for no reason other than the doctor's convenience and will equally lower the threshold for cesarean deliveries (Chapters 4, 6). These practices inevitably harm their patients' health. Women should realize that the current provider-centered system was never designed for and is not aimed at their best interests, nor does it benefit obstetricians for that matter; both sides suffer greatly under this system.

> *The emperor of the traditional, provider-centered care model has no clothes.*

26.3.2 Current crisis in obstetrics services

Hectic and unpredictable working hours, topped by the stifling legal climate, are increasingly causing gynecologists to retire or cut back on OB services. Job dissatisfaction is not anecdotal but structural; evidence exists for a marked increase in fatigue, substance abuse, poor personal relationships, and burnout.[5–10] Clearly, this is of no service to any pregnant woman.

Little wonder that the number of medical graduates choosing a career in obstetrics and gynecology has recently dropped markedly.[11,12] Apparently, medical students rotating through obstetrics mainly observe stressed or demotivated practitioners and understandably decide that there must be a better way to make a living. Future work capacity is jeopardized and the dwindling workforce recruitment aggravates all problems even further, completing the vicious circle. Clearly, the need for grassroots reforms of the obstetric system is acute.

> *As it goes now, both access to and the quality of obstetrical care are in real jeopardy. The provider-centered system must therefore be replaced by a new system that is patient-centered in design.*

26.3.3 Societal changes

Fortunately, major sociocultural reforms have occurred throughout all western societies in the past decades, including a gradual gender transformation of academic professionals. This trend did not pass by the domain of obstetrics and gynecology; today, more than 70% of all residents are female. Undoubtedly, the greatest benefit to accrue from this change is a heightened sensitivity to "women's issues" in the training programs and practice of medicine, such as the need to balance the demands of work and raising a family.[13,14] This has triggered permanent changes. No longer are doctors – of either gender – willing to work 70–80 hours a week while personal and family life suffer. The new lifestyle demands exclude a practice with 24/7 availability and continuous personal commitment. Solo practices become increasingly unpopular and most obstetricians now practice in groups that provide their members with reasonable call schedules and duty hours. Even part-time practice has now become possible. The new function of laborist-obstetrician, whose job is restricted to working in the labor and delivery ward, is becoming increasingly popular and benefits both doctors and patients.[15] Surely, most patients in labor prefer the personal attention and time of a devoted obstetrician who is constantly there above their "own" doctor, who is there only occasionally and always in a rush. The new breed of obstetrician-laborists fits perfectly in the ideal organization of the delivery unit.

> *Physicians want a reasonable work/family balance, just like all other people, including women who happen to be pregnant. Today the majority of patients accept this as a matter of course.*

By now, patients are used to seeing different doctors and understand the inevitability thereof. They only disapprove when reorganization is primarily aimed at making things better for doctors rather than for patients. Patients' dissatisfaction does not result from doctors' discontinuity but from frustrating inconsistencies in information by different practitioners and annoying discrepancies between information and actions. The problem is not the group practice but non-cooperating egos who refuse to adapt to commonly established guidelines. The opportunity for major breakthroughs is often missed, for it is exactly the joint practice that finally opens possibilities for genuine improvement of all standards of care including patients' satisfaction. To this end, of course, the prerequisites of a common strategy of care, meaningful cooperation, and consistent patient information must be met.

> *Patients' dissatisfaction with large practices does not result from disruption of doctors' continuity, but from inconsistencies in information and disappointing discrepancies between information and actions.*

26.3.4 Refocusing obstetric practice

The final logical step is to refocus the specialty of obstetrics on what the discipline originally was meant for: the pathology of pregnancy and child-birth. In contrast, the care for normal pregnancy and childbirth are the specialty of well-trained and legally certified midwives. The evidence shows that it is inherently unwise and often even unsafe for healthy women with normal pregnancies to be cared for by obstetric specialists, even if the required staffing is available.[16] Besides, obstetricians – caring for women with both normal and abnormal pregnancies – because of time constraints have to make an impossible choice: to neglect the normal pregnancies in order to concentrate their care on those with pathology, or to spend most of their time supervising biologically normal processes. In that case they rapidly lose their specialist expertise. We had better refocus our identity as medical specialists rather than as primary care providers. The benefit will be the reemergence of the specialty we all chose and love to practice: a technical and surgical profession. The challenge is to restrict the application of these operative skills to those who really need it.

> *Obstetricians should refocus on their primary task: the care and treatment of pathological pregnancy and labor and delivery disorders.*

26.3.5 Primary care

Yet it is still the physicians who provide almost all antenatal care and who deliver more than 90% of all babies in the USA.[17] In the majority of other countries most babies are delivered by hospital midwives, but it is no secret that cooperation with the physicians is far from ideal, mainly because an integrated and mutually agreed concept of normal childbirth is often lacking. In those countries, too, a lot still has to be improved.

Every childbearing woman wants personal attention for "rosy issues" that consume a lot of time, something most medical specialists do not have. The more reason to leave primary care for normal pregnancies to the experts in this field – well-trained and legally certified midwives – provided, of course, that they wholeheartedly keep to the principles of *proactive support of labor*, just as medical-specialist staff should do. That implies that midwives and obstetricians must work closely together both at the antenatal clinics and in the delivery ward, ideally in one collective enterprise.

A joint practice guarantees instant consultation and a care continuum if complications arise. Strict division into two independently operating echelons of care simply does not work, as the current system in the Netherlands clearly shows (Chapter 5). Patients' preferences and needs are much more complex and contain many elements of both midwifery and medical styles of care, both of which should be honored at all times.[18–20] A recent systematic review of the international literature on the efficiency and effectiveness of integrated perinatal care confirms the crucial importance of organizing modalities that aim to support woman-centered care and cooperative clinical practice.[21]

> *Primary care is best provided by midwives who are fully integrated into the system, who know the boundaries of their expertise, and who have instant access to help from cooperating obstetricians.*

Reorganization cannot neglect more earthy issues; the collective of obstetricians and midwives should make new financial arrangements with the health insurers, eliminating improper incentives to direct care. In fact, the much more demanding efforts to promote spontaneous delivery should be better paid than the resolution of preventable labor problems by a quick but unnecessary cesarean delivery. Reforms should therefore be neutral or positive to the incomes of all participating obstetricians and midwives. A guaranteed and fair income ultimately enhances quality of care and reduces consequent overall costs. In our experience most health insurers are glad to cooperate.

26.3.6 Home deliveries and emotions

The final issue that needs to be addressed is home birth, an endless source of conflict and strong emotions. Women's preference for home birth originates in sociocultural values or reflects fear of hospitals and opposition to overmedicalized hospital birth (Chapter 5). As it is now, rejection of medical birth care by women's health groups and home birth activists is often all too well-founded on women's adverse hospital experiences (Chapter 4). Views are particularly polarized in the USA, with activists on the barricades for home births and hospitals denying independent midwives access when problems arise at home, so that they are forced to smuggle their patients into the ER and leave. Many US hospitals even deny midwives a job when they are also involved with home births.[22] Clearly, there is a lot of rancor there.

> *Experiences with overmedicalized, impersonal and even harmful hospital care will continue to arouse reactionary calls for home births, sometimes even in chancy circumstances. Who is to blame?*

Despite decades of political and academic debate, the relative merits of home versus hospital birth and vice versa remain unproven.[23] This is likely to remain so, as comparisons that are sufficiently unbiased and large enough to address crucial safety issues are unlikely to be forthcoming.[24] Be that as it may, women will continue to choose to give birth at home for a variety of reasons and these women and their babies are equally entitled to effective hospital back-up if problems should arise. It is therefore much wiser to listen to women's wishes and women's health movements, to elaborate and agree on strict selection criteria and safeguards for home births, to define mutual responsibilities, and to monitor the results.

Entrenched positions, by either party, only make women suffer.

26.3.7 Integration

Broadening women's options involves moving from the preconceived biomedical or midwifery notions of appropriate care into a patient-based and multi-option setting. This reorientation holds for all aspects of in-hospital as well as out-of-hospital care. The most logical and the ideal answer to the sociocultural pressures would be to integrate both services into one collective system, based on a common plan. A joint practice of obstetricians and midwives can offer the possibility of safe home births in selected cases, attended by the midwives who also work in the hospital. The integrated practice guarantees consistent policies, a continuum in care, instant access to the hospital if needed, and a good collaborative relationship between the home-attending midwives and the hospital.

Mutual trust is a matter of fundamental importance on which all else ultimately depends and this requires mutual respect and undivided adherence to all components of a central plan both in the hospital and at home. In a collective initiative there is no place for competition; like all other professionals, independently operating midwives will have to sacrifice (a part of) their autonomy for the sake of the common good, join the collective practice, adopt the common policies, share its profits, and subject themselves to peer review. This is the acid test of goodwill on the part of midwives.

> *Women's preferences and needs contain many elements of both midwifery and medical styles of care. These wishes should be met by integrating out-of-hospital and in-hospital care.*

Honoring women's choices means that there should be no pressure for or against planned home birth after a normal pregnancy. As it is now, both biomedical obstetrics and the women's health movement's critique of it share a belief in the ability to control childbirth so that there will be a positive and rewarding outcome. This emphasis on happy endings – whether believed to be the result of medical intervention or women's natural inborn powers to give birth – actually exacerbates the adverse experiences of those women whose happy expectations do not come true.[25] Obstetricians' emphasis on risks may disempower women, but homebirth activists' emphasis on the "dream delivery" and the importance of women being in control of their own bodies equally surely contributes to disappointment and women's self-blame when delivery is not completed at home.[26,27] Clearly, both attitudes should be abandoned. The best practice is to provide low-risk women with data-driven information, replacing anecdotal horror stories of "what might happen" at home or in the hospital. Only constant and unbiased evaluation allows for meaningful bilateral cooperation.

> *There should be no pressure for or against planned home birth in low-risk pregnancies.*

26.3.8 Case selection for home birth

The authors work in a highly developed western country where, uniquely, home birth is still valued as a cultural heritage (Chapter 5). Currently, we are in the middle of the challenging process of merging formerly independent midwife practices into a collective system with the hospital. As a result, more and more midwives in our region increasingly work both in the hospital and at home. Their activities at home are somewhat narrowed while their facilities in the hospital are increased. As a result, home birth is not considered as a goal per se any longer by these midwives but as a responsible option in strictly selected cases. We have agreed on the following:

1. Home births remain restricted to uneventful, singleton pregnancies with a normal fetus in the cephalic presentation and with a gestational age between 37 and 42 weeks.

2. VBACs are not allowed at home. If the cesarean section and the postoperative recovery have been uneventful, VBAC is accepted in the hospital.

3. Stripping of membranes at 41-plus weeks, to induce a home birth before the 42-week limit is passed, should no longer be practiced.

4. The transfer-time to the hospital in case of complications should never exceed 30 minutes, taking into account the usual traffic conditions. Patients living farther away deliver in the hospital.

5. The midwife attending home birth takes full responsibility. The hospital guarantees instant medical back-up.

6. The midwife at home keeps the obligatory partogram. She breaks the membranes whenever indicated, even at 1 cm dilatation if needed. Whenever progress remains unsatisfactory, the patient is transferred to the hospital in time to allow effective corrective action. The midwife continues attendance in the hospital and remains responsible for the accelerated labor.

7. The midwife stays at the home throughout the entire birth process and fetal heart beat is counted every 15–30 minutes. In case of any abnormality, including passage of meconium, the woman is immediately transferred and the obstetrician takes over responsibility.

8. To enhance mutual understanding and respect, all residents and nurses in training should attend a few planned home births.

Intensive audit continues to refine and enforce the system. Initially, most midwives were inclined to stretch the time criteria, but constant peer review clearly identified such expectancy as a contributor to higher operative delivery rates and women's dissatisfaction. On the basis of constant review of their own data, most midwives in our region now agree that timely amniotomy and timely transfer for augmentation with oxytocin reduce overall interventions in first labors. The scale advantage of the collective practice increasingly facilitates the midwives staying with their clients at home throughout first-stage labor. Constant audit does not reveal any adverse fetal outcomes, if protocols are followed, that could have been prevented had the patients been in the hospital from the onset. When strict criteria are met, the integrated facility of home births proves to be safe.

> *Under strict conditions, an integrated in- and out-of-hospital practice can responsibly provide facilities for safe home births.*

In our region, between 30% and 35% of all nulliparas currently opt for a home delivery and are given this chance. Approximately 60% of them succeed in doing so, which is actually a greater percentage than the Dutch average, thanks to timely amniotomy in early labor at home. However, since nulliparity includes a 40% chance of intrapartum transfer to the hospital – which is actually lower than the 50% national average (Chapter 4) – an increasing number of our associated midwives now label a first delivery at home as inadvisable. Freedom from adverse effects on their income and constant review of results made them discover this by themselves, which is the only way that will work. On the other hand, the percentage of parous women planning births at home increased markedly to 45–50%, partly owing to improved mothers' first birth experiences and thus increased self-confidence, and in part because of the decreasing number of parous women with a cesarean scar. Although no goal in itself, on balance the overall percentage of women giving birth at home increased to nearly 35% in our region. The overall low operative delivery rates will be discussed in Chapter 29.

> *Home birth should not be an escape from the overmedicalized childbirth services that still exist in many hospitals. Home delivery should be the optional bonus for parous women who experienced high-quality hospital care throughout their first childbirth and gained the ultimate prize of vaginal delivery.*

26.4 Benefits for all

Apart from locally colored debates on the desirability of home birth facilities, grassroots systematic reforms of childbirth services prove to be of great benefit for all involved. The patient-centered system based on the principles of *proactive support of labor* effectively restores the balance between natural and medicalized childbirth. Women's satisfaction with their childbirth experience increases markedly as now continuous personal attention is guaranteed and prolonged labor is effectively prevented. Most importantly, all women finally get the maximal chance to deliver their baby safely by their own efforts. The system normalizes work hours and work pressure for all care providers, thereby greatly increasing job satisfaction. The nurses and midwives focus on *care* and the efforts of obstetricians remain restricted to *cure*. Obstetricians can now concentrate on their specific medical expertise and certified midwives, who love to extend their chances for conducting the birth process properly, regain the pivotal role in the supervision of normal pregnancy and childbirth.

26.5 Summary

- Poor labor ward organization is the rock on which most good intentions founder.
- Sound organization involves strict labor room rules and a redefinition of the working relations and mutual responsibilities between nurses, midwives, and physicians.
- In most maternity care systems it is the organization that directs the content of care, whereas the desired care content should rather determine the organization.
- Provider-centered care should be replaced by 24/7 woman-centered care.
- Patients' preferences and needs are complex and contain many elements of both midwifery and medical styles of care, both of which should be honored by means of an integrated obstetric-midwifery childbirth service.

- The only way to lower undue operative delivery rates and to improve women's satisfaction with their childbirth experience is to implement organizational reforms that will allow caregivers to execute all components of a central, high-quality birth-plan: *proactive support of labor.*

REFERENCES

1. Nelson EC, Batalden PB, Godfrey MM. *Quality Design: A Clinical Microsystems Approach.* New York: Wiley; 2006.

2. Godfrey M, Wasson J, Nelson E, *et al. Clinical Microsystem Action Guide*; 2002 (available at: www.clinicalmicrosystem.org/images/PDF20%Files/cmsactionguide.pdf).

3. O'Driscoll K, Meagher D, Robson M. *Active Management of Labour*, 4th edn. Mosby; 2003.

4. Hodnett ED. Pain and women's satisfaction with the experience of childbirth: a systematic review. *Am J Obstet Gynecol* 2002; 186: S160–72.

5. Spickard A, Gabbe SG, Christensen JF. Mid-career burnout in generalists and specialist physicians. *JAMA* 2002; 288: 1447–50.

6. Defoe DM, Power ML, Holzman GB, *et al.* Long hours and little sleep: work schedules of residents in obstetrics and gynecology. *Obstet Gynecol* 2001; 97: 1015–18.

7. Storr CI, Trinkoff AM, Anthony JC. Job strain and non-medical drug use. *Drug Alcohol Depend* 1999; 55: 45–51.

8. Myers MF. Don't let your practice kill your marriage. *Med Econ* 1998; 9: 78–87.

9. Maulen B. Depression, divorce, malpractice, bankruptcy: why do so many physicians commit suicide? *MMW Fortschr Med* 2002; 144: 4–8.

10. Kravitz RL, Leigh JP, Samuels SJ, *et al.* Tracking career satisfaction and perceptions of quality among US obstetricians and gynecologists. *Obstet Gynecol* 2003; 102: 463–9.

11. Queenan JT. The future of obstetrics and gynecology. *Obstet Gynecol* 2003; 102: 441–2.

12. Gibbons JM. Springtime for obstetrics and gynecology: will the specialty continue to blossom? *Obstet Gynecol* 2003; 102: 443–5.

13. Pearse WH, Haffner WHJ, Primack A. Effect of gender on the obstetric-gynecologic work force. *Obstet Gynecol* 2001; 97: 794–7.

14. Frigoletto FD, Greene MF. Is there a sea change ahead for obstetrics and gynecology? *Obstet Gynecol* 2002; 100: 1342–3.

15. Weinstein L. The laborist: a new focus of practice for the obstetrician. *Am J Obstet Gynecol* 2003; 188: 310–12.

16. Kitzinger S, Shearer M, *et al.* Social, financial, and psychological support during pregnancy and childbirth. In: Chalmers I, Enkin M, Keirse MJ, eds. *Effective Care in Pregnancy and Childbirth.* Oxford: Oxford University Press; 1998.

17. Ventura S, Martin JA, Curtin SC, *et al. Births: final data for 1999.* National vital statistics reports; 49. Hyattsville, MD: National Center for Health Statistics; 2001.

18. Lyon DS, Mokhtarian PL, Reever MM. Predicting style-of-care preferences of obstetric patients: medical vs midwifery model. *J Reprod Med* 1999; 44: 101–6.

19. Huntley V, Ryan M, Graham W. Assessing women's preferences for intrapartum care. *Birth* 2001; 28: 254–63.

20. American College of Obstetricians and Gynecologists. *Frequently asked questions about having a baby in the 21st century.* Washington; 2001 (availale at www.acog.org/from_home/publications/press_releases/nr12–12-01-4.cfm; accessed May 5, 2005).

21. Rodriguez C, des Rivières-Pigeon C. A literature review on integrated perinatal care. *Int J Integrated Care* 2007; 7: 1–15.

22. Declercq ER, Sakala C, Corry MP, *et al. Listening to mothers: report of the first national US survey of women's childbirth experiences.* New York: Maternity Center Association; 2002.

23. Olsen O, Jewell MD. Home versus hospital birth. *Cochrane Database Syst Rev* 2000; (2): CD000352.

24. MacFarlane A. Trial would not answer key question, but data monitoring should be improved. *BMJ* 1996; 312: 754–5.

25. Laynne LL. Unhappy endings: a feminist reappraisal of the women's health movement from the vantage of pregnancy loss. *Soc Sci Med* 2003; 56: 1881–91.

26. Christiaens W, Gouwy A, Bracke P. Does a referral from home to hospital affect satisfaction with childbirth? A cross-national comparison. *BMC Health Services Research* 2007; 7: 109–17.

27. Rijnders M, Baston H, Schönbeck Y, *et al.* Perinatal factors related to negative or positive recall of birth experience in women 3 years postpartum in The Netherlands. *Birth* 2008; 35(2): 107–16.

27

Continual audit and feedback

Promoting normality of labor is as much about caregivers' (re)education as about changing behaviors, and neither can be accomplished in a haphazard manner. Indeed, altering practice patterns of highly educated professionals is not an easy task. It requires clinical leadership, careful planning, and ongoing maintenance. The first step is to identify the most sensitive areas of care and to standardize the general outline of procedures.[1,2] These matters have been addressed in the previous chapters under the headings diagnosis of labor, prevention of long labor, continuous support, organization, etc. A continual cycle of audit should then be introduced, leading to step-by-step improvements in labor conduct, labor support, and overall care. This chapter discusses the crucial internal audit and feedback systems required for successful implementation of the overall policy.

27.1 Internal audit by strict peer review

The key factor to achieving enduring success is an ongoing system of close peer review within the hospital, weaving all medical and non-medical components of *proactive support of labor* into an overall pattern of practice. The main platform for an effective audit cycle is the daily morning report, attended by all obstetricians, midwives, residents, and interns.

The morning report
Daily evaluation of all the medical and non-medical processes involved is the most important factor in establishing and maintaining the practice of proactive support of labor.

27.1.1 Content

Instead of the team rushing through the operative deliveries, each woman operatively delivered during the previous 24 hours should be made the object of scrutiny. Insistence on the precise use of well-defined terms and diagnoses is a matter of prime importance (Chapter 11). Thus, undefined observations such as "dystocia" or "non-reassuring CTG" should no longer be accepted. Instead, the underlying cause of each problem and exact diagnoses (as listed in Chapters 17 and 21–24) should be assessed and the timing and nature of corrective actions taken must be analyzed.

Although there will always be some subjective elements in clinical diagnosis, a collective judgment on the appropriateness of diagnosis and treatment can be reached in almost every case provided that the details of each labor have been carefully documented. Omissions in relevant information should be exposed. The final diagnosis, or combination of diagnoses, should be recorded in the patient's chart as well as in the institutional files. Through these plenary sessions the whole staff, including all consultants, become actively involved in the regular analysis of labor as never before and the morning reports gain enormously in substance, relevance, educational value, and fun.

> *A strict diagnosis of labor disorders and close analysis of the corrective measures taken are critical for meaningful medical audit and continuing education of all care providers involved in childbirth.*

Adherence to a uniform, disciplined approach which includes fail-safe procedures is a fundamental feature of *proactive support of labor*. The biomedical quintessence is the correct diagnosis of labor and the timing of interventions, whether these be amniotomy, use of oxytocin, pain relief, or operative delivery. Reasons for any departure from protocol should be motivated and defended. Initially, practitioners and midwives may feel threatened by these rigorous reviews, but experience shows that their job satisfaction and prestige improve markedly with the quality of care. Prerequisite for an effective learning curve is that an open, professional atmosphere is nurtured. Peer review should not be directed to assigning blame to individuals or to deflecting criticism from others but should be aimed at enhancement of the general fund of knowledge in the basic requirements for normal labor and delivery and promotion of new standards and expectations. An honest review looks at what could have been done differently in the timing of intervention (*prompt*), the amount of labor support (*sufficient*), and the type of corrective measures or treatment (*appropriate*). Cause and effect need to be determined if progress is to be made.

> *Local peer review must be detailed, inspiring, ongoing, and high profile.*

27.1.2 Leadership

Strong clinical leadership is critical. Analysis of the guideline movements shows that formal guidelines issued by professional associations or government agencies have limited, if any, effect on overall practice, mainly because of a lack of committed local leadership.[3,4] Likewise, many "active management programs" have failed in the past because of a lack of authoritative direction and daily peer review. As labor management decisions are "local," activities to bring about practice change have to be driven locally and such initiatives are destined to fail in the absence of committed leadership. Authority should be based on professional knowledge and the ability to inspire and motivate all co-workers. Physician and midwife behaviors and practice patterns are unlikely to change in the absence of recognition, praise, public accord, and private admonishments by senior staff.

> *Initiatives for altering practice patterns require committed clinical leadership and "peer pressure."*

27.1.3 Commitment to low intervention rates

Patients and professionals should be encouraged to consider spontaneous birth positively, so creating disincentives for unnecessary interventions in pregnancy and childbirth is important. To this end, every individual indication for termination of pregnancy – be it induction of labor or prelabor cesarean delivery – has to be discussed and carried at the plenary morning report. Just the strict peer review of indications effectively reduces the number of these interventions and their related iatrogenic complications. Since the aim of labor induction is to effectuate a vaginal delivery, each cesarean birth after priming/induction should be reported as "failed induction" (Chapter 23). This very assessment proves to be an eye-opener to many doctors and further reduces the local induction rate.

> *Each proposal for priming/induction and for prelabor cesarean section should be reviewed at the plenary morning report. The same goes for the outcomes.*

27.1.4 Regular perinatal audit

Changing practice patterns serves no useful purpose if the reduction of interventions is achieved at the expense of perinatal outcomes. Therefore, formal feedback from the pediatricians to the midwives and physicians must be provided at least every fortnight. In these regular meetings the obstetric details of every case with suboptimal neonatal outcome should again be markedly subjected to careful scrutiny. In our experience, following low-risk pregnancies, adverse outcomes such as perinatal infection, trauma, and asphyxia are almost always exclusively the result of protocol violations.

> *A continuous, multidisciplinary audit system ensures that every important aspect of maternity care is kept under constant review.*

27.1.5 Regular nursing audit

The labor ward nurses play the pivotal role in *proactive support of labor*. That is why the nurses should be encouraged to hold regular meetings to discuss the art, skill, and science of labor support on the basis of mutual experiences, nursing studies, and structured feedback from patients.

27.1.6 Patient debriefing and personal feedback

Standard debriefing six weeks after delivery by the childbirth educator/nurses evaluates women's satisfaction with their childbirth experience (Chapter 19). These structured interviews provide indispensable information – both positive and negative – for meaningful feedback to individual labor ward nurses, midwives, and physicians about their attitudes and care in labor. In fact, intensive use of patient feedback is the most effective tool to improve professional bedside manners.

> *Continual audit of interventions linked to neonatal and maternal outcomes and constant*

> *evaluation of women's childbirth experiences are the very foundation of proactive support of labor.*

27.1.7 Hospital year reports

A current account of interventions must be maintained on a regular basis and the overall year results of the unit should be discussed in plenary. It is difficult to address what "a good induction rate" or "a good cesarean birth rate" is for a given hospital, since not every maternity center is dealt the same cards. Sociocultural and medical characteristics of the population may vary widely between hospitals. What is obligatory, though, for any institution and health insurer, is to know the level of these interventions and to have an opinion on whether or not they are appropriate.[5] That is the subject of the next chapters.

27.2 Summary

- Promoting normality of labor involves a simultaneous process of constant (re)education and changing behaviors of physicians and midwives.
- Practice patterns can only be altered with strong physician leadership and the intensive use of local audit, "peer pressure," and personal feedback.
- Only detailed analysis of labor, on a daily basis, identifies the shortcomings in current care processes, giving clear and constant direction to structural improvements.
- Meaningful audit depends on complete reporting of all relevant details of labor and delivery, both medical and non-medical, and on the assessment of strict diagnoses.

REFERENCES

1. Nelson EC, Batalden PB, Godfrey MM. *Quality Design: A Clinical Microsystems Approach*. New York: Wiley; 2006.

2. Godfrey M, Wasson J, Nelson E, *et al. Clinical Microsystem Action Guide*; 2002 (available at: www.clinicalmicrosystem.org/images/PDF20%Files/cms actionguide.pdf).

3. Lomas J, Anderson GM, Dominick-Pierce K. Do practice guidelines guide practice? The effect of a consensus statement on the practice of physicians. *N Engl J Med* 1989; 321: 1306–11.

4. Gates PE. Think globally, act locally: an approach to implementation of clinical practice guidelines. *Jt Comm J Qual Improv* 1995; 21(2): 71–84.

5. Robson MS. Classification of cesarean sections. *Fetal and Maternal Medicine Review* 2001; 12: 23–39.

28

Quality assessment

Every woman in labor deserves high-quality professional care. While no-one is likely to disagree with this principle, there may be marked disagreement about what constitutes a high quality of care (Section 1). Unfortunately, the debate is more often about choice of caregiver or place of birth than about the content of intrapartum care. And whenever the latter does come up, disputes arise from differences of opinion about the objectives of intrapartum care and the best means of achieving them. Objectives, or the relative emphasis placed on particular objectives, may range from women's enjoyment of childbirth to shaving another fraction of a percentage point off the perinatal mortality rate, no matter what the costs. Consequently, methods of care currently range from a highly expectant approach that dogmatically eschews intervention to strongly interfering approaches with standard use of technology and major interventions. This diversity in approaches explains the disparate indicators used to claim "quality" of birth care and the disagreement about the value of "evidence" advanced to support or criticize the diverse types of care. Points of view are predominantly ideologically driven, with means and objectives mixed up and women's preferences taken for granted or forgotten in both camps. Obviously, more clarity on these issues is needed and fruitless disputes should be settled for the sake of all women. That is the purpose of this chapter. In fact, most controversies can be successfully bridged by the introduction of *proactive support of labor*.

> *Childbirth is the same physiological process worldwide. Therefore, universal criteria for the quality of care in childbirth can and should be assessed, regardless of the place of birth.*

28.1 Quality criteria

Evidently, all birth professionals – obstetricians and midwives alike – have a dual responsibility: the welfare of both the mothers and their unborn babies, especially during labor and delivery. Some procedures and outcomes of labor care can be objectively assessed, allowing inter-hospital comparisons. These include induction rates, prelabor and intrapartum cesarean rates, instrumental vaginal delivery rates, and perinatal mortality rates. However, the most important outcome – maternal satisfaction – does not lend itself to objective quantification for inter-hospital comparisons and must therefore be assessed personally and evaluated locally (Chapter 27).

> *Not everything that counts can be counted, and not everything that can be counted counts. –* Albert Einstein

28.1.1 Objective outcome measures

Since the vast majority of operative deliveries are performed to resolve problems of first labors, and since maternal birth injuries are almost exclusively related to these surgical interventions, operative delivery rates in "standard" nulliparas (Chapter 29) are currently the most realistic, objective measure of the standard of care afforded to mothers, replacing maternal mortality rates, which are outmoded for this purpose in western countries. With regard to the neonates, perinatal mortality must continue to serve the same purpose until such time as neonatal morbidity rates are sufficiently clearly defined. By these combined criteria, quality of care can be markedly improved in many places.

> *The rate of spontaneous vaginal deliveries in "standard nulliparas" is the most objective benchmark for overall quality of obstetric care afforded to mothers. With regard to the babies, perinatal mortality rates must continue to serve as the measure of quality of care.*

28.1.2 Sense of proportion

O'Driscoll et al.,[1] criticizing the rapidly expanding cesarean rates in the early 1990s, summarized the problem: "In the light of the extraordinary increase in the number of women who are subjected to major abdominal operations which are of no direct benefit to themselves, the detached observer might reasonably assume that the benefits conferred on their offspring could be shown to be overwhelming. Alas, this is far from being the case." There is indeed no evidence that the staggering increase in cesarean rates seen over the last 25 years has made any improvement to overall perinatal mortality rates. Rather the reverse is true (Chapter 2). Most striking in this respect are practice variation studies showing that countries, hospitals, and doctors vary markedly for cesarean rates – with some at or below 15% – although at the same time having similar perinatal mortality rates.[2] Governmental agencies, professional associations, consulting groups, and managed care organizations have all struggled with this issue for more than 20 years.

This resulted in "The Healthy Person 2000 Project" aimed at a reduction of the US national cesarean rate to 15%.[3] But none of the initiatives has approached this Year 2000 goal, which has been attacked as "unrealistic" or "unsafe for babies." It should be pointed out, however, that this goal is to be applied to the whole population, not to individual obstetricians who may to some extent have adverse patient selection.

Change of practice to reduce improper cesarean delivery rates has to be brought about locally at hospital level (Chapter 27) and, evidently, the Healthy Person 2000 goal of a 15% cesarean rate remains a valid target level for any standard maternity unit. To this end, many an institution needs to reform its practices. The aim is a new balance between spontaneous and operative deliveries and between fetal and maternal outcomes. It was O'Driscoll who showed us the way to do it: *proactive support of labor* serves the best interests of both mothers and their babies (Chapter 29).

> *The Healthy Person 2000 goal of a 15% national cesarean rate remains a valid target.*

28.1.3 Duration of labor

Of course, major interventions without a formal indication cannot be defended in any circumstance, but objections against minor interventions, such as amniotomy and use of oxytocin, originate in the unfounded assumption that women reject effective measures to prevent long labor. Still, few caregivers would disagree that a common complaint is that a labor was "too long." Thus, the length of labor should be regarded as an important independent outcome (Chapter 15). In fact, all aspects of care and all outcomes including maternal satisfaction deteriorate with overly long labor. Indeed, prevention of long labor is the key to patient satisfaction. In our hospital about 97% of all women give birth within the time frame of 12 hours.

> *The length of labor should be regarded as an important independent quality parameter.*

28.1.4 Maternal satisfaction

Although women's satisfaction with childbirth should be considered as the principal measure of quality of care, few obstetricians and midwives evaluate this outcome in their practice on a systematic basis. Consequently, their impressions of women's attitudes to (minor) interventions in labor might easily be colored by reactions of (ill-informed) patients/clients with strong views or complainants who may not be representative. Caregivers' general ideas about women's preferences and desires may therefore be quite biased and reinforced by self-selection. Yet generalizations are readily made and strong opinions are often defended without any serious attempt at systematic verification with their patients/clients after delivery.

Maternal satisfaction was addressed extensively in Chapters 18 and 19, emphasizing the need for prelabor information that corresponds with actual practice. Our childbirth educators have yet to meet the woman who fundamentally disagrees with the offered birth-plan. The importance of structured postpartum debriefing is also evident (Chapters 19 and 27). In our practice, very few women complain afterward of the method of care, as long as the clear policies were fully executed, the promises about intensive labor support were kept, and the reasons for any intervention were clearly explained. Of course, 100% maternal satisfaction with the childbirth experience will never be reached, but patients' dissatisfaction, if critically analyzed, nearly always proves to originate in disappointing mismatches between expectations and actual practice. This emphasizes the importance of strict adherence to the agreed birth-plan, facilitated by clear patient education and sound organization, and constantly reinforced by continual audit of all procedures and relevant outcomes, as well as by structured feedback from all patients six weeks after delivery.

> *Continuous evaluation of maternal satisfaction is precisely the hallmark of practicing* proactive support of labor.

28.2 Summary

- Quality improvement initiatives need to be driven locally.
- Quality of childbirth needs to be evaluated as much in physical as in emotional terms.
- Quality assessment is as much about evaluation of objective labor outcome data as about constant audit of labor procedures and structured evaluation of maternal satisfaction.
- Criticism of the proposed policies is generally advanced by doctors and midwives who do not evaluate women's satisfaction with childbirth in their own practice on a regular, structured basis.

REFERENCES

1. O'Driscoll K, Meagher D, Robson M. *Active Management of Labour*, 4th edn. Mosby; 2003.
2. Main EK. Reducing cesarean birth rates with data-driven quality improvement activities. *Pediatrics* 1999; 103: 374–83.
3. US Department of Health and Human Services, Public Health Service. *Healthy People 2000*. DHHS Publication No. 91–50213. Washington DC: US Government Printing Office; 1991: 378–9.

29

Hospital statistics

Although quality assessment of an obstetric service involves much more than just reporting operative delivery and perinatal mortality rates (Chapter 28), all care providers within one institution should know the institutional intervention and outcome data. An effective initiative to rekindle professionals' desire to have a good spontaneous delivery rate is provision of each obstetrician with his/her individual operative delivery rates on a regular basis.[1] But in comparisons the populations must be comparable. Some obstetricians will complain that their intervention rates are relatively high because of their "skewed population" with a higher proportion of multiple gestations, breech presentations, and patients with complicated diabetes, early-onset preeclampsia, HIV, etc. These conditions will have to be verified and taken into account when comparing overall intervention rates between doctors.

29.1 Problems and pitfalls in inter-hospital comparisons

Unfortunately, there still is a lack of standardized information allowing meaningful comparisons of hospital annual reports. Operative delivery rates may be affected by several demographic, obstetric, and fetal factors, as well as childbirth-system related issues – such as whether hospitals cover the entire regional pregnant population or only a part because of out-of-hospital deliveries attended by independent midwives. These factors are beyond the control of obstetricians and for this reason the "raw" cesarean birth rate of a hospital is unsuitable for assessing the labor and delivery skills of its birth professionals.[2] To complicate matters further, hospital year reports vary widely in patient stratification. They report parity-based or mixed-parity data, with breech and multiple pregnancies included or excluded, and use subdivisions into varying gestational age groups as well as arbitrarily defined subsets of low-risk, medium-risk, and high-risk pregnancies, to name just a few confounders. Several suggestions have been made for risk-adjusted algorithms to facilitate inter-unit comparisons,[1–5] but so far none of these concepts has gained general acceptance. What is more, the incidences of "dystocia" and "fetal distress" currently reported in hospital reports are merely statements of the number of cesarean deliveries included under those headings on an arbitrary basis. The same holds true for national databases. Such data relay nothing about the care processes involved. For evaluation of labor and delivery skills, far more sophisticated diagnoses and labor management strategies should be reported (Chapter 27), but most hospitals are unable to give such detailed data.

> *Blunt comparison of overall operative intervention rates between hospitals is meaningless. The motto for intervention reduction programs should be: "Think nationally, but act locally."*[6]

29.2 Comparing apples with apples

Despite these problems in inter-unit comparisons, the authors report the intervention and outcome data of their joint obstetric-midwifery practice (as explained in Chapter 26) to demonstrate that the concept of *proactive support of labor* actually works. The concept is exclusively intended for term women carrying a singleton in the vertex presentation. The data of these "standard" pregnancies are therefore presented, subdivided into "standard nulliparas" and "standard multiparas." Well-defined conditions such as prematurity, breech presentation, multiple pregnancies, and presence of a cesarean uterine scar have been excluded. To avoid debates on arbitrary definitions and for ease of comparison with other hospitals, all so-called "high-risk" pregnancies complicated by intrauterine growth restriction (IUGR), preeclampsia, diabetes, HIV, PROM, postmaturity and so forth, have been included, as well as the "low-risk" labors concluded out of hospital by our affiliated midwives (overall roughly 30%: about 25% of all standard nulliparas and about 40% of all standard multiparas, see Chapter 26). These aggregated data should be eligible for comparison with those of any standard hospital catering for the entire pregnant population of a region (no home deliveries) as is the case in most western countries.

29.2.1 Standard nulliparas

The concept of *proactive support of labor* is specifically designed to improve professional labor and delivery skills and these are best assessed by the intervention and outcome data of standard nulliparas (Table 29.1). In all survey studies "dystocia" in first labor and repeat cesarean delivery are the dominant indications for cesarean delivery; each accounts for approximately one-third of cesarean births (Chapter 2). Clearly, the management of "dystocia" in first labors has the greatest opportunity for quality improvement. In our hospital the cesarean rate for "dystocia" in first labors is 4.5%: in about 1% of standard nulliparas "mechanical

dystocia" is diagnosed – 0.5% malpresentation and 0.5% cephalopelvic disproportion (Chapter 22) – and in about 3.5% therapy-resistant "dynamic dystocia" is diagnosed, of which nearly half are "failed inductions." There is no plausible reason why these results should not be reproduced in other centers. It all depends on strict diagnoses and clearly defined labor and delivery procedures.

29.2.2 Standard multiparas

Labor policies in parous pregnancies are subject to liability concerns in case of a cesarean scar. For this reason we report our data on "standard multiparas": ≥37 weeks' gestation, singleton, vertex, and no previous cesarean births (Table 29.1). Again, these figures also include the high-risk parous patients with preeclampsia, IUGR, diabetes, HIV, PROM, postmaturity, etc. The data clearly demonstrate that a first vaginal birth results in low intervention rates in the next pregnancy. Clearly, the best way to avoid problems in parous childbirth is to avoid a cesarean delivery first time around.

29.2.3 Population context

For reasons of clarity and transparency some key characteristics of our total population need to be illuminated (Tables 29.2 and 29.3). Our joint obstetric-midwifery practice caters for about 2000 mixed-risk pregnancies per year with an average Western European population. Roughly 15–20% are first- or second-generation non-European in origin. These overall obstetric data illustrate the background against which the data of the "standard" pregnancies (Table 29.1) must be interpreted.

29.2.4 Practice versus ideal

Although these data compare favorably with those of most other centers with similar patient population characteristics, the concept of *proactive support of labor* has not yet reached its full potential, even in the authors' hospital, and it probably never will. Constant review continues to identify gaps

Table 29.1. Pooled data from the obstetric-midwifery collaboration at the St. Elisabeth Hospital in Tilburg, the Netherlands in a five-year period (2002–2006), focused on labor management. It should be emphasized that all so-called "high-risk" singleton pregnancies with vertex presentation at term are included

	Standard nulliparas ≥ 37 weeks' gestation, singleton, vertex		Standard multiparas ≥ 37 weeks, singleton, vertex, no uterine scar		Total	
Babies born	4 329	**(100%)**	3 877	**(100%)**	8 206	**(100%)**
Labor induction	595	(13.7%)	402	(10.4%)	997	(12.1%)
Prelabor cesarean	108	(2.5%)	97	(2.5%)	205	(2.5%)
Spontaneous labor onset	3 626	(83.8%)	3 378	(87.1%)	7004	(85.4%)
Spontaneous deliveries	3 312	(77%)	3 667	(94.6%)	6 957	(84.8%)
Vacuum/forceps delivery	649	(15%)	35	(0.9%)	684	(8.3%)
Intrapartum cesarean	260	(6%)	78	(2%)	338	(4.1%)
Epidural analgesia	429	(9.9%)	81	(2.1%)	510	(6.2%)
Perinatal mortality[a]	4	(0.1%)	2	(0.05%)	6	(0.07%)

[a] Possibly labor- and delivery-related perinatal mortality: intrapartum and neonatal deaths within 28 days of birth, prelabor intrauterine deaths, and lethal congenital malformations excluded

Table 29.2. Pooled data of the obstetric-midwifery collaboration at the St. Elisabeth Hospital in Tilburg, the Netherlands

The entire population (2002–2006)		
Overall ≥ 24 weeks	**Total**	**Percentage**
Pregnancies	10 424	100(%)
Overall cesarean sections	1 388	13.3
Multiple pregnancies	226	2.2
Babies born	10 671	**100(%)**
Premature babies (≥24 weeks and <37 weeks)	714	6.7
Babies born ≥37 weeks and <42 weeks	9 410	88.2
Post-term babies (≥42 weeks)	547	5.1
Perinatal mortality (≥24 weeks)[a]	69	0.6
Multiparas with cesarean scar	545	**100(%)**
Successful VBACs	350	64.2
Repeat cesarean	195	35.8
Breech presentations	581	**100(%)**
Vaginal breech delivery	142	24.4
Cesarean delivery	439	75.6

[a] Fetal deaths plus neonatal deaths within 28 days of birth, congenital malformations included

Table 29.3. Cesarean rates, overall and divided into subgroups, expressed as percentages of all pregnancies and as percentage of all cesarean deliveries

Cesarean deliveries (2002–2006)			
Total of pregnancies (≥24 weeks)	10 424	**100%**	
All cesarean deliveries of which:	1 388	13.3%	**100%**
"standard" pregnancies	543	5.2%	39%
Breech presentation	439	4.2%	32%
Repeat cesarean	195	1.9%	14%
Rest: complications <37 weeks; multiple pregnancies; etc.	211	2%	15%

between the ideal and practice. An estimated 10–20% of our operative deliveries in standard nulliparas are still being judged in retrospect to be "most likely preventable." There are several explanations. First, the integration of in- and out-of-hospital care (Chapter 26) is still in its infancy, though rapidly growing and improving. Not all community-based midwives in the region share the initiative and some continue to transfer patients to the hospital far too late. Of course, these patients cannot be refused. Second, the volume of deliveries in the hospital is still slightly too small to permit the optimal employment of personnel (Chapter 26). To address this problem, hospital management is presently working on merging the obstetric unit with that of a neighboring hospital. Third, as in all other teaching hospitals, residents and fellows – often previously trained elsewhere in conventional labor care – come and go, straining compliance with the system. Likewise, there is a considerable turnover in student midwives and nurses who need to adapt to radical practice changes compared with what they learned elsewhere. In our experience it takes at least half a year for new team members to become fully acquainted with the integrated concept of *proactive support of labor*, inevitably making mistakes along the way. This emphasizes the importance of unstinted education and ongoing, rigorous audit. While the early augmentation protocol is the easiest aspect to teach to new co-workers, it is far more difficult to instill the overall conceptual approach to childbirth and to make the appropriate mindset their own. It takes time to learn to understand the importance of consistency in information and conduct and the mutual dependency of all the biomedical and psychological processes involved. It also takes a while to master the proper, positive attitude marked by avoidance of black cloud psychology (Chapter 4). In this respect, many patients need to be reeducated as well and that is, in fact, the greatest challenge of all. However, the more the system is spread the easier this will be.

> *The creation of optimal birth care is a continuously evolving process that must be maintained by a careful audit of all its components.*

29.2.5 Safety

Like the intervention rates, the perinatal outcome data outlined above compare favorably with those of other centers. Yet some aspects need further explanation. All suboptimal fetal outcomes in our hospital are reviewed on a regular basis, and all

perinatal deaths are also reviewed by independent experts from out of hospital. As anywhere else, errors in risk assessment continue to play a role in a few cases, but no case of prelabor fetal demise could be attributed to the restrictive induction policy. In the subset of "standard nulliparas and multiparas," three out of the six cases of perinatal mortality were judged to be definitely avoidable but unrelated to the labor management or the fetal surveillance protocols. On the contrary, the protocols had been severely violated. In fact, there has not been a single cause to date to question fetal safety in terms of the protocols.

> *The protocols of* proactive support of labor *prove to be entirely safe for babies.*

29.2.6 Obstetric quality ranking and league tables

The low intervention rates outlined above cannot be explained by specific characteristics of our population, since operative delivery rates of most other Dutch hospitals are significantly greater. A sophisticated risk-adjustment algorithm was introduced nationwide in the Netherlands in 1994, based on 17 risk factors (intervention predictors) identified by logistic regression of the aggregated obstetric data from all Dutch hospitals on an annual basis.[7] This system adjusts individual hospital data for relevant patient population characteristics, thus providing a basis for an honest and more meaningful inter-hospital comparison of intervention and outcome data. This so-called "National Obstetric Peer Review" provides every Dutch hospital, in a confidential annual report, with its *expected* and *observed* rates of interventions and outcomes in three gestational age groups, as well as the hospital's ranking on the national percentiles for risk-adjusted intervention rates.[8]

For many consecutive years our hospital has ranked at the bottom of the national, risk-adjusted league tables for prelabor and intrapartum interventions at term: induction plus prelabor cesarean rates much less than the 10th percentile and intra-partum operative delivery rates (cesareans plus instrumental vaginal deliveries) much less than the 10th percentile. Conversely, for years on end one of the highest spontaneous vaginal delivery rates has been achieved (much greater than the 95th per-centile). At least as important, of course, is that the number of perinatal deaths *observed* in our hospital has been consistently equal to or lower than what would be *expected* on the basis of the national, risk-adjusted comparisons.[7] These combined data clearly demonstrate the balance that has been struck between maternal and fetal outcomes.

> *Risk-adjusted inter-unit comparisons provide the ironclad evidence that* proactive support of labor *can keep operative delivery rates low without any adverse effects on fetal outcomes.*

Because the evidence suggests that the spiraling operative delivery rates in most other centers are ineffective if not downright harmful (Chapter 2), the ball is in their court to provide good evidence to justify the continuation of their practice.

29.3 Summary

- To allow inter-hospital quality comparisons, populations must be comparable.
- The concept of "standard nulliparas" and "standard multiparas" permits a fair comparison of labor and delivery skills between doctors and between hospitals.
- The best reflection of institutional obstetric performance is the hospital ranking on risk-adjusted league tables of interventions in "standard nulliparas" and "standard multiparas."
- In our hospital a new balance has been struck between maternal and fetal outcomes, marked by the nationally highest spontaneous delivery rates in "standard nulliparas" as well as in "standard multiparas" without any detrimental effects on perinatal outcomes.

REFERENCES

1. Main EK. Reducing cesarean births rates with data-driven quality improvement activities. *Pediatrics* 1999; 103: 374–83.
2. Robson MS. Classification of cesarean sections. *Fetal Maternal Med Rev* 2001; 12: 23–39.
3. Cleary R, Beard RW, Chapple J. The standard primipara as a basis for inter-unit comparisons of maternity care. *Br J Obstet Gynaecol* 1996; 103: 223–9.
4. Elliott JP, Russell MM, Dickason LA. The labor adjusted cesarean section rate: a more informative method than cesarean section "rate" for assessing a practitioner's labor and delivery skills. *Am J Obstet Gynecol* 1997; 177: 139–43.
5. Lieberman E, Lang JM, Heffner LJ. Assessing the role of case mix in cesarean delivery rates. *Obstet Gynecol* 1998; 92: 1–7.
6. Gates PE. Think globally, act locally: an approach to implementation of clinical practice guidelines. *Jt Comm J Qual Improv* 1995; 21(2): 71–84.
7. Elferink-Stinkens PM, Van Hemel OJ, Hermans MP. Obstetric characteristics profiles as quality assessment of obstetric care. *Eur J Obstet Gynecol Reprod Biol* 1993; 51: 85–90.
8. Elferink-Stinkens PM. *Quality Management in Obstet-rics: Reporting population adjusted intervention and mortality rates. Academic thesis*, University of Nij-megen, The Netherlands; 2000.

30

Sum of the parts

Proactive support of labor is an all-embracing concept of birth care, firmly rooted in the basic physiology of birth and strongly supported by clinical evidence for each of its components. Throughout the previous chapters it was constantly emphasized that all ingredients of the program need to be addressed if real progress is to be made. None of them can be ignored. Lessons should be learned from the confusion raised by "active management" programs – mostly deceptively so-called – whereby practice change remained restricted to intensified use of oxytocin while O'Driscoll's other propositions – strict diagnoses, consistent policies, personal attention, organizational reforms, and continuous audit – were virtually ignored (Chapter 12). Predictably, such a stripped version does not work. This final chapter discusses the misunderstandings pervading the literature about "active management," from which *proactive support* has been derived, separating the wheat from the chaff.

30.1 The interventional component

Doubts have been cast on the value of amniotomy and oxytocin because some controlled trials failed to demonstrate a reduction in cesarean rates (Chapter 17). Although these studies were strictly focused on the subject of augmentation, meta-analyses and editorial comments simply concluded that "the active management of labor" does not work.[1–4] This is a typical example of how "evidence-based" data may lead to misplaced extrapolations and false conclusions. Desktop scientists questioning the system by focusing on one single part are "like a mechanic trying to decide which component of a car's engine makes it go."[5] They fail to see that it is the sum of the parts. But there is more. Firstly, a meta-analysis can be no stronger than the studies that contribute to it. And in the light of the heterogeneity of the study groups, the absence of information about co-interventions, and the importance of the timing and dose of oxytocin, many questions about the studies meta-analyzed can and should be raised (Chapter 17). Secondly, one of the most influential biases in the acquisition of evidence is the choice of the question, and the best evidence in answer to the wrong question is useless; cesarean rate is neither the only relevant outcome parameter nor the only measure of quality of care (Chapter 28). As a matter of fact, early labor augmentation alone has never been claimed to reduce cesarean delivery rates. That does not alter the fact that judicious use of oxytocin effectively prevents prolonged labor and consequently contributes significantly to maternal satisfaction (Chapter 17). Most importantly, prevention of long labors makes all the other elements of high-quality care possible at last: it permits the permanent presence of a labor companion throughout the entire birth process as well as personal continuity and commitment of all staff in attendance. All the ingredients of good practice are closely intertwined. Besides this, none of the trials included in the meta-analyses was able to demonstrate any increase in operative delivery rates or adverse fetal outcomes. In conclusion: all attempts to discredit the use of amniotomy and oxytocin for failure to progress in early as well as advanced labor prove to be unfounded.

> *Prevention of long labor is an integral part of and a precondition for high-quality care.*

30.2 The whole package

Few readers will question the importance of adequate prelabor education, psychological support, continuous personal attention and commitment, and good communication throughout the entire process of labor. And few will doubt the benefits of sound labor ward organization and the need for continual audit and feedback. One should realize, however, that none of these critical elements of high-quality care can be truly met if a well-defined policy for the conduct of birth is not implemented as well, including a clear diagnosis of labor and early detection and correction of dysfunctional labor. Prevention of prolonged labor is an integral part of the program and, in fact, a precondition for all the other aspects of high-quality care.

> Proactive support of labor
>
> *It is the sum of the parts that makes the system work.*

30.2.1 Inconclusive controlled trials

In general, randomized controlled trials have greatly improved the quality of evidence guiding clinical practice, but when applied to complex phenomena they have important limitations.[6] *Proactive support of labor* is a mindset, and given the interaction between the biomedical, psychological, and organizational aspects of the proposed childbirth system the concept does not lend itself well to randomized controlled trials, as pointed out

by Impey and Boylan.[7] It is in fact impossible to conduct such a trial free from bias, as became painfully clear from previous attempts to examine the active management of labor.[8-11] Firstly, in most of the controlled trials claiming to have tested the whole package, up to 50% of the eligible nulliparas were not included, mainly because of inductions. This means that one of the most important recommendations – curtailed use of induction – was not implemented and thus not examined. Secondly, in all trials but one, women were only randomized once "active labor was established," so that the key component of the policy – strict (early) diagnosis of labor and repudiation of the "latent phase" – were also not taken over or studied. Equally disappointingly, the other key element – one-on-one nursing – either was not strived for or was evenly realized in both study arms of the trials. Another prominent omission from all trials was the use of continuous review. Added to this, in all trials there were sizable spill-over effects from the intervention groups onto the randomized control groups, which by the way did considerably better than the historical controls. Even worse, the protocol compliance in most studies was markedly poor: in one study up to 40% of the study group was not attended to according to the study protocol "because the midwives considered the active management protocol to be medical interference and thus contrary to the philosophy of midwifery" (sic) as the authors commented.[11] It is rather an achievement that they succeeded in getting the study published, for what remained is that only an intention to routine amniotomy and early augmentation was compared with a control group that proved on closer examination to have had practically the same treatment and care. That no significant effect on outcomes was found – except for a shorter duration of labor in the study group – is not surprising; a half full bottle differs little from a half empty bottle. Despite claims, none of these trials examined the integral concept of care as proposed by O'Driscoll, and the same goes for their meta-analyses.

Deceptively, these (pseudo-)controlled trials continue to be cited to criticize the concept of active management [1–5] and, by inference, *proactive support of labor*, even though none of them could reveal any adverse effects, however poor the design and execution of the study. Robson *et al.*[12] commented: "Before further large, expensive, and often inconclusive trials are performed it might be better to ensure that experienced staff work in labor wards and that continual local audit is used to determine standards and expectations; then appropriate changes in management could be instigated."

> *Clinical studies on birth care concepts can give meaningful results only when applied to the whole of the package, delivered appropriately by expert staff.*

Clearly, the integral concept of *proactive support*, directing all medical and non-medical aspects of childbirth, cannot be examined by a classical randomized controlled trial. Much more interesting is the finding that cesarean rates in the trials discussed above decreased markedly during the study period in comparison with previous years. The intensified interest in labor appeared to have affected obstetric care providers and affected care of all patients in both research arms, a classic example of the Hawthorne effect.[13]

30.2.2 Convincing clinical evidence

O'Driscoll's original ideas have been adopted in many different practice settings around the world, invariably producing positive results.[7,14–24] These observational studies are difficult to ignore, as are our results (Chapter 29) and the carefully documented data from the National Maternity Hospital in Dublin, the birthplace of this form of conceptual care, whose database now nears 300 000 deliveries.[25]

The most successful initiatives have tended to be those that operated protocols closest to the original concept, including the key element of regular audit of procedures and outcomes. With regard to cesarean delivery rates, for instance, Turner *et al.* observed over 1000 consecutive labors managed actively and found a reduction from 14.5% to 10.8%. Changes in rates of operative and normal delivery had significance values of between $p < 0.05$ and $p < 0.0001$.[14] Robson *et al.* achieved an overall cesarean reduction from 12% to 9.5%, with the cesarean rate for nulliparous women in spontaneous labor falling from 7.5% to 2.4% with an active management program including rigorous peer review. Both results were highly significant ($p < 0.0001$).[15] With a similar approach in a private hospital in California, the overall cesarean rate fell from 31.1% to 15.7% and nulliparous cesarean rates from 17.9 to 9.8% over 6 years.[24] Akoury *et al.* found a cesarean section reduction from 13% to 4.3% after introduction of an active management program.[16] These data may be observational and non-randomized but they cannot be dismissed. To quote Bloomfield: "The implication that changes of this order of significance arose as the result of some factor other than changes in practice, when entire obstetric populations were studied, strains credulity to its limits."[26] Those seeking to explain the observational data often quote the Hawthorne effect: cesarean section was under greater scrutiny when the policy was introduced in a maternity unit. However, this scrutiny should be continuous (Chapter 27). In the words of Buist: "If cesarean reduction is the result of the Hawthorne effect entering day to day clinical practice then that is fine: it is the end result that matters."[27]

> *Strong albeit inferential evidence shows that the integral approach of* proactive support of labor *effectively reduces operative delivery rates and enhances women's childbirth satisfaction without any negative effects on perinatal outcomes*
> *(Evidence level B–C).*

It bears repetition that *proactive support of labor* is designed not with the sole intention of reducing overall operative delivery rates but rather to enhance professional labor and delivery skills, promoting high-quality labor care that facilitates short, safe, and spontaneous delivery in low-risk pregnancies. Improvement of women's satisfaction with their childbirth experiences is in fact the most beneficial and rewarding outcome (Chapter 27).

30.3 General conclusion

Proactive support of labor is a carefully orchestrated expert team approach aimed at a safe and rewarding normal delivery, based on the best possible evidence. It is the sum of all parts that makes it a highly sophisticated form of maternity care. The system involves an ongoing cycle of prelabor education, personal psychological support, a well-defined birth-plan including strict diagnoses and timely corrective measures in abnormal labor, and constant peer audit of all procedures. The conceptual framework effectively enhances professional labor and delivery skills, providing the expertise for preventing or adequate handling of dystocia, which is the root cause of the cesarean pandemic. The method is based on a thorough understanding of the natural biophysics of normal birth and the pathophysiology of abnormal labor. The all-embracing system combines the best of obstetric, midwifery, and nursing expertise and promotes sound organization, congenial collaboration, and good communication in labor. The guiding principles and protocols guarantee optimal intrapartum fetal care, thereby effectively preventing poor fetal outcomes and related malpractice litigation without resorting to harmful defensive medicine. *Proactive support of labor* strikes a new balance between natural birth and intervention and invariably enhances women's satisfaction with their childbirth experience.

In conclusion: *proactive support of labor* is of great benefit to all pregnant women, their babies, and the providers who care for both of them. The ability to offer real and supportive help at the beginning of life is both a challenge and a privilege.

REFERENCES

1. Olah KS, Gee H. The active mismanagement of labour. *Br J Obstet Gynaecol* 1996; 103: 729–31.
2. Smyth RM, Alldred SK, Markham C. Amniotomy for shortening spontaneous labour. *Cochrane Database Syst Rev* 2007; (4): CD006167.
3. Thornton JG. Active management of labour; it does not reduce the rate of caesarean delivery. *BMJ* 1996; 313: 378.
4. Thornton JG. Active management of labour. *Curr Opin Obstet Gynecol* 1997; 9(6): 366–9.
5. Stratton JF. Active management of labour: Standards vary among institutions. *BMJ* 1994; 309: 1015.
6. Kotaska A. Inappropriate use of randomised trials to evaluate complex phenomena: case study of vaginal breech delivery. *BMJ* 2004; 329: 1039–42.
7. Impey L, Boylan P. Active management of labour revisited. *Br J Obstet Gynaecol* 1999; 106: 183–7.
8. Lopez-Zeno JA, Peaceman AM, Adashek JA. A controlled trial of a program for the active management of labor. *N Engl J Med* 1992; 326: 450–4.
9. Frigoletto F, Lieberman E, Lang J, *et al*. A clinical trial of active management of labor. *N Engl J Med* 1995; 333: 745–50.
10. Cammu H, van Eeckhout E. A randomised controlled trial of early versus delayed use of amniotomy and oxytocin infusion in nulliparous labour. *Br J Obstet Gynaecol* 1996; 103: 313–18.
11. Sadler LC, Davidson T, McCowan LME. A randomised controlled trial and meta-analysis of active management of labour. *Br J Obstet Gynaecol* 2000; 107: 909–15.
12. Robson MS. Active management of labour. Continual audit is important. *BMJ* 1994; 309: 1015.
13. Roethlisberger FJ, Dickenson WJ. *Management and the worker: an account of a research program conducted by the Western Electric Company, Hawthorne works, Chicago*. Cambridge, MA: Harvard University Press; 1939.
14. Turner M, Brassil M, Gordon H. Active management of labor associated with a decrease in the cesarean section rate in nulliparas. *Obstet Gynecol* 1988; 71: 150–4.
15. Robson MS, Scudamore IW, Walsh SM. Using the medical audit cycle to reduce cesarean section rates. *Am J Obstet Gynecol* 1996; 174: 199–205.
16. Akoury H, Brodie G, Caddick R, McLaughlin V, Pugh P. Active management of labor and operative delivery in

nulliparous women. *Am J Obstet Gynecol* 1988; 158: 255–8.

17. Boylan P, Frankowski R, Roundtree R, Selwyn B, Parrish K. Effect of active management on the incidence of cesarean section for dystocia in nulliparas. *Am J Perinatol* 1991; 8: 373–9.

18. Boylan P, Parisi V. Effect of active management on latent phase labor. *Am J Perinatol* 1990; 7: 363–5.

19. Ward A. *Introducing active management to Nigeria.* Presented to the Society of Gynaecology and Obstetrics of Nigeria; 1977.

20. Masoli P, Picó V, Pellerano 1. Manejo activo del parto. Experiencia en el hospital Gustavo Fricke. *Rev Chil Obstet Ginecol* 1986; 51: 223–30.

21. Vengadasalam D. Active management of labour: an approach to reducing the rising caesarean rate. *Singapore J Obstet Gynecol* 1986; 17: 33–6.

22. Hogston P, Noble W. Active management of labor: the Portsmouth experience. *J Obstet Gynaecol* 1993; 13: 340–2.

23. Glantz JC, McNanley T. Active management of labor: a meta-analysis of cesarean delivery rates for dystocia in nulliparas. *Obstet Gynecol Surv* 1997; 52: 497–505.

24. Lagrew DC, Morgan MA. Decreasing the cesarean rate in a private hospital: success without mandated change. *Am J Obstet Gynecol* 1996; 174: 184–91.

25. O'Driscoll K, Meagher D, Robson M. *Active Management of Labour*, 4th edn. Mosby.

26. Bloomfield TH. Active management of labour. Non-randomised studies cannot be ignored. *BMJ* 1994; 309: 1016.

27. Buist R. Active management of labour. Commitment to low intervention rates with audit of outcomes is important. *BMJ* 1997; 314: 606–7.

Index